To Susana
with thanks.
Hope you
Enjoy

Tarek

Healthy *Bytes...*

Digital-Age eSkills & Tools for Weight-Loss
Because Motivation alone is not Enough

Tarek K.A. Hamid

ISBN: 978-1-48356-531-6

TABLE OF CONTENTS

PART I

A RISING TIDE THAT's LIFTING ALL...
WEIGHTS

CHAPTER 1

The Heavy Burden of
A Heavy-Weight

You're *not* Alone

It's no secret: Americans have become way fatter than what medical science recommends. While we may debate the *why* and *what can we do about it*, there seems to be little debate on one thing: our weights have not been increasing because we are consciously trying to gain weight. Indeed one of the major perplexities of the obesity epidemic is that more and more people are getting fatter even in the face of broad publicity about the risks, tremendous pressure to be thin and a titanic struggle by tens of millions of people to manage their weight. The fact that Americans spend more than $50 billion annually on weight-loss products and services, with thousands willing to "stomach" expensive and grueling procedures such as liposuction—making it the most popular cosmetic surgery procedure in the land—shows that they can hardly be happy with the status quo.[1]

Beyond the "cosmetic" consequences of weight gain—which is what most people continue to obsess over—excess weight, as we shall see, is strongly linked to a wide variety of deleterious health effects and thus should be viewed (and treated) as a serious health problem. It's why there is legitimate (and growing) worry that if this trend is not reversed, it could wipe out much of the progress that has been made in preventing some of the other major chronic health problems such as heart disease, diabetes and certain cancers.[2]

How did we get ourselves into this mess? And what can we do to get out of it? These are the important questions that I aim to tackle in this book.

The book is organized into three major parts. In Part I, we will focus on the environmental forces that triggered this (modern) problem and continue to perpetuate it. While the basis of obesity—positive energy balance—could not be more simple from a physiologic point of view, the behavioral, cultural and environmental factors affecting this energy imbalance are varied and complex.

We will understand—and it is important that we do— that the problem is far more than absence of willpower or a case of moral failure. Because eating is under conscious control—one can always decide not to put fork to mouth— weight has always been seen as a very individual, very personal thing. And being overweight, in turn, a matter of an individual's decisions—or, rather, of a failure to make decisions.[3] That is perhaps why most people believe that every overweight person can achieve slenderness and should pursue that goal, why obese people are stereotyped as lacking in self-control, and why being obese elicits scorn as often as sympathy.[4] *But human behavior is never expressed in a vacuum.* Our physical and social environments provide the context within which people live their lives—what they eat and how they work, play, and move around. All of these affect energy intake and expenditure. For example, our choice of foods is not only a matter of personal preferences, but is also very much a function of what food is available in the variety of food outlets we have access to in our communities—the restaurants, supermarkets, and vending machines. And how our neighborhoods are built—with/without bike paths, foot paths, street lighting, and public transport—has a great influence on our choice to use, for example, active transport (walking, cycling) versus motorized transport (cars).

To mitigate the risk—as a society, as individuals, as parents—we need to recognize and better understand the environmental pressures (economic, cultural, technological) surrounding all of us in modern societies that triggered the upsurge in obesity and continue to fuel it.

A key message of the book is that successful weight management requires more than motivation. Managing our health—and our bodies—is not unlike managing any complex system, a task that requires skill and the right tools. In Parts II and III we turn our focus inwards—onto our body's system of weight/energy regulation. The goals are twofold. First we'll seek to gain a better understanding of the workings of the body's system of weight/energy regulation—how energy consumption and expenditure are regulated and how the two processes influence one another and are influenced by the external environment. *Understanding* is the focus of Part II.

Understanding without a capability to predict the system's behavior—to devise treatment strategies and/or assess treatment outcomes—is of little practical utility however. Hence, our second goal is better prediction. Effective prediction of treatment outcomes (e.g., pounds lost from a diet) is critically important in managing any aspect of personal health. In the case of weight management, effective prediction is key to setting *attainable treatment goals*. If one's goals are unrealistic, then failure is inevitable regardless of how hard one tries. Failure, in turn, saps motivation, undermines beliefs in self-efficacy, and drives people to give up.

The two skills –understanding and prediction—are needed together.

In Part III, I discuss the challenge of "personalized" prediction. We'll understand that the overweight are *not* a homogeneous lot and that response to weight loss intervention can vary greatly between people. Hence, reliance on simplistic one-size-fits-all tools such as the ubiquitous energy balance equation—also known as the 3500 kcal per pound rule—is a bankrupt strategy that must be abandoned in favor of more intimate tools that actually fit.

But first, let's see how big of a mess we, as a society, are in.

America's Obesity Tsunami!

According to the centers for Disease Control and Prevention (CDC), approximately two thirds of all adults in the U.S. over the age of 20 are overweight, with a body mass index (BMI) of more than 25—calculated as weight in kilograms divided by the square of the height in meters. This means that, currently, there are more than 140 million Americans who are overweight enough to begin experiencing health problems as a direct result of that weight. Even more concerning, close to half of them (approximately 78 million Americans) are heavy enough to count as clinically obese (with a BMI greater than 30)—that's being so overweight that their lives will likely be cut seriously shorter by excess fat. A BMI of 30 (the threshold to obesity) roughly means being 30 pounds overweight for an average-height woman and 35 to 40 pounds overweight for an average-weight man.[5]

But what is perhaps most ominous of all is the rise of obesity rates among children and adolescents. Most of today's obese adults were not obese children, accumulating their extra pounds only after they were 25 or 30 years old. But now we have more and more young people who are already obese at the age of 10,

15, or 20.[6] Today there are nearly twice as many overweight children and almost three times as many overweight adolescents as there were in the 1980s. The latest government data show that 30 percent of children and adolescents—about 25 million—are overweight or are at risk of becoming so.[7] That's the highest number ever recorded. All these overweight kids are on a course to fuel an even bigger national health problem as they mature into obese adults. Because of the deleterious (and lifelong) health effects associated with obesity, public health experts believe that today's children may well be the first generation of Americans whose life expectancy will be shorter than that of their parents.[8,9]

Not only has the speed at which obesity escalated in the population been alarmingly impressive, but so has its breadth—geographically, demographically, socio-economically. A study of obesity's dispersion in the U.S. found that "... the rate of American obesity was increasing in every state and among both sexes, regardless of age, race, or educational level".[10] It seems hard to believe that a chronic condition like obesity could spread with the speed and breadth of a communicable disease epidemic. But it has.[11]

Even Fido and Fluffy are not immune! A 2012 survey by the Association for Pet Obesity Prevention indicated that approximately 50 percent of dogs were overweight or obese while 60 percent of cats were, literally, "fat cats."[12] And the experts are saying our pets are gaining weight for many of the same reasons people do. "They're living longer ... are often fed too much ... and are increasingly confined to fenced-in suburbs with shrinking yards. Guilty owners, meanwhile, are showing their love not with walks, but snacks."[13,14]

If the rate of obesity in the general population continues to increase at the same pace it has for the past two decades, the *entire* U.S. adult population (and their pets) could be overweight within a few generations.[15]

"Globesity"

The problem is no longer just an *American problem*. The situation is nearly as dismal around the globe, as country after country follows the American lead and grows heavier.[16] According to Dr. Stephan Roessner, a past president of the International Association for the Study of Obesity, "There is no country in the world where obesity is not increasing. Even in developing countries we thought were immune... the epidemic is coming on very fast. In some areas of Africa, overweight children outnumber malnourished children three to one."[17] If its prevalence continues on its current trajectory, by 2030 the number of overweight and obese persons is projected to exceed three billion worldwide—arguably making them the largest patient population in existence. [18]

In her annual message, Dr. Gro Harlem Brundtland, the Director-General of the World Health Organization, was clearly alarmed:

> These are dangerous times for the well being of the world... Too many of us are living dangerously—whether we are aware of that or not... Either because we have little choice, which is often the case among the poor, or because we are making the wrong choices in terms of our consumption and our activities.[19]

The Heavy Burden of a Heavy Weight

All this would matter less if being overweight were beneficial or, at the very least safe. But in most cases it is neither. While the complications of obesity may not be as dramatic as those of HIV, for example, its burden can affect more people and is a source of far more deaths. According to the Centers for Disease Control (C.D.C.), obesity now kills five times as many Americans as "microbial agents"— that is, infectious diseases.20 Recently published assessments indicate that obesity results in an estimated 300,000 premature deaths each year.[21] (Worldwide, according to a 2014 McKinsey Global Institute study, obesity is responsible for about 5 percent of all deaths.[22]) Experts predict that if current trends continue—with Americans smoking less but continuing to get fatter—obesity will soon overtake smoking as the primary preventable cause of death among Americans.23

In a new study, a group of Dutch researchers sought to quantify the mortality risk people face from being overweight. Specifically, they sought to assess the "Years of Life Lost" (YLL) due to obesity—that is, the difference between the number of years one would be expected to live if obese versus not obese. The study was one of a few that actually tracked a group of individuals over an extended period and that helped identify the deleterious effects of obesity on health and longevity in ways that cannot be revealed by "snapshot" type studies that look at a cross-section of the population at one point in time. Their findings, based on a study of the health history of more than three thousand people over four decades (between 1948 and 1990) were portentously straightforward: getting fat, indeed, kills. And as the degree of overweight increases, the life spans contract. Somewhat of a surprise was the finding by the Dutch researchers that even moderate amounts of excess weight "conferred a noticeable diminution in life expectancy." 24

Here are some sobering findings from this important study:

- Nonsmokers who were overweight but not obese (which roughly means being 10 to 30 pounds above a healthy weight) lost an average of three years off their lives.
- Obese people (with BMI greater than 30) died even sooner
    o Obese female nonsmokers lost an average of 7.1 years
    o Obese male nonsmokers lost 5.8 years.
- For those who were obese *and* smokers, the double burden caused the loss to be significantly higher
    o Obese female smokers died 7.2 years sooner than normal-weight smokers and 13.3 years sooner than normal-weight nonsmoking women.
    o Obese male smokers lived 6.7 years less than normal-weight smokers, and 13.7 years less than normal-weight nonsmokers.

To put these figures into perspective, just consider that completely eliminating all kinds of cancer in America would add only about three-and-a-half years to life expectancy![25]

Obesity, it is becoming increasingly clear, exacts such a heavy toll on longevity because it increases the risk of developing many chronic diseases at surprisingly low levels of excess fat—as little as five to ten pounds above desirable body weight.[26] That's because surplus body fat—which was once thought of as little more than an inert storage depot—is, metabolically, a highly active organ, producing hormones and chemical substances that can flood the body, damaging blood vessels, causing insulin resistance, and promoting cancer-cell growth.[27]

A growing number of studies are now allowing us to quantify the links between obesity and coronary heart disease, diabetes, hypertension and selected cancers—which are the major ailments most frequently associated with obesity.[28] In one recent study, for example, obese individuals were 1.7 times more likely to have heart disease, twice as likely to have hypertension and three times as likely to have diabetes compared to normal-weight people.[29] Another study that investigated cancer risk found that excessively heavy men and women were three times as likely to develop kidney cancer compared with those of healthy weight, while obese post-menopausal women faced up to a 50-percent-higher chance of developing breast cancer than non-obese women.[30]

As science marches ahead and the methods for studying disease become more sophisticated, we can expect the news about weight and health to grow even worse.[31] New research, for example, already points to a link between excess body weight and the risk of death from most cancers. A recently published study by the American Cancer Society found that the higher a patient's body-mass index (BMI), the greater the risk of cancer death. The researchers attributed the higher death rates in obese cancer patients to several possible causes. For some patients, the cause was delay in diagnosis. That's because the cancers of obese patients may be under layers of the body fat and, thus, can be harder to detect (a person's fat can literally be too dense for X-rays or sound waves to penetrate). It was also recently found that in men, excessive body fat can suppress P.S.A., the blood protein used to diagnose prostate cancer in its early stages. The resulting delay in diagnosis explains why in obese men, prostate cancer tends to be diagnosed in more advanced forms.[32] For others, the culprit can be biological mechanisms associated with obesity, such as increased levels of certain hormones (sex steroids, insulin and Growth Factor I) that are believed to stimulate the growth of nascent cancer cells in various organs.[33]

For Older Americans, however, the Future is *Now*

For obese people in their fifties and sixties, the physical burden of carrying excess weight can interfere with even the most routine activities. Physical tasks—such as climbing stairs, maneuvering into an automobile, finding comfortable chairs, and walking any distance can become difficult and sources of pain and embarrassment.[34] A recent study to assess disability among older Americans (aged 50 to 69) found that difficulties in performing tasks such as bathing, eating, dressing and getting in or out of bed rises by 50 percent in men who are moderately obese and threefold in those who are severely obese (BMI greater than 35). In women, the likelihood of such problems doubles with moderate obesity and quadruples with severe obesity.[35]

As baby boomers get older and fatter, they're also more likely to develop one of the double burdens of age and weight: arthritis. Survey data from the Centers for Disease Control and Prevention suggest that the likelihood of experiencing arthritic pain increases fivefold in very obese people aged 60 and older compared to those who are underweight.[36]

Putting on extra weight may also be far riskier for cognitive dysfunction than most people have imagined. Recent scientific studies have determined that weight gain may lead to degenerative changes in the aging brain and, quite possibly, Alzheimer's—a disease that many elderly—and their families—fear more than death itself.[37]

Such findings fly in the face of widely-held assumptions that older Americans are getting healthier and that their disability rates are dropping. Instead, obesity-related ailments may very well be wiping out the recent health gains that the elderly have heretofore enjoyed from reduced exposure to infectious diseases and advances in medical care.

And then… there is the Socio-Cultural Burden

Obesity not only affects long-term health and longevity, it is unique among chronic disease risk factors in that it also carries a socio-cultural burden.[38] Indeed, to most of its victims it is through psychological pain that obesity has its most noxious effects.[39] The full public health burden of the obesity epidemic must thus be measured not only by the traditional measures of morbidity and mortality, but also by the psychological and social consequences experienced by those who suffer and by those around them.[40]

Using an imaginative new method they called "owning one's disability," two University of Florida (Gainesville) researchers, Rand and MacGregor,[41] sought to quantify the heavy psychological toll that obesity exerts on the psyche. They had patients answer a series of forced-choice questions as to whether they would prefer their current disability to a number of other handicaps.[42] In a sample of formerly severely obese patients who had undergone gastric surgery, Rand and MacGregor found that every single one of the patients they interviewed would prefer to be deaf, dyslexic, diabetic or to suffer from very bad heart disease than to return to their morbidly overweight status. All patients preferred to be of normal weight than to have "a couple of million dollars" when given a hypothetical choice.

The extensive research done on obese people's quality of life suggests that the obese live in a world that often treats them with notable antipathy.[43] Some observers have gone so far as to characterize the disparagement of overweight and obese individuals as the last socially acceptable form of prejudice.[44] The last, perhaps, but certainly not the latest. "History shows that prejudice against obese individuals is not simply a product of society's current worship of a thin ideal. As early as the 12th century, Buddhists stigmatized obesity as the karmic consequence of moral failing."[45]

The frightening thing is that even small children are not immune from prejudice against the obese. Researchers have found that children "learn" at a very early age to associate obesity with undesirable personal characteristics. In one study, when children as young as six to nine years of age were shown a fat person's silhouette and asked to describe the person's characteristics, they said: "lazy, lying, cheating."[46,47] And when shown black-and-white line drawings of an obese child and children with various handicaps—including missing hands and facial disfigurement—the participants singled out the obese child as the one with whom they least wished to play.[48] It's no wonder that "among the most prevalent consequences of obesity in children is the discrimination that overweight children suffer at the hands of their peers."[49] Such discrimination is effectively robbing those overweight kids of their childhood, preventing them from doing the same kinds of activities that their leaner peers do.[50]

As children grow older, discrimination against the obese becomes more institutionalized.[51] Society's negative attitudes toward the obese take the form of discrimination in areas such as employment opportunities, college acceptance, and even marriage. In a study of college students, as an example, the eligible bachelors and bachelorettes rated embezzlers, cocaine users and shoplifters as more suitable marriage partners than obese individuals.[52] Other studies found that obese young women were far less likely to marry than non-obese women, and those who did marry were more likely to marry "down"—that is, to marry someone of a lower social status—than were non-obese women.[53]

Feeling obesity's economic pinch can be even more direct, however. Insurance premiums, for example, rise in proportion to one's girth and could easily be double, triple or up to five times the normal premium, even if one is otherwise in perfect health. And some severely overweight people may be declined insurance coverage altogether. To add insult to injury, this "fat tax" often falls on a slender wallet.[54] Studies consistently show that overweight job candidates are less likely to be hired than non-overweight candidates (even when perceived to be equally competent on job-related tests).[55] And when hired, they often earn less.[56]

The physical and psychological consequences of obesity have profound economic ramifications for the nation as a whole. These economic ramifications take the form of direct costs—these include the costs incurred on preventive, diagnostic and treatment services related to overweight and obesity such as on physician visits, hospital care, and medications—as well as indirect costs that accrue to the wider economy because of time and productivity lost to sickness and premature mortality.[57] A recent study conducted partly by the federal Centers for Disease Control and Prevention estimated that obesity-related health conditions cost the nation more than $150 billion annually or close to 10 percent of all health care spending—an amount that's comparable to the entire gross national product of countries such as Portugal, Ireland or Argentina.

How Did We Get into this Mess?

Of the numerous diseases that have struck humanity throughout history, never has there been a disease as common as obesity. Many diseases were more deadly, for sure, but none as common. This suggests two things: First, that "...obesity develops through a mechanism which, unlike plague, tuberculosis, or AIDS, is induced by exposure to factors surrounding all of us in modern societies,"[58] and second, that heretofore our strategies for managing the risk have been ineffective.

How to engineer a turnaround?

For starters—as already argued—we need to acquire a deeper understanding of the societal drivers that created the problem and continue to perpetuate it. (Understanding *why* you are *not* alone.) This would provide us great leverage in mitigating our personal risks—for ourselves and our families. Gaining such understanding is our task in the next three chapters.

CHAPTER 2

Unbalanced Act

From a physiologic point of view, the basis of weight-gain is no mystery: it is induced by positive energy balance. The human body, like all systems—whether technological or biological—obeys the laws of thermodynamics, which define the immutable principle of energy conservation. Body weight can increase only if energy intake exceeds expenditure. The upward trend in the population's weight, thus, suggests that recently the amount of calories consumed is exceeding those burned-off by a growing proportion of the population. The burning question is why this is happening now—when for thousands of years humans were (naturally) in energy equilibrium?

To understand the why we'll need to back—way back—into our human history and evolution.

"Civilization is but a filmy fringe on the history of man"

By this, the Canadian physician and historian William Osier meant that the past few millennia of human civilization represent a tiny fraction of the time since our human ancestors first appeared on earth.[59] For most of our long existence as a species, humans lived as hunter-gatherers. Archaeological data suggest that it was not until approximately 12,000 years ago that some human groups started to shift from a food-foraging mode of existence to one of food production. This shift was driven primarily by ecological pressures from population growth and food scarcities. And it would prove to be of great consequence, as it was this relatively recent economic transformation that would ultimately allow for the evolution of complex societies and of civilization itself.[60]

But before that "filmy fringe on our history" and for hundreds of thousands of years, humans lived as hunter-gatherers dependent for their nourishment on the supply of game and on whatever fruits, nuts, berries, roots, leaves, and other vegetable matter was available.[61] While their diet was qualitatively adequate, food was scarce and the next meal unpredictable. In most prehistoric societies, starvation was a constant threat.[62]

Our understanding of life in the hunter-gatherer societies of antiquity is based not only on the abundant archaeological evidence that we've accumulated, but also on the anthropologic study of *contemporary* hunter-gatherer populations. In what would surely qualify as a *Believe It or Not* story, there are today—in the 21st century—some contemporary non-industrial societies that are, in fact, "good approximations" of late Stone Age humans of about 20,000 years ago. Not one or two… but a hundred or more.

Not surprisingly, they have all been the focus of intensive study by anthropologists. A cross cultural ethnographic survey of a sample of more than a hundred such societies found seasonal food shortages for all of them—the same type of pattern that archaeological studies of excavated skeletal remains have revealed about the prehistoric hunter-gatherer societies. Shortages occur annually or even more frequently for roughly half of the societies and the shortages are "severe" (approaching starvation-level) in nearly a third of them.[63]

That's the bad news. The good news, however, is that these best approximation surrogates for our human ancestors experience slow population growth, enjoy high-quality diets (when food is available), maintain high levels of physical fitness, and are generally healthy. They are healthier, in fact, than many of the third-world populations currently undergoing the process of economic modernization or westernization.[64]

This is no Accident

The interaction between a species—any species—and its food supply is one of the most important influences affecting biological adaptation and cultural evolution.[65] Because the struggle for survival of the human species has been driven by a lack, not an excess, of food, the human body has developed over the years to defend itself actively against this threat.[66] And it has succeeded.

In the hunter-gatherer mode of existence, where a high level of physical activity was required for daily subsistence and the food supply was inconsistent, the challenge to the body energy-control system was to provide a strong drive to eat to keep pace with energy expenditure and to rest when physical exertion was not required.[67] And because starvation was not only real, but also a periodic threat, the greatest survival rates were among those who not only ate voraciously when food was plentiful, but who also stored the excess energy efficiently as a buffer against future food shortages.[68] Such individuals built up stores of fat that increased their survival prospects during famines, and they passed on these traits to their progeny, who, similarly, were more likely to survive.[69] For the females— whose reproductive fitness depended on their ability to withstand the nutritional demands of pregnancy and lactation—greater energy reserves provided a selective advantage over their lean counterparts in withstanding the stress of food shortage, not only for themselves but for their fetuses and nursing children.[70,71]

It should not surprise, then, as Sharman Russell writes in his informative book *Hunger: An Unnatural History*, that since human beings evolved to survive chronic threats of famine, we've grown afflicted by "chronic, troubling urges to gorge, grab and hoard."

Our taste buds are also rooted in our evolutionary past. When, thousands of years ago, humans were hunting wild game and gathering wild plants for food, their primary food sources contained limited sugar, fat, and salt. But because these are essential to the proper functioning of the human body, it was always good for people to eat as much of them as they could find. In another adaptive response to human dietary needs, evolution equipped us with a nearly insatiable appetite for fat, salt, and sugar to encourage us to eat these foods. These strong taste preferences have been genetically passed on to us over the generations—and to good effect (until now).

> Fatty foods helped our ancestors weather food shortages. Salt helped them maintain an appropriate water balance in their cells, helping avoid dehydration. Sugar and the sweetness associated with it helped them distinguish edible berries from poisonous ones. By giving us the taste for fat, sugar, and salt, our genetics led us to prefer the foods that were most likely to keep us alive. It also led us

to want to eat a wide variety of foods. The more types of foods we could eat, the more we were likely to consume the wide range of unknown nutrients we needed. Our natural inclination for variety made sure we got enough of these nutrients without us needing to know the difference between Vitamin C, riboflavin, and a complex carbohydrate.[72]

In this evolutionary context, the usual range of human metabolic variation would have produced many individuals with a predisposition to become fat, but chronic food scarcity and vigorous physical exertion ensured that they never would.[73] Skeletal remains indicate that our human ancestors were typically more lean and muscular than we are today. And studies of contemporary hunter-gatherer populations are consistent with this. For example, studies of the !Kung San tribe in the Kalahari Desert show them to be lean, with skin fold thicknesses approximately half those of age-matched North Americans and suffering no obesity problem.[74,75]

This suggests that, despite seasonal fluctuations in food availability and a mode of existence characterized by vigorous physical exertion, the caloric intake and output of our hunter-gatherer ancestors were balanced over time.[76] Eating whatever animals they could kill or scavenge and whatever fruit and vegetable matter they could take from plants, early humans kept enough fat stores to make it through the occasional lean times, but not so much that it slowed them down significantly. Further, control of their body weight was largely accomplished through innate physiological processes and required little conscious effort. They did not have to think about how much to eat in order to maintain a desirable weight. Their bodies told them.[77]

Our current predicament, it turns out, is a direct byproduct of our early successes. Let's see how.

Asymmetric Physiology

As mentioned, feeding behavior was a function that humans accomplished largely unconsciously and automatically. Given that obesity was not a common health problem throughout most of human history, it is not unreasonable that people instinctively believe that the body's regulatory system strives to maintain stability at some "natural" body weight, defending against both weight loss and weight gain.[78] Such a system would be symmetrical, defending against both positive and negative energy balances that threaten to cause weight change.

Unfortunately, this is a fundamental misconception that, because it remains quite common, seriously undermines (as we shall see in later sections) prevention efforts.

In reality, humans are endowed with a system of weight regulation that is *asymmetrical*. Because survival in a food-scarce environment is more acutely threatened by starvation than by obesity, evolution has selected our physiology and behavior to favor over-consumption rather than balanced consumption. And to build and protect our (long-term) energy reserves, our regulatory system has been organized by evolutionary selection to galvanize to deficiencies in energy intake and stores in a more robust way than to excess energy.[79]

Before we see how this is accomplished, let's contemplate for just a moment the alternative: that of a *symmetrical* system that defends *equally* against weight loss or gain, while striving to maintain stability at some "normal" body weight. In a food-scarce environment, such a system would have probably led to extinction. That's because lower-than-average food levels would have led to a drop in weight to below "target." That's the downside. But an abundance of food would have exceeded the regularity system's "needs" (and capacity) to store it, leading to a maximum weight equal only to the target weight. This provides no upside to balance the downside.

Professor Sam Savage of Stanford University provides an interesting analogy that demonstrates how such a symmetric model would similarly lead to bankruptcy (cash starvation?) in business. Consider a hypothetical case of an entrepreneur considering building a manufacturing facility for a new product. She did extensive market analysis for her new product and expects average annual demand to be 100,000 units. A further analysis of construction and operating costs suggests that building and running a manufacturing facility with a 100,000 capacity would yield a healthy $10 million annual profit. What would happen if the demand of 100,000 units is indeed the correct average, but with year-to-year fluctuations between say 50,000 ("famine" market conditions) and 150,000 units ("feast" market)? Intuitively, most people would expect that profit would still average out to $10 million: Some years it would be below, but those would be compensated for by other years when it's above. Right? Wrong. Lower-than-average demand clearly leads to profits of less than $10 million. That's the downside. But greater demand exceeds the capacity of the new plant (at 100,000 units), leading to a ceiling on profit of $10 million. There is no upside to balance the downside. The result: an average profit much lower than the "target," perhaps leading to bankruptcy (extinction).

Snatching Balance from the Jaws of Imbalance

So how did our hunter gatherer ancestors manage to maintain relatively stable body weights despite an asymmetric physiology that favored overconsumption?

While this might seem paradoxical—an asymmetric physiologic system maintaining a stable body weight— "snatching balance from the jaws of imbalance" is actually a "trick" commonly played by nature. Organisms, both simple and complex, adapt to asymmetric stresses in their external environments by evolving internal asymmetric structures and/or processes that cleverly compensate for— even exploit—rather than fight the external environmental asymmetries.[80] Nature evolves such "solutions" and humans have also learned to invent them.

To see how, let's consider a simple "home improvement" analogy: a self-described carpenter building a dining table for his new home. His goal, naturally, is to design a dining table that provides a leveled tabletop. There is one complication: the carpenter's new house is on a hill, and the dining room floor is sloping. Not a problem. To achieve a level tabletop, he builds an *asymmetric* table (and possibly chairs)—that is a table with legs that are shorter on one side—like so (Figure 2.1):

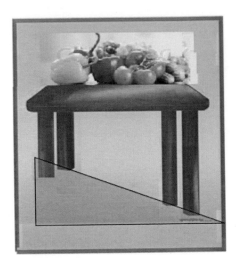

Figure 2.1: An *asymmetric* table on a sloping floor

That'll work!

Balance of the table top is achieved by compensating for (counteracting) the imbalances in the environment (the sloping floor) by designing-in asymmetry into the table (its support subsystem). "Fighting" external asymmetry with internal asymmetry is akin to fighting fire with fire—or (more abstractly) in arithmetic of obtaining a *positive* result from multiplying two *negative* numbers.

Analogous to our enterprising carpenter, natural selection works (albeit at a much slower pace and over many generations) to mold the characteristics of species so as to attain optimal equilibria vis-a-vis their living environments. Specifically, in the case of human energy regulation, "natural" body-weights could be maintained long-term—despite an asymmetric food environment characterized by chronic food shortages—by endowing humans with an asymmetric physiology that (slightly) favors positive energy balance. The optimal system that evolved is one that *slightly* favored overconsumption *by just enough* for our hunter-gatherer ancestors to build enough fat reserves to make it through the occasional lean times, but not so much that it slowed them down significantly.

The sketch below (Figure 2.2), while admittedly highly simplified, aims to (graphically) demonstrate how our *asymmetric* system of energy regulation would have worked throughout most of human history to maintain long-term stability by compensating for an *asymmetric* food environment.

Our asymmetric energy regulation system meant that we had a built-in drive to overeat in order to build up fat reserves in times of abundance—as in point "A" (A for abundance). Given the chronic boom-bust cycles in food availability in the hunter-gatherer environment, such fat stores would be called upon at least every two to three years during periods of famine. During these periods, body weight would drop, as in point "S" (S for starvation) in the insert sketch, but not for long and typically without adverse consequences. As good times eventually returned, body weight and energy reserves were restored. And so it went.

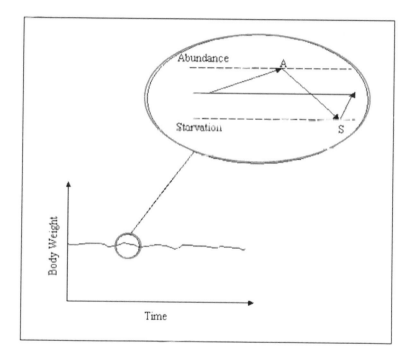

Figure 2.2 Body weights fluctuate but stable long-term

As suggested above, in this asymmetric food environment, a *symmetrical* energy regulation system that defends *equally* against weight loss or gain, while striving to maintain stability at some "normal" body weight would have probably led to extinction. Figure 2.3 compares the performances of the two designs. On the left is the asymmetric system just as described above. The system's performance—under the same boom-bust scenario—is compared to a symmetric design shown in the right panel. In the symmetric system (a system that defends *equally* against weight loss or gain, while striving to maintain stability at some "normal" body weight), the initial state of food abundance would have led to a maximum weight equal only to the target weight... to point "small a" in the figure. When this is followed by a lower-than-average food availability, body weights would have to drop to levels below S (the low point in the cycle for the scenario on the left)... say to point D (for death). (As indicated in the figure, I am assuming the amount of weight loss during the food shortage period is approximately the same.)

The "design flaw" in the symmetric system design is that the good times do NOT provide any upside to balance the downside. As can be seen in Figure 2.3, during food shortages weight drops below "target,"—that's the downside— while during periods of food abundance energy stores rise to target level but no higher—providing no upside to balance the downside. The inevitable result: over time *average* weight is significantly below target. The probable result: extinction.

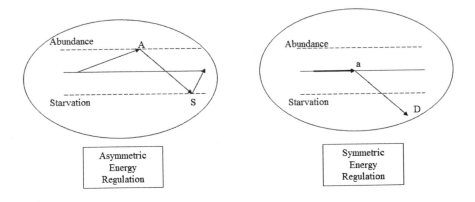

Figure 2.3 Asymmetric vs symmetric energy regulation

(For the interested reader, a multi-year simulation of this dynamic is played out and analyzed in an academic paper published by this author, titled: *Eureka... Insights into Human Energy and Weight Regulation from Simple—Bathtub-like— Models*. The paper presents a case study of seasonal variation in food availability and subsistence strategies of a contemporary hunter-gatherer population—the Hiwi hunter-gatherers of southwestern Venezuela.)

From this we arrive at the interesting insight: in order to maintain stable long-term weights and energy reserves, nature successfully *evolved an energy regulatory system that does NOT shoot for stability* per se. That is, in order to attain optimal balance in an unbalanced food environment, nature compensated and equipped us with an asymmetric regulatory system. And it worked. The fact that obesity wasn't a realistic possibility for our hunter-gatherer ancestors was a result of the "fit" between this asymmetrical design and their food-scarce environment—not the goal of the body's weight and energy regulation system.

Balance Breaking

The dining table on the sloping floor and hunter-gatherer populations in a food scarce environment are two very different examples of how different systems (biologic and man-made) can adapt or be designed to attain stable equilibrium by (cleverly) evolving internal asymmetric mechanisms that compensate for the asymmetries in their external environments.

It is important to emphasize, though, that in such successful adaptations where "balance is snatched from the jaws of imbalance," the population's (or table's) equilibrium state is not absolute but *relative* to the environmental conditions. And this means that if the environment were to change, there is every reason to suspect that the morphology or asymmetric design may not be adaptive under the new conditions—resulting in disequilibrium. (In Physics, this not uncommon phenomenon, where a balanced system becomes unbalanced, is called *symmetry breaking*.)

Devising internal asymmetric adaptations to compensate for external environmental asymmetries may, thus, be clever and functional... but it comes at a price: inherent vulnerability. And that's because if the system's asymmetric environment should change, the balanced "deal" is disrupted as the internal asymmetric "solutions" that were functional become dysfunctional. In nature this often is not a problem. Because most natural systems can *continuously adapt*, the disruption simply induces pressure for a new accommodative design. Such continuous change and adaptation is, in fact, a primary engine of change in nature. It is why it is often said that even as nature seeks and often attains equilibrium and symmetry, much of the *dynamic* texture of the world is due to mechanisms of symmetry breaking!

But the re-adaptation dance requires synchricity. If the tempo at which change occurs in the environment is different (e.g., faster) than the capacity of the system to adapt, problems arise and re-adaptation breaks down. This is what is happening with regards to human energy regulation. The tempo of man-made cultural/socioeconomic change is much faster than nature's tempo of biological adaptation.

To clarify the dynamic, consider the analogy below of two interacting gears. On the left, the two gears are colorfuly in sync (white on top, blue at bottom). This state of colorful synchronicity is disrupted if the gears rotate. Because of the different sizes, the rates of rotation will not be the same. On the right we see that as the smaller faster gear (think socio-economic environment) completes exactly half a revolution, the slower/larger gear (think human physiology) completes less than half a revolution. The result: the colorful lockstep is broken.

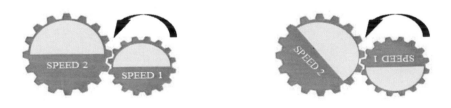

Figure 2.4: "Now you *sync*, now you don't"

That's analogous to what's been happening with regards to human energy regulation. The two processes—biological adaptation by nature (gear 1) and cultural/socioeconomic change by human intervention (gear 2)—progress at vastly different tempos. In the case of biology, the evolutionary process is a relatively slow process, often with a long lag time between environmental change and evolutionary adaptation. Indeed, our current physiology reflects evolutionary experience extending millions of years into the past. The tempo of cultural and socioeconomic change, on the other hand, is much faster—where dramatic changes have occurred in mere decades. It is this very substantial difference that has, in effect, knocked the heretofore well tuned "biology-behavior-environment" symphony out of tune.

The vulnerability—and inevitable imbalance—that result from *symmetry breaking* are perhaps easier to see in a simpler physical system... such as our table example. Figure 2.5 depicts the resulting (messy) disequilibrium when the asymmetry of the floor (the table's environment) changes from high-on-left to high-on-right. (Analogous to a shift in our modern food environment from one that is food-poor activity-rich environment to one that is food-rich activity-poor.) The environmental change exposes the built-in asymmetry, breaks the table-floor "fit," and ultimately knocking the system out of its happy equilibrium.

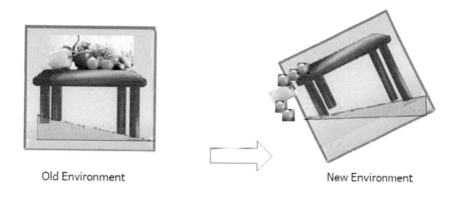

Old Environment   New Environment

Figure 2.5: The *asymmetric* table on floor with reversed slope

The failure of the dining table in the new environment is analogous to what is happening with regards to human energy regulation. Our asymmetric hard-wired physiology (evolved to nudge us to eat voraciously when food is plentiful and efficiently stored the excess energy as a buffer against future food shortages) is dysfunctional in today's food-rich activity poor environment. In a world of high-calorie, high fat foods, always in plentiful supply, our bodies are socking away a few extra calories day after day, year after year for a famine that never comes. Furthermore, with a paucity of opportunities for physical exertion, our under-active lifestyle contributes to the positive energy imbalance. This persistent imbalance of energy intake and output was not anticipated by biology, and given the capacity of the human body to adjust to excess calorie intake by adding body fat, the upside potential for gaining weight in the population was enormous.

Because physiology/environment asymmetries—that were in sync for millennia but now aren't—are at the root of our obesity problem, and thus are crucial to fully understand, I devote the next chapter to providing a deeper insight into their *how's*: (1) How asymmetry in human energy regulation was engineered by nature; and (2) how age-old asymmetries in our environment are being reversed.

CHAPTER 3

Modern Environment... "Flintstones' Physiology"

The long-term energy balance for our hunter-gatherer ancestors, we now understand, arose *not* out of a symmetric regulatory process or living in a stable environment, but from an asymmetric process that compensated for their unstable and food-scarce environment. (Hence the analogy with the carpenter's dining table on a sloping floor [Figure 3.1].)

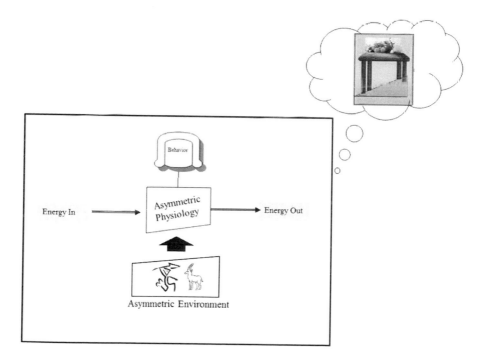

Figure 3.1: Hunter gatherer *asymmetric* physiology and environment

And while for thousands of years this system was (naturally) in equilibrium, the recent upward trend in the population's weight suggests the balance has been broken. Specifically, that (in our modern environment) the amount of calories consumed is *consistently* exceeding those burned-off for a growing proportion of the population.

In the remainder of this chapter, we will explore how the balance was broken as a result of swift (in evolutionary terms) socioeconomic transformations affecting what we eat and how we work and play—transformations that are mismatched with our "legacy" hunter-gatherer physiology. The discussion of the environmental transformations will be presented here from a *global* high-level perspective. In Part II, I will then provide a more in-depth case study of the U.S. experience. That discussion will detail how (and why) the eating and physical activity habits of Americans started to change in the 1950s and 60s (as the U.S. economy shifted from an emphasis on the production of goods to the provision of services) in lockstep with the recent escalation in obesity.

The Energy Input Side of the Equation

As mentioned, humans lived as hunter-gatherers foraging for food for more than 90 percent of their existence as a species. The food supply environment for humans started to fundamentally change approximately 12,000 years ago when some human groups started to shift from a food-foraging mode of existence to one of food production through farming. This shift was driven primarily by ecological pressures from population growth and food scarcities.[81] And it would prove to be of great consequence, as it was this relatively recent economic transformation that would ultimately allow for the evolution of complex societies and of civilization itself.[82]

Unfortunately… it would also lead to obesity.

(Indeed), obesity seems not to have appeared until after the development of agriculture and never to have affected more than a small percentage of any population until recently, when industrialized economies have created a luxurious living environment unlike anything ever seen before.[83]

The development of farming allowed for the production of a reliable surplus of food, but initially productivity was modest and food production was strenuous. This started to change in the late eighteenth century as industrialization mechanized food production (farming) and progressively improved agricultural productivity. This changed the environment to one in which food is significantly more abundant (and affordable) and food production not as strenuous.[84] These technological changes accelerated even more in the last century. Advances in mechanization and increasing availability of chemical inputs led to ever-increasing economies of scale.

> Agriculture in developed countries has undergone startling change in the past 100 years. Vastly increased crop yields; reduced price of production; irrigation of previously unusable land; genetic engineering; and widespread use of fertilizers, pesticides, and antibiotics have transformed the basic economics of food.[85]

As a result, food has become more abundant and much more affordable. For example, in the United States, the share of average household income spent on food fell from 42 percent in 1900 to 30 percent in 1950 and to 13.5 percent in 2003.[86] Food abundance in the United States, and in many other industrialized countries, afforded their populations an opportunity that humans had not previously had: "to eat food merely for pleasure and to consume more than the body needed to survive."[87]

The Energy Output Side of the Equation

The recent rise in the population's caloric intake could very well have been stifled had there been a balancing increase in energy expenditure. Unfortunately, the population's increased energy intake has been accompanied by a decline in energy output—further exacerbating our collective energy surplus. It is a trend that most experts expect will continue.[88]

For most of our existence as a species, humans lived as physically active hunter-gatherers—a mode of existence in which energy input (food) and energy expenditure (physical activity) were inextricably linked. But thanks to technological advancement, this natural balance has now been disturbed.

> The convenient modern world has virtually eliminated the evolutionary connection between energy expenditure and calorie ingestion. The "search and pursuit" time [to hunt, gather, forage, and fish] are minimized, while the caloric payoff is almost unlimited. Today, the acquisition of massive amounts of calorie-dense foods and beverages requires minimal energy expenditure. This systematic and pervasive disconnect between energy intake and energy expenditure inherent in modern cultures is a fundamental factor in the obesity epidemic.[89]

In gradual, often subtle ways, physical exertion continues to be technologically engineered out of our modern lifestyle. Whether in the farm, factory, office, or home, technology increasingly performs the tasks our bodies once performed. It is all adding up to an environment where fewer of us are expending the energy necessary to maintain a grip on our growing appetites.[90]

The drivers underlying these trends are not just technological; they are economic as well. As is often said, "Economics craft institutions into energy-saving enterprises."[91] In many industries, minimizing physical labor and replacing it with technology has certainly been an effective strategy to save cost. While (on balance) this has been good for our pocketbooks, it has had profound (and unintended) consequences on the economic incentives that drive us to burn calories.

Simply put, when work was strenuous, we were, in effect, being *paid* to exercise. Today, as more and more jobs become increasingly sedentary, we must *pay* for physical activity[92]—not only in the money we pay to get into the gym, but in foregone leisure time.[93] To expend serious calories in our society today often involves a choice between going to the gym and spending time with our spouse or kids.[94]

In the home, increasing reliance on prepared foods and the proliferation of labor-saving appliances—such as washing machines, dishwashers, microwave ovens, self-propelled lawn mowers, and automatic garage door openers—have caused household-related work to also markedly decline, further compounding the problem.[95]

A Sad Irony

In toto, the emerging picture is that of a confluence of multiple factors—agriculture, technology, socioeconomic forces—that are working together, enforcing each other to change our environment from one in which work was strenuous and food is scarce to one in which energy expenditure is low and food is abundant (Figure 3.2).[96]

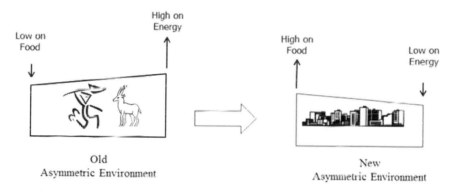

Figure 3.2: From one form of *asymmetry* to another

It is a sad irony. This modern environment that we toiled so hard to create for ourselves, while a very comfortable one, is one that our body's energy-regulating systems were never designed for. And an increasing number of people are paying the price.[97]

A Mismatch with our *Asymmetric* Physiology

Food abundance in the United States, and in many other industrialized countries, has afforded their populations an *opportunity* to consume more than the body needed to survive. While a *necessary* condition, food abundance is not, however, a *sufficient* condition for over-consumption. Abundance, in other words, does not necessarily lead to increased consumption.[98] Obesity and abundance are sort of analogous to lightning and thunder. Though related, lightning is not what *causes* thunder. Rather, both lightning and thunder are caused by an electric discharge (the fundamental cause) that we perceive first visually and then aurally.

In a similar sense, the "cause behind the causes" of the global obesity epidemic is *balance-breaking*—a result of mismatch between our modern environment and an asymmetric energy regulation system that evolved to help us survive in earlier times of privation, when the challenge to the body energy-control system was to provide a strong drive to eat in order to endure the periodic threat of famine and to maintain the high level of physical exertion needed to stay alive. And to accomplish that, our weight regulation system needed to be *asymmetric*.

As I explain below, it is in fact three-way asymmetric—not only in energy input but also in energy expenditure and storage.

Asymmetry in Energy Input. On the energy input side, asymmetry in energy regulation means we are "wired" to compensate aggressively (quickly and completely) for caloric deprivation but exhibit more tolerance for increases in caloric intake. As already argued, selecting our physiology and behavior to asymmetrically favor over-consumption rather than under-consumption constitutes an adaptive advantage since survival in a food-scarce environment is more acutely threatened by starvation than by obesity.

Asymmetry in the system is achieved by the fact that the neuronal and endocrine factors generated to stimulate feeding when fat stores decrease (as a result of a negative energy balance) are more potent than are the inhibitory signals generated when fat stores increase.[99] This was demonstrated more than twenty years ago in a series of experiments designed to assess differences in how humans compensate for increases/decreases in the energy content of their diet. In the experiments, Mattes et al.[100] surreptitiously diluted and then boosted the energy content of meals offered to free-living experimental subjects and observed how they compensated over a two week period. What they found was that when the experimental subjects received meals (lunches) containing 66 percent fewer calories than customary, they tended to compensate fully for the deficit by ingesting additional calories in subsequent meals. As a result their total energy intakes over the two week period did not decrease. In contrast, when the subjects were covertly provided meals containing 66 percent more calories than customary, they did not adjust their energy intake downward in subsequent meals to compensate. As a result, total energy intake was significantly higher. Humans, these results suggest, are "wired" to compensate for (significant) caloric dilution but not the reverse, exhibiting more tolerance for increases in caloric intake.

The cloning of the *ob* gene in 1994 and the discovery of leptin has helped delineate the biological underpinnings of the asymmetry in human energy regulation, allowing researchers to decipher the signaling mechanism between the body's fat stores and the brain centers that control eating.[101](Leptin, a hormone that is the product of the *ob* gene, is synthesized in fat cells and secreted into the blood stream in concentrations that are proportional to total fat stores. In this way, changes in leptin's plasma level concentration indicate to the brain alterations in the state of the body's aggregate energy reserves. That is, increased levels of leptin signal increased body fat, and, conversely, a drop in leptin reflects a depletion of fat stores.[102]) For example, it has been shown experimentally that when a person's fat stores shrink, the drop in leptin production leads to an increase in appetite and a decrease in metabolism.[103, 104] By contrast, increases in leptin production subsequent to significant weight gain does little to inhibit appetite.[105] The much more limited role that leptin plays in preventing weight gain is thought to be due to increases in cellular resistance to the leptin signal—possibly another evolutionary adaptation to promote fat storage.[106] (Leptin resistance—like insulin resistance in the development of diabetes—would explain why obese people sustain their high body weights, even though they have higher-than-normal levels of leptin in their bodies.[107])

In summary, these findings provide prospective dieters with two crucial insights:

> Firstly . . . biological processes exert a strong defense against under-eating which serves to protect the body from an energy (nutritional) deficit. Therefore, under-eating must normally be an active and deliberate process. Secondly, in general biological defenses against over-consumption are weak or inadequate. This means that over-eating may occur despite efforts of people to prevent it.[108]

To adequately manage our energy reserves, it is not enough for the body's regulatory systems to manage the amount of energy input into the body. Just as in managing the financial budget of a business or a household, one needs to keep an eye on both sides of the ledger—what is coming in and what is going out. And so with human energy regulation, the system needs to also oversee how energy is stored and consumed.

Asymmetry in Energy Expenditure (EE). The To stay alive, humans, like all living organisms, need to continuously expend energy—literally every second of every day, whether we are awake or asleep. Total energy expenditure can be divided conceptually into three components. The smallest component (about ten percent of daily energy expenditure) is the amount of energy expended in processing the food we eat—its digestion and absorption. A second component is the energy expended for muscular work. This typically accounts for 15 to 20 percent of daily energy expenditure, but can increase by a factor of two or more with heavy physical exertion.[109] The third and largest component is basal energy expenditure—also known as maintenance (or resting) energy expenditure (MEE)—which is the maintenance energy required to keep us alive. This is the amount of energy required for the basic maintenance of the cells, maintaining body temperature, and sustaining the essential physiological functions (e.g., keeping the lungs inhaling and exhaling air, the bone marrow making new red blood cells, the heart beating 100,000 times a day, the kidneys filtering waste, etc.). For most of us the MEE makes up about 60 to 70 percent of total energy expenditure.

As with the energy input side, the body's regulatory system for energy expenditure evolved to protect us against the frequent peril of food shortages—and associated energy deficits—rather than energy surplus. The system evolved to complement the over-consumption bias (explained above) with the capacity to reduce the body's metabolic rate in response to negative energy balance and a bias toward conserving energy when physical activity is not required.[110] As Polivy and Herman[111] argue, it is an effective strategy that best ensures that the body's fuel reserves are conserved in lean times:

> If there is a dearth of food available, the organism is better served
> by physiological adjustments that render what *is* available more

useful—by means of what has come to be known as a *thrifty* metabolism—rather than by promptings to acquire more food when there simply is no more to be acquired, or when the energy expended in acquiring more might well exceed the energy content of the food itself. In short, in an ecology of scarcity, we are better served by metabolic adjustments than by behavioral adjustments.

As soon as the body senses an energy deficit, basal metabolism drops quite dramatically in order to conserve energy and restrain the rate of tissue loss. This is achieved chiefly through hormonal mechanisms that operate to decrease the metabolic activity at the cellular level, in essence enhancing the tissues' metabolic efficiency— akin to the body changing its light bulbs to fluorescent lights to save energy.[112] (For example, muscle biopsies taken before, during and after weight loss show that once a person drops weight, their muscle fibers undergo a transformation, making them more like highly efficient "slow twitch" muscle fibers that burn 20 to 25 percent fewer calories during everyday activity.[113]) This homeostatic mechanism acts as a first line of defense against energy imbalance—a buffer, if you will, that helps spare the body's fat reserves in lean times. While, today, that may be bad news for dieters (because it limits weight loss), the survival value of an energy-sparing regulatory process that aims to limit tissue depletion during food scarcity is obvious.

The body's regulatory mechanisms work in reverse when confronted with a positive energy balance. Sort of. When a period of sustained positive energy balance induces weight gain, the body's maintenance energy expenditure (MEE) does rise. But, experimental studies of human energy regulation have demonstrated that in this less-threatening case, the body's biological signals are relatively "muted."[114] That is, while the body does adjust its MEE level upward when in positive energy balance, the adjustments do not increase energy expenditures enough to fully compensate for the imbalance.

The system clearly is not as robustly organized to galvanize in response to surplus energy balances (which are not particularly threatening to survival) as it is in responding to deficits (which are very threatening). This asymmetric bias in energy expenditure is in sync with the one we saw earlier on the energy intake side. Working in concert, these two limbs of our body's energy regulation system have effectively evolved us into what we are today: "exquisitely efficient calorie conservation machines."[115]

Asymmetry in Energy Storage. Beyond the asymmetry in regulating energy input/expenditure rates, there is a third form of asymmetry relating to energy storage: a bias in the system favoring the build-up (and against the depletion) of the body's energy reserves.

The food we eat—which is our primary source of energy—provides us with three energy-yielding macronutrients: protein, carbohydrate, and fat. The primary task of proteins is to provide the major building blocks for the synthesis of body tissue.[116] By contrast, fat and carbohydrate serve as the primary fuels to the body—fueling biologic work and physical activity.

Initially, when food is ingested, the chemical energy trapped within the bonds of the food nutrients is stored in its chemical form within the body's tissues. There, it is transformed into mechanical energy (and, ultimately, heat energy) by the action of the musculoskeletal system, or it is used to build body structures. If we eat too many calories or are too inactive relative to the calories we eat, the excess energy is stored in the body's energy reserves.

By a large margin, the primary form in which the body stores excess food energy is fat in the fat cells—called adipocytes. That's no coincidence since fat is the more efficient way to store energy. When stored as fat, energy is stored at about nine kilocalories (kcal) per gram of adipose tissue, which is almost two and one-half times as many calories of energy as each gram of glycogen (the form in which carbohydrates are stored in the body). "In lean adults, fat reserves typically amount to some 10 kg, an energy reserve of 90,000 kcal, enough to survive about two months of near total food deprivation."[117] By contrast, the average person has only about 2,500 calories of carbohydrate reserves—stored mostly in liver and muscle.

Our fat stores allow us to store energy efficiently and in a compact form, making it possible for us to carry a substantial energy reserve without being slowed down. That's an enormous benefit when an individual (or an animal) must be highly motile to survive.

Fat tissue in the human body, we now understand, is not just a static "spare tire" of energy around our waist. Rather, it is a highly dynamic tissue that's continuously secreting active substances (e.g., leptin) that play important roles in the body's weight-regulating system. And, as we have seen above, when it comes to its fat reserves, the human body is decidedly biased: with defenses against the depletion of its fat reserves that are more potent than the inhibitory signals it generates when fat reserves increase (as a result of over-feeding). There is a second asymmetry in the regulation of fat stores in humans: *when body fat is shed during weight loss, the size, but not the number, of fat cells dwindles.*[118]

The total amount of fat in a person's body is dependent on two factors: the number and the size of the fat cells in the body. When a person experiences a positive energy balance and starts to gain weight, initially the excess energy gets stored in the body's existing stock of fat cells, increasing them in size. Fat cells can expand in size a long ways, but not forever—they have a biologic limit. When the cells approach maximal or "peak" size, a process of adipocyte proliferation is initiated, increasing the body's fat cell count. Thus, obesity develops when a person's fat cells increase in number, in size, or, quite often, both. Once fat cells are formed, however, the number seems to remain fixed even if weight is lost.[119]

This means that the number of fat cells tends to ratchet up over time. And because (according to fat-cell theory) the body strives to maintain normal fat-cell size, the increased number of fat cells that invariably accompanies excessive weight gain results not only in an elevation of body weight but in the defense of that body weight.[120] (The details of this mechanism are explained in Part II.)

The System in Action… then and Now

In earlier times of privation, when the challenge to the body energy-control system was to provide a strong drive to eat in order to endure the periodic threat of famine and to maintain the high level of physical exertion needed for survival, an *asymmetric* system of energy regulation drove early humans to eat voraciously when food was plentiful and store the excess energy with great efficiency, aiding survival. Yet, throughout most of human history, obesity was never a common health problem. The boom-bust cycles in food availability coupled with a mode of existence characterized by high-energy throughput, (naturally) balanced the caloric intake and output over time.[121] Like in arithmetic when a *positive* result is obtained from the multiplication of two *negative* numbers, maintaining a healthy "normal" body weight was, thus, a result of the "fit" between this asymmetrical design and the food-scarce environment of our hunter-gatherer ancestors—not the goal of the body's weight and energy regulation system.

Today, we are not always so lucky. The same physiologic adaptations that kept us alive and in good form in a hunter-gatherer environment are resulting in a maladaptive response in our modern food-rich, activity-poor environment. Our pro-consumption physiological system is still intact, still encouraging us to over-eat. And with constant access to an abundant supply of high-calorie, high-fat food and a sedentary lifestyle that has reduced our energy requirements, there is constant pressure on the system towards positive energy balance (and weight gain).

The sketch below, while admittedly highly simplified, does capture these key distinctions between *the way it was* and *the way it is*. Both then and now, the strong drive to overeat and efficiently store excess energy builds up fat stores and body weight in times of abundance—as in point "A" in both figures. Given *the way it was*, such fat stores would be called upon at least every two to three years during periods of famine. During these periods, body weight would drop, as in point "S" in the left sketch, but not for long and typically without adverse consequences. As good times eventually returned, body weight and energy reserves were restored. And so it went.

In today's environment, our bodies are socking away a few extra calories day after day, year after year for a famine that never comes.[122] Furthermore, with a paucity of opportunities for physical exertion, our under-active lifestyle contributes to the positive energy imbalance—pushing weights even higher, to point "A+" (in the "The Way it is" sketch).

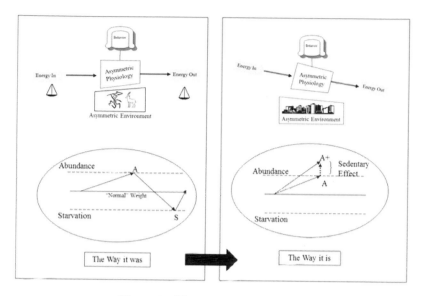

Figure 3.3 The way it was… and is

The current epidemic of weight gain in many cultures, thus, is an understandable function of a changed relationship between biology and the environment.

> Living in a world of high-calorie, high-fat foods, always in plentiful supply, and with labor-saving devices that keep us from having to exert ourselves too much, sometimes our finely tuned internal machines fail us. They tell us to eat more than we need for a healthy, normal weight, and, if we listen to their advice, we get fat. This makes maintaining a healthy weight a very different matter than it was intended to be. Instead of it being a task that is accomplished unconsciously and automatically, it becomes something we have to think about.[123]

It means we'll have to teach people to override their biological instincts with their cognitive abilities. And here's the really hard part: not for a week, or a month, but for a lifetime.

Postscript: Déja vu?

It is interesting (or perhaps alarming) to note that this is not the first time that human behavior disrupts a heretofore natural boom-and-bust (oscillatory) cycle that endured for millennia. We are doing it to the carbon dioxide level in the earth's atmosphere.

For almost the entire span of human civilization—roughly the last 8,000 years—the CO_2 level remained relatively stability... albeit cyclical. From studying air bubbles trapped in Antarctic ice, scientists know that going back 800,000 years, the carbon dioxide level oscillated in a tight band, from about 180 parts per million in the depths of the ice ages to about 280 during the warm periods between. But since the Industrial Revolution, a mere geological instant, the burning of fossil fuels has caused a 41 percent increase in the heat-trapping gas. And scientists say the climate is beginning to react. As shown in the Figure 3.4 (and reported in the New York Times), the level of carbon dioxide (the most important heat-trapping gas in the atmosphere), has passed a long-feared milestone, escalating beyond its "natural" cyclical band and reaching a concentration not seen on the earth for millions of years.[124]

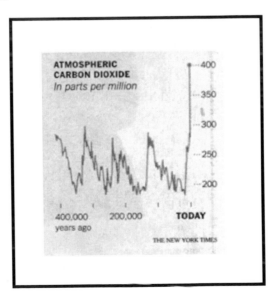

Figure 3.4: Recent disruption of long-running carbon
dioxide oscillatory cycle

CHAPTER 4

Wrong Ideas

The speed and spread of the obesity epidemic—unprecedented among the numerous diseases that have struck humanity throughout history—suggests two things: First, that obesity develops through a mechanism which, unlike plague, tuberculosis, or AIDS, is induced by exposure to factors surrounding all of us in modern societies; and second, that our strategies to manage the risk have (so far) been inadequate. The focus in Chapters 2 and 3 was on the former—the mismatch between our (hunter-gatherer) physiology and our modern (obesogenic) environment. In this chapter we now focus on the latter.

Prisoners to more than Hunter-Gatherer Physiology

Unlike the air we passively breath, personal energy balance is a product of deliberate lifestyle choices about how much and what to eat, and how much energy to expend and how. So, while the interactions between people and their environment (physical and socioeconomic) define our opportunities, options and incentives, ultimately it is human *decision making* (e.g., about food, work and play) that modulates such interactions.[125] Let's face it: There are no laws legislating less exercising/physical exertion, and no fast food chain can force us to gobble up that chocolate cake instead of picking an apple.[126]

Despite the pressures of our modern obesogenic environment, the recent rise in the population's positive caloric imbalance could very well have been stifled had we been smart enough to cognitively override our wired-in hunter-gatherer feeding drives—to eat to our physiological limits when food is readily available and selectively focus on foods high in fat and sugar. (In Part III, we will see how smart selection of foods with low energy density allows us to moderate energy intake while maintaining satiety.) So, why have we failed?

In this (and coming chapters) I'll argue that our choices (what and how we eat) are based on *mental models*. And just like our physiology, our hunter-gatherer mental models have not changed—reflecting behavioral (feeding) instincts that no longer apply. That is, today, people are prisoners not only to the physiology that was vital to our Pleistocene-era ancestors, but also to hunter-gatherer instincts that no longer apply. And what's most disturbing is that too many people remain unaware of this situation—and are paying the price.

Mental Models

People analyze many situations and make hundreds of decisions every day while at home, at school, at work, or on the road. Rarely, however, do we stop to think about *how* we think. No one's head contains a family, city, or business. All human decisions are based on models, usually mental models (of family roles and relationships, a city's layout of streets and neighborhoods, the power hierarchy in a business organization, etc.) created out of each person's prior experience, training and instruction.[127] They are the deeply ingrained assumptions, generalizations, or even pictures or images we form of ourselves, others, the environment, and the things with which we interact. These cognitive constructs are not simply repositories for past learning; they also provide a basis for interpreting what is currently happening, and they strongly influence how we act in response.[128]

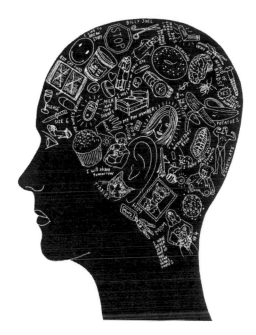

Figure 4.1

(Illustration courtesy of Peter Arkle)

We like to think (and most us believe) that well-adjusted individuals possess relatively accurate mental models—or perceptions—of themselves, their capacity to control important events in their lives, and their future. Unfortunately this isn't the case. And, what is more disturbing, most people are unaware of this situation.[129] A great deal of research in cognitive psychology has revealed that mental models are only simplified abstractions of the experienced world and are often incomplete, reflecting a world that is only partially understood.[130]

In the remainder of this chapter, I explain some of the mental conceptions that may have served us well in the past but are failing us in the current environment. And explain why mental models are often hard to correct.

I'll start with…

The Mother of all Misconceptions

When it comes to energy and weight regulation, the one misconception that is perhaps the most concerning is the mistaken belief that it is O.K. (normal?)

to defer to the body's wisdom and "cruise" on automatic feeding control. That is, to regulate feeding behavior in accordance with our body's biological drives—which drive us to eat to our physiological limits when food is readily available and selectively focusing on foods high in energy density.

It is not surprising that such a misconception remains pervasive... and stubbornly entrenched. Humans after all have learned to rely on and trust their bodies' self-regulatory mechanisms to maintain many aspects of their bodies' internal environment (e.g., body core temperature, body fluid volume and tonicity, blood glucose, etc.). In feeding, humans have similarly learned to instinctively regulate behavior in accordance with the body's biological states of need: eat when hungry (when the body signals an energy deficit) and stop eating when feeling full (when the body senses the energy depots are replenished). And, for most of our history, we did not have to think about how much to eat in order to maintain a desirable weight. Our bodies told us.

And it worked. These wired-in instincts helped our hunter-gatherer ancestors maintain enough fat stores to make it through the occasional lean times, but not so much that it slowed them down significantly. And despite seasonal fluctuations in food availability and a mode of existence characterized by vigorous physical exertion, the caloric intake and output of our hunter-gatherer ancestors were balanced over time.[131] Which is why it's perfectly reasonable for people to instinctively believe that the body's "automatic control" system is symmetric—defending against both weight loss and weight gain while striving to maintain stability at some "natural" body weight.

Unfortunately, this is a fundamental misconception that, because it remains quite common, seriously undermines prevention efforts. For, as we've seen, our weight regulation system is asymmetric—not only in energy input but also in energy expenditure and storage. The built-in asymmetries in human energy regulation mean that continuing to instinctively cruise on "automatic feeding control" in our modern obesogenic environment puts us at the risk of sustained positive energy balance... and weight gain.

The fundamental reason why some automatic-control mechanism—whether biologic or mechanical—that works admirably in one environment can lead us astray in another relates to the idea of vulnerability in balance breaking.

As we saw, when internal asymmetric structures or processes evolve (or are engineered) in organisms to compensate for asymmetries in the external environment and maintain equilibrium, the state of balance achieved is never absolute but *relative* to the environmental conditions. And this means that if the environment were to change, there is every reason to suspect that the morphology or asymmetric design may not be adaptive under the new conditions... resulting in disequilibrium.

Examples of automatic-control mechanisms that work admirably in some environments but become dysfunctional when the environments change are many and varied. Because man-made systems are often less complex and are more transparent to illustrate I'll use a relatively familiar example of a *dynamic* system whose management has interesting parallels to managing the dynamics of weight gain/loss: the autopilot that steers a boat.

The "Biased" Autopilot that Works

The torrent obesogenic pressures that are affecting all of us in our modern environment has often been compared to fast and furious sea currents that sweep all ships in a turbulent sea.[132] In many ways, it is a very apt analogy, and one that underscores several intriguing similarities. It aptly conveys, for example, how exposure to factors surrounding all of us in modern societies induces obesity in the population just as a raging current can carry all ships out at sea. The analogy also nicely explains how and why our built-in asymmetric system for energy regulation worked for us so well and for so long but is failing us now.

Our hard-wired physiologic system of energy regulation that is "steering" us towards over-consumption and that defends against negative energy balances can be likened to an automatic steering system (an autopilot) that helps steer a ship at sea. In the case of energy regulation, our *asymmetric* system keeps us in good form in an environment in which food is scarce and the next meal unpredictable. And that would be like relying on an *asymmetric* autopilot—one that's rigged to steer slightly to the left or to the West of North—to safely steer ships that sail on a body of water with a West-to-East cross current. While heading for the lighthouse (see Figure 4.2), the biased autopilot steers the boat on course B (slightly left of the mark). But because of the current (from left to right), the boat actually moves on the correct course "A"... ultimately arriving as intended at the lighthouse.

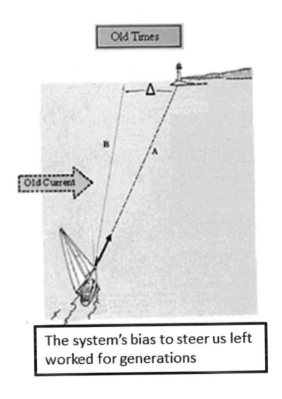

Figure 4.2: Biased autopilot steers boat to destination
in West-to-East current

This type of boat with this type of (biased) autopilot would safely make it *in this type of environment...* just as for thousands of generations our ancestors did with their energy "autopilots." Success, in both cases, arises from an *asymmetric* (biased) regulatory process that compensates for an unbalanced (biased) environment.

Now, let's take this analogy a step further. It is no longer a stretch, nor is it hypothetical—it is sad to say—to contemplate how human intervention may alter the weather environment in some significant or dysfunctional way. (Global warming, of course, comes readily to mind.) So—with a relatively straight face—we keep our nautical analogy going and consider what happens if human intervention causes winds—and the associated wind-driven sea currents—to reverse direction, becoming East-to-West.

The figure below depicts what happens *if we continue to steer by automatic control.* We'll be blown out to sea (along course "C").

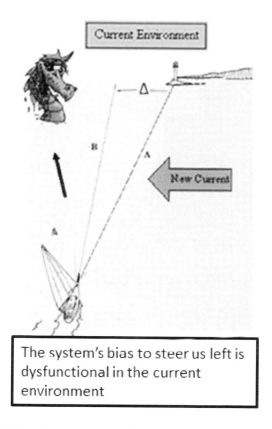

Figure 4.3: Biased autopilot steers boat off-course in East-to-West current

In an analogous manner, our innate asymmetric physiologic drives are "steering" us to higher weights in our current food-rich activity-poor environment. On the ocean, the solution requires a shift in strategy—disengaging automatic control, and assuming control of the helm. Similarly, most of our population will maintain a healthy body weight only by replacing the passive model of involuntary (automatic) energy regulation and asserting cognitive control to proactively resist the "obesifying" aspects of the current environment.

"Essentially," says James Hill, director of the Center for Human Nutrition at the University of Colorado, and a leading researcher in the obesity field, "we have to teach people to override their biological instincts with their cognitive abilities."[133] And-here's the really hard part—it's not for a week, or a month, but for a lifetime.

Seeing is Believing or Believing is Seeing?

Our mental models not only inform decision-making (e.g., to steer by autopilot or manually or to override our wired-in urges "to gorge, grab and hoard"), they also operate like "cognitive goggles" through which we view the world, others, and even ourselves. In sensing the world (both the physical and intellectual), we are rarely passive-objective observers; instead, our brains *actively construct* (model) our world, affecting what we see.[134]

While it may be comforting to believe that our senses reveal the world as it is, that's not how it works in reality. A great deal of research in cognitive psychology has revealed that our mental models are often biased by needs and emotions. Prior expectations and self-serving interpretations weigh heavily into how we view the world, and people's predictions of what will occur often corresponds closely to *what they would like to see happen* or to what is socially desirable, rather than to what is objectively likely.[135,136]

Below are two health-related examples on how people misperceive the risk/evidence (1) around them and (2) in them.

Example 1: The Illusion of Unique Invulnerability

One example of how people often distort the drivers of disease risk <u>around them</u> and, as a result, underestimate their own risk is the "it won't happen to me" illusion that many people succumb to. It is a serious impediment to disease prevention.

The "it won't happen to me" illusion is an example of how people often distort the drivers of disease risk <u>around them</u> and, as a result, underestimate their own risk. It is a serious impediment to disease prevention.

Research studies consistently show that "… people display an unrealistic optimism (also labeled *illusion of unique invulnerability*) in their assessment of perceived risk of occurrence of a variety of potential negative health and safety outcomes."[137] This optimistic bias is commonly defined as the mistaken belief that one's chances of experiencing a negative event are lower than that of one's peers. Such perceptions of relative invulnerability (the "it won't happen to me" notion) have been found across a wide range of diseases, hazards, and catastrophic events. For example, "when asked to assess their chances of experiencing a negative event such as getting cancer or having a heart attack, being sterile or being involved in an automobile accident, it is found that most people consider their chances are less than others."[138]

Research in clinical and developmental psychology suggests that such positive illusions serve a wide variety of cognitive, affective, and social functions. For example, the illusion of unique invulnerability is often an attempt to avoid the anxiety one would feel from admitting a threat to well-being—a form of defensive denial. Illusions about unique invulnerability can also enhance a person's self-esteem. People may believe that vulnerability (say to tooth decay) is a matter of their constitution, so if the problem has not appeared, their bodies must be super-resistant. In problems like obesity or drug addiction, which many believe to be caused by behavior or personality, people may feel invulnerable because they would like to believe that they do not have the weakness of character that allows it to develop in them.[139] In short, even the well-adjusted individual appears to have the enviable capacity to distort reality in a way that enhances self-esteem and promotes an optimistic view of the future.

While the capacity to develop and maintain positive illusions may help make each individual's world a warmer place in which to live, it can be a risky business. Unrealistic optimism in matters of health and disease often leads people to ignore legitimate risks in their environment and avoid taking the necessary measures to offset those risks.[140] This, of course, can become a significant impediment to preventing conditions such as obesity. If people convince themselves that they (and their kids) are invulnerable to obesity, then they are unlikely to take measures to reduce their risk of gaining weight no matter how educated they are about the dire consequences of obesity. The "it won't happen to me" mindset gets in their way: why protect yourself from an event that will not occur?

Example 2: Misperceiving the Evidence <u>In Us</u>

While distorting *future* risk may be excusable—even understandable—and, therefore, not uncommon, surely you would think distorting *current* reality would not be. Wrong! This second example is about how people misperceive the evidence in them... and why it is a serious impediment to *treatment*.

It would seem that educating people to acknowledge, and accurately assess, their overweight status would surely rank among the most achievable health education goals—an assured public awareness "homerun." And yet, a number of studies have demonstrated significant gaps between people's assessment of their weight status and their actual status. In one recent study, researchers sifted through data from the third National Health and Nutrition Examination Survey (NHANES III, 1988-94) to assess the degree of agreement between individuals' *actual* weight status, as measured by their body mass index (BMI), and their *perceptions* of their weight status. They found that substantial numbers of overweight and obese people underestimate their weight status and believe themselves to be of a healthier weight than they actually are. Interestingly, overweight men, not women, were the major culprits—with 43 percent of the overweight male subjects failing to correctly perceive that they were overweight and, instead, reporting themselves as being "about right" or underweight.[141] Significantly, for both the men and the women, the mistakes were not just at the margin (when weights were a few pounds over the overweight cut-off point); many of the mistaken perceptions were of quite large discrepancies.

A possible reason why weight misperceptions occur is because overtime obesity may have become 'normalized'. As exposure to obesity increases, perceptions of what is a 'normal' weight are likely to change and this may result in overweight and obese people being perceived as healthier weights than they actually are.

This would constitute a form of anchoring effect, whereby individuals use the weight of the people they see around them to determine what a 'normal' weight looks like, and then only perceive people above this anchor to be overweight.[142]

Nevertheless, such misperception is cause for concern because if people misperceive their weight, it is likely to affect whether a person feels they should try and lose weight.

Another potentially serious distortion is the finding that parents of overweight children systematically underestimate their children's weight.[143] In a recent systematic review of the literature that was conducted to identify differences between parental perception and the actual weight status of children, revealed that a large proportion of parents fail to recognize the overweight weight status of their especially in young children. Specifically, only a third of the overweight children were perceived as being overweight by their parents. It is a disturbing but also a surprising finding given the recent focus on the prevention and treatment of overweight in children.[144]

Misperceptions about weight obviously have direct implications on people's perceptions of risk—for themselves or their children. Such misperceptions, health experts agree, are formidable roadblocks to prevention and treatment efforts. In the case of childhood obesity, the issue of parental misclassification of child weight status is immensely important because parent involvement is a key component in treatment and prevention. In order to recognize that their overweight child needs help, parents must first identify their child as overweight or obese.[145]

How to de-fog our "Cognitive Goggles"?

To many the answer is obvious: "It's the information… stupid."

Indeed, many public health officials and academics continue to believe that the key to clearing the public's misconceptions and reversing obesity's escalation *is* information—offering the public more and better information such as about healthy food and lifestyle choices. Most government programs aimed at weight control are based on this principle. This viewpoint relates to what the philosopher Karl Popper used to call "the bucket theory of the mind." When minds are seen as containers, and public understanding is viewed as a function of how much scientific facts are known, the focus naturally is on how much scientific facts public minds contain.[146]

That bucket-filling strategy hasn't worked.

An irony of America's obesity epidemic is that despite the drumbeat of educational campaigns and broad publicity about the obesity problem, widespread fundamental misconceptions (such as about "symmetric" energy regulation, invulnerability, and weight status) persist. [147,148] And meanwhile, Americans keep piling on the pounds.

Although the notion that knowledge shapes beliefs and behavior seems reasonable, the evidence to-date suggests that merely providing information does not have much effect on changing health beliefs and behavior.[149,150] And neither have mass-media-type educational campaigns (such as distributing copies of the *Dietary Guidelines for Americans* or the many similar educational materials on nutrition and exercise) proven effective in correct entrenched mental models.[151,152] While this may surprise many people and must surely frustrate policy makers, it is no mystery to cognitive psychologists.

Research in human cognition has repeatedly demonstrated that many of us tend to use information as a drunken man uses lampposts—for support rather than for illumination.[153] For example, people often (unconsciously) seek out information that supports their existing instinct or point of view, while avoiding information that contradicts it—a behavior that psychologists call confirmation-seeking bias. This "not only affects where we go to collect evidence but also how we interpret the evidence we do receive, leading us to give too much weight to supporting information and too little to conflicting information."[154]

The result: access to more information tends to increase *confidence* in judgment—as people assume that their decisions are good because they can find information to support them—but it does not necessarily increase the *quality* of judgment. For example, "All that many people did on low-fat and fat-free products was gain weight because they figured that fat-free gave them license to eat as much as they wanted, without regard to serving size and calories per serving."[155]

Interestingly, this applies not only to "ordinary" folks, but to scientists and professionals, as well. Professor John Sterman, of MIT, provides some fascinating—and, perhaps, troubling—examples in the science and public policy domains. One example relating to global warming is particularly interesting because, like the obesity epidemic, it is a phenomenon with potentially grave consequences for humanity.

The first scientific papers describing the ability of chlorofluoro-carbons (CFCs) to destroy atmospheric ozone were published in 1974. Yet much of the scientific community remained skeptical, and despite a ban on CFCs as aerosol propellants, global production of CFCs remained near its all-time high. It was not until 1985 that evidence of a deep ozone hole in the Antarctic was published. . . . The news reverberated around the scientific world. Scientists at NASA . . . scrambled to check readings on atmospheric ozone made by the Nimbus 7 satellite, measurements that had been taken routinely since 1978. Nimbus 7 had never indicated an ozone hole. Checking back, NASA scientists found that their computers had been programmed to reject very low ozone readings on the assumption that such low readings must indicate instrument error. The NASA scientists' belief that low ozone readings must be erroneous led them to design a measurement system that made it impossible to detect low readings that might have invalidated their models. Fortunately, NASA had saved the original, unfiltered data and later confirmed that total ozone had indeed been falling since the launch of the Nimbus 7.[156]

Sterman's summary of the lessons learned is both poignant and succinct: "[S]eeing is believing *and* believing is seeing."

"It's (NOT) the Information... Stupid"

A shift in emphasis is desperately required.

To achieve a turnaround, we'll need to move beyond the so called knowledge *accretion* model in health promotion and education—where we aim to stuff people's "mental buckets" with nutritional guidelines and food pyramid images—to a more enlightening knowledge *restructuring* model. By that I mean challenging people's deeply ingrained assumptions and misconceptions (about their bodies and health risk) and providing them with the skills (and the tools) needed to effectively exercise personal control over their health/bodies.

Knowledge accretion—or the accumulation of facts as in learning a new vocabulary word or the spelling of an already known word—is the easy form of learning.[157] The deeper but more difficult form of learning is *restructuring*, in which we use new knowledge to form a new (more effective) conceptual structure of a problem or a situation. Learning in this deeper sense is discovery—discovery of mental maps and decision rules that are more appropriate to the decision task— and that can be much harder. (In upcoming chapters, *you* will discover new mental maps and decision rules that are more appropriate for managing body weight.) While accretion is often relatively easy, even automatic, acquiring new conceptual understanding is neither easy nor automatic. And as cognitive scientist Donald Norman has argued, it often requires tools "to reflect; to explore, compare, and integrate."[158]

That's what I'll try to do in the remainder of this book.

CHAPTER 5

Step on *U.P.*

It seems paradoxical, but the wondrous advances in health care over the last century—a period historians hail as the time of the "great flowering of medicine"—have made the task of managing *personal* health more critical—and complex—not less. Improved medical care and the elimination of infectious diseases have increased life expectancy so that minor dysfunctions due to personal mismanagement have now more time to morph into chronic ailments later in life. A good (bad?) example of the challenges—and the mismanagement—is the growing obesity problem. A century ago, when the life expectancy was only 40, gaining 30 or 40 pounds at the age of 20 or 30 would not have been too much of a concern. A century later, the life expectancy of the United States population has nearly doubled, from 40 to almost 80 years (although the trend may be reversing), which means that there is ample time for those 30 or 40 pounds to translate into serious ailments (including hypertension, heart disease, type 2 diabetes, even cancer).[159]

Today, what we desperately need is a "second great flowering" in *personal* health management, one that promotes the customization of healthcare and where medicine seeks not just to cure disease but to develop our capacities to prevent it. The ticket, many in public health increasingly believe, is the growing—and synergistic—entwinement of the healing and personal digital technologies.

An expanding repertoire of personal information technologies is engendering enormous possibilities for empowering ordinary people with the learning and decision-making tools they need to better manage personal health and well-being. Particularly exciting is how easily (and economically) these new generation *e*tools can be tailored to each person's health needs, lifestyle (why they do or do not do), and even style of thinking. (In Part III I will discuss several such tools that specifically support personal health regulation—tools that can help you look back to diagnose and monitor [e.g., how many calories you burn and how you burn it] as well as to look forward when planning some intervention [e.g., optimizing the frequency and intensity of exercise or the composition and size of a diet].)

To catalyze this digital transformation, you—the consumer—will need to step up and lead the way. "Without the active participation of consumers in this revolution, the process will be inexorably slowed."[160] And for this to happen, people must come to realize that in managing their health—and their bodies—they are decision makers who are managing a truly complex and dynamic system: the human body. And that effective self-regulation requires *skill*... and the right decision-support tools. Motivation alone is not enough.

And the First Step to Take... is *U.P.*

U.P. is the acronym I'll use (in Part II) to designate two fundamental skills we'll need to acquire to be effective: <u>U</u>nderstanding and <u>P</u>redicting how our body works as a system.

Research in control theory and behavioral decision making suggests that effective regulation of any complex system—whether it is the energy regulation of our bodies or the energy regulation of an atomic reactor—requires that we do two things well: (1) *understand* how and why the system (our body) behaves the way it does; and (2) *predict* how it will behave in the future (e.g., in response to our interventions).

By *understanding* is meant acquiring *structural knowledge* about the system—that's knowledge of how the system's variables (such as the energy consumed and expended in the case of weight regulation) are structured (related) and how they influence one another and are influenced by the external environment. (The terminology reflects the engineering roots of these concepts and appropriately so, since it was the engineers who long ago learned to how to build and manage complex technological systems.) *Understanding* how the human energy and weight regulation system works, why it works that way, and how to better manage it will be the focus of the book's Part II. We will see then how the human weight and energy regulation system is truly a fascinating conglomerate of interrelated and interdependent control processes and subsystems that work in concert to regulate appetite, energy expenditure, body composition, etc. And we'll learn how the system's varied processes do not operate in isolation but rather are highly interdependent, interacting in complex ways with each pushing on the others and being pushed on in return. (A good case in point is energy intake/expenditure processes which replenish/consume the body's energy stores and are simultaneously regulated by them.) Such mutual interdependencies mean we cannot voluntarily change one part of the system, say decrease energy input, and expect that the other parts (energy expenditure) will hold steady and, thus, are important to understand (and properly account for) when devising treatment interventions.

Understanding alone is *not* enough, however, when managing complex systems. Understanding without a capability to *predict* the system's behavior—e.g., when devising treatment strategies and/or to assess treatment outcomes—is of little practical utility. The ability to infer system behavior is essential if the decision maker—*you*—is to know how actions taken will influence the situation or system and is therefore essential in devising appropriate interventions for change. In managing personal health, effective prediction of treatment outcomes is critically important because people's expectations about treatment (e.g., pounds lost from a diet or an exercise regime) can affect their self-efficacy and long-term commitment.

The two skills—understanding and prediction—are thus needed *together*. Understanding helps us *look back* to diagnose and interpret what is happening, while prediction helps us *look forward* to prevent or to devise treatment strategies.

It is important to note that while understanding and prediction are interdependent, they are conceptually different skills.[161] For example, while one may be able to explain how the eclipse of the sun occurs, most of us would not be able to predict when the next eclipse will occur. On the other hand, a person may accurately predict the rattling sound that occurs every time he/she depresses their car's gas pedal, but may not be able to explain it.

Furthermore, recent experimental studies of human decision making performance have revealed rather interesting asymmetries in how we tackle understanding-versus-prediction tasks. They indicate, for example, that while people (both lay and professional) are generally adept at acquiring structural knowledge (i.e., grasping what the key variables are in some system and how they are interrelated), they are usually unable to accurately determine the dynamic behavior implied by these relationships.[162] Being able to "run" our mental model of some system or situation to project its future behavior, in other words, is a much more difficult task for us. (You will have a chance to experience this first hand using a simple exercise in Part II.) This obviously presents a serious challenge in managing body weight as we shall see.

Luckily for us, that's precisely where computer tools can help. Unlike mental (or intuitive) simulation, a computer model can reliably and efficiently predict the dynamic implications of a messy maze of interacting variables. And it can do so tirelessly, reliably and efficiently. Computer modeling is thus well suited to fill the gap where human cognition is most suspect—prediction.

Hence, a key takeaway message from the book is this: that we cannot—should not—rely on intuition alone in managing a system as complex *and important* as our bodies. With its many interrelated subsystems and processes (some counteracting, some reinforcing) the human body is simply too complex to effectively manage by human intuition alone. Furthermore, in matters of health and disease some consequences may be hard if not impossible to reverse, which makes trial and error or learning from experience a risky business. To effectively manage a system as complex as our body, a reliable (and efficient) system of dynamic "bookkeeping" is required. The digital computer (on your desk or in your phone) provides that functionality.

But what if we do not?

Making Do

For concrete examples of the inherent pitfalls in relying on intuition and raw judgment when managing personal health and wellbeing we must wait until later in the book when we've had a chance to explore the intricacies of the body's system of weight/energy regulation. For now, we have to settle for a sneak preview. To provide that, I revisit the analogy I drew earlier between "steering" our bodies toward health (in the current obesifying environment) and steering a boat (in torrent seas). Recall the interesting parallels between these two complex systems: both the boat and the human body are complex yet delicate machines. And both are subject to personal control as well as to uncontrollable environmental forces.

Furthermore, in both cases, *individual characteristics* matter a great deal. The analogy is particularly handy to invoke here because, in contrast to the internal (and still opaque) processes of weight and energy regulation—such as metabolism, hormonal signalling in appetite regulation, macronutrient ingestion/absorption, fat cell pruliferation—the forces and structures regulating a boat's performance—sea, wind, sails—are easy to discern and visualize (even by non-sailors).

The Direct-versus-Crooked Course to a Target

Consider the challenge of steering a boat towards some desired destination—say to a lighthouse to the North—when sailing through a body of water where there is a strong cross current (as depicted in Figure 5.1.). (The dieting parallel: steering our body towards a lower target weight in an obesifying environment with pressures to eat more and move less.)

As with managing other complex systems success here requires both *understanding* and *prediction* skills. Specifically, the skipper needs to understand that in order to safely and efficiently make it to the lighthouse she needs to make due allowance for the estimated effect of the current. This means that the boat should be steered on a course somewhat *into the current*—and to the east of the direct course to the lighthouse. Specifically, to sail the most direct course to the lighthouse the trick is to chart a course "X" with an offset to the east that precisely compensates for the current's push to the west. If the skipper successfully pulls this off, the counter-balancing effects would cause the boat to sail in a *straight line* towards the lighthouse.

Understanding all of that is crucial... but still is *not* enough however!

The reason: figuring out the angle Δ for course "X" is a non-trivial navigation problem that requires *predicting* the net effect of many different factors relating to the boat's performance and sea state. Because different boats perform differently, this course calculation needs to be "personalized" to reflect the boat's unique performance characteristics (a function of things like the boat's hull shape, keel design, sizes and configuration of sails, etc.). Further, the boat's performance will depend on a proper assessment of the environmental conditions—in this case, on factors such as the strength and direction of wind and current. Accounting for all these factors is a rather formidable computational task.

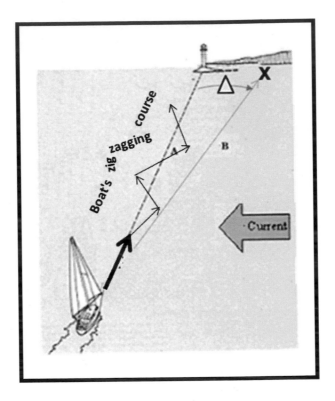

Figure 5.1: What course to the lighthouse?

The good news: modern route-planning software can now tackle this formidable computational task and reliably compute the direct most efficient route to the lighthouse (route "B" in Figure 5.1). And yet—not unlike dieters who opt to manage body weight and personal health by intuition and raw judgment—there are "old salts" around who still feel they can rely on their seat-of-the-pants navigation skills. A bad idea! To appreciate the inherent pitfalls let's return to the water… and sail along such a seat-of-the-pants skipper.

Lacking the leverage of a computational tool to account for all the interacting factors, our skipper will rely on a series of action-and-adjustment steps to take her progressively to the destination. Such an action-and-adjustment approach is a strategy we routinely deploy to tackle many of our daily chores (including managing personal weight), and in this case it would work as follows: the skipper makes an intuitive determination on the appropriate angle to steer her boat (i.e., determines what's a reasonable offset to the east of the direct course to steer), proceed to sail on that best-guess course, and then continuously monitor the boat's progress so as to make adjustments when/as necessary.

What's the most likely outcome of this seat-of-the-pants strategy? It is *not* going to be a straight-line course to the lighthouse, but rather an inefficient zigzagging course such as the one depicted in Figure 5.1. After the skipper points the boat's bow slightly to the east of the lighthouse and starts sailing, initially, the boat may sail in the desired direction *towards* the lighthouse, but before long it will start drifting with the current and wander off course. It might take little time, but eventually the skipper would notice that she'd deviated from the desired course, and would take action to correct it by re-setting the boat's heading. And then the performance-feedback-correction cycle would start again: sailing for a while, drifting off course, detection by the skipper, and correction.

Obviously, the resulting zigzagging course is not the fastest (most efficient) course to the lighthouse. In systems with even longer time delays between action and reaction and where effects are irreversible—as in the case of human health and disease—such an action-and-adjustment strategy can fail even more spectacularly.[163]

This sailing analogy serves to demonstrate the challenges and pitfalls of steering our body to health in a turbulent obesifying environment. It demonstrates that understanding of system structure—even "perfect" understanding—is no guarantee for proper prediction of system behavior. And the consequences of *improper* prediction. The inefficient zigzagging course when naively steering a boat by feedback has intriguing parallels to the weight cycling ("yo-yo dieting") phenomenon that many dieters experience… and loathe (Figure 5.2).

The figure shows the results of a study that tracked the weight of 31 women over a 25-year period. Over that extended period, this group of women (whose average age was 40 years) dieted an average of five times.

Source: (Wadden et al., 1992)

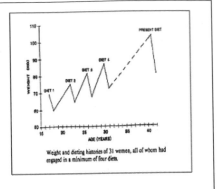

Figure 5.2: Weight cycling ("yo-yo dieting")

eSteering our Bodies to Health

Engineers, of course, long ago learned to use computer models to manage and predict the behavior of complex technological systems. So have pilots, who rely on computer-based flight simulators to learn how to manage and predict the behavior of advanced new aircraft. Well, our bodies are as complex as (if not more complex than) many of our most advanced technological systems. Why then not use the same approach engineers and pilots use, and create and use models of our physiology to learn about and better manage ("fly") our bodies?

We should… and indeed we will (when our focus turns to *prediction* in Part III).

Deploying computer models to manage our bodies and personal health is no futuristic vision or wishful thinking. All the technological building-blocks to build tailored tools for personal health management are available… here and now. For example, thanks to the great advances in medical and computational sciences, we already have the models to predict with greater fidelity how the human body regulates its energy and mass. And thanks to the availability of affordable, high-quality computing capabilities (such as in phones and tablets) and increasingly user-friendly software interfaces we can "tame" these models so that ordinary people can use them effectively and easily.

A concern often stated is that the average person's knowledge and skill is grossly insufficient for properly using models of a system as complex as the human body. But what justification can there be for the apparent assumption that ordinary people do not know enough to use models of their health, but believe that they do know enough to directly intervene in managing their weight and energy regulation? I contend (and substantial supporting evidence is beginning to accumulate) that people do know enough to use such models. Indeed, Americans of all ages have already shown an uncanny ability to make use of computers as routine tools for study, communication and entertainment. And as digital technology becomes an ever-increasing part of our lives, computer-based health regulation will not only be appropriate, but perhaps even requisite for an increasingly tech-savvy population.

Furthermore, the timing may be just right. The explosive growth of computer-based electronic communication is converging with another powerful trend· the increase in public initiative in taking greater responsibility for their well-being. This is opening enormous possibilities for empowering people with the tools they need to more effectively manage their well-being with potentially far-reaching transformative consequences.

So, please get ready to step *U.P.*!

PART II

WE CAN'T MANAGE WHAT WE DON'T UNDERSTAND

CHAPTER 6

Change your Mind

Progress is impossible without change, and those who cannot change their minds cannot change anything.

George Bernard Shaw

Albert Einstein once observed that the significant problems we face cannot be solved at the same level of thinking we were at when we created them. That we'd have to shift to a new level, a deeper level of thinking, to solve them.

Going back in history even further, the Greeks had coined a wonderful word for the mental "jumps" to new ways of thinking and acting that we often need to make: *metanoia*. It means a fundamental shift of mind or, more literally, transcendence *("meta"*—above or beyond, as in "metaphysics") of mind ("noia," from the root "*nous*," of mind).[164]

It may be time for a "metanoic" jump in addressing our overweight problem. In this book I argue for, and present, a different perspective for thinking about and managing our bodies: a *Systems Thinking* perspective.

It is a different way of thinking.

Understanding How Your Body Works as a *System*

A major shortcoming in much of the current debate on obesity has been the inability to integrate our knowledge of the multiple dimensions of the problem—such as behavior, biology, and environment—into an integrated whole. Treatments of the problem, whether in academic circles or around kitchen tables, invariably emphasize one aspect or problem area: nutrition, individual responsibility, metabolism. There is much attention on the separate mechanisms of human weight and energy regulation, but little on the whole psychobiological system as an integral operating system.

This fragmentation of knowledge is not a reflection of the way the world (and our body) works, but rather is the result of the analytic lens we impose—our natural predisposition when confronting a difficult problem to take things apart and treat the parts separately. In the case of obesity, this takes nutrition out of the context of lifestyle, biology out of the context of behavior, and behavior/lifestyle out of the context of the environment.

While breaking things apart is integral to the process of simplification—an effective (divide-and-conquer) strategy that scientists use to find points of entry into what may otherwise be impenetrably complex problems—we often forget that it is only a lens.[165]

> The difficulty arises when the method itself is reified into... a 'true' and 'complete' representation of reality (i.e., 'the world is like the method' rather than 'the method helps us understand some aspects of the world').[166]

The performance of any system (whether it is an oil refinery, an economy, or the human body) obviously depends on the performance of its parts, but a system's performance is never equal to the sum of the actions of its parts taken separately. Rather, it is a function of their interactions.[167] These interactions (and their properties) are destroyed when the system is dissected, either physically or theoretically, into isolated elements. It's why breaking a system into its component pieces and studying the pieces separately is usually an inadequate way to understand the whole.

No matter how exhaustively one studies a particular component in isolation, there is usually no way to know what its true properties will be when it's put back in association with other parts of its ensemble.[168] For example, the properties of water are not easily derived from understanding the behavior of hydrogen and oxygen molecules. An important, if not the most important, aspect of a part's performance is how it interacts with other parts to affect the performance of the whole. Forgetting that can only be at our peril. Even death. In medicine, for example, the effect of one chemical frequently depends on the state of another, as when each of two medications may be helpful, but exposure to both in combination could be fatal.

It is important to emphasize that what I am saying here goes beyond the popular phrase, "The whole is greater than the sum of its parts." When dealing with systems, whether living or technological, the whole is *different from*, not *greater than*, the sum of the parts. That's because the essential properties of a system are properties of the *whole*, which none of the parts have.[169] For example, no part of an automobile can transport people, not even its motor. Therefore, when an automobile or any system is taken apart, it loses its defining function, its essential properties. "A disassembled automobile cannot transport people, and a disassembled person does not live, read, or write."[170]

The emergence of systems thinking in the middle of the last century was a profound revolution in the history of Western scientific thought. The great shock of twentieth-century science has been that systems cannot be understood by analysis.

> To understand things systematically literally means to put them into a context, to establish the nature of their relationships. . . . This is, in fact, the root meaning of the word 'system,' which derives from the Greek *synhistanai* ('to place together')... Thus the relationship between the parts and the whole has been reversed. In the systems approach the properties of the parts can be understood only from the organization of the whole.[171]

The challenge to us today in addressing the obesity epidemic—indeed, many of our persistent societal problems—is to "put things back together" again, after they have been examined in pieces. It's a callenge the medical community is just starting to embrace. In its recently published guidelines on obesity prevention policies and programs, the authoritative Institute of Medicine (IOM) recommends, "... (looking) at obesity from a systems perspective in order to fully understand it as a complex, population-based health problem."[172] Such a holistic perspective does not imply denying the independent roles of the separate factors (nutrition, psychology, metabolism), but rather entails integrating them into a broader framework that incorporates the interactions between them—interactions that tend to get lost when the individual mechanisms are examined in isolation.

In this book, we will view and understand how the human weight and energy regulation system is a conglomerate of interrelated and interdependent control processes and subsystems. Taken together, they constitute a complex and dynamic marvel of system integration, where changes in one subsystem can be traced throughout the entire body. A good example is appetite: a phenomenon arising out of and maintained by a biopsychological system that includes the external environment (cultural and physical), the behavioral act of eating, the processes of ingestion and assimilation of food, the storage and utilization of energy, body composition, and the neuro-humoral system.[173] All these various factors are interconnected, pushing on each other and being pushed on in return. Appetite shapes body weight, and body weight influences appetite. Weight reflects activity levels (which are also shaped by the socioeconomic environment), and activity levels reflect weight. And on and on.[174] Though all of these influences are always there, they are usually hidden from view. And, because we are part of that lacework ourselves, it's doubly hard for us to see.[175]

Explaining things in terms of their context means explaining them in terms of their environment, and thus we can also say that all systems thinking is environmental thinking.[176] This contrasts with the atomistic and individualistic perspective in the analytical paradigm, in which objects are viewed as separate from their environments and people as separate from each other and from their surroundings.[177]

A strength of the systems approach lies in its capacity to integrate variables that otherwise would be isolated from each other and to examine the interactions between them—such as between the physiologic and the behavioral, and between people and their external environment. Applying such a systems perspective will (I am hoping) usher a sea change in the approach we take as a society to problems like obesity—to look less to the individual alone for answers, and more to the symphony of "behavior-biology-environment" interactions.

Though the tools associated with systems thinking (such as computer modeling tools used on large systems studies) are new and advanced, the underlying worldview, as we are about to see in the next chapter, is extremely intuitive. Even young children can learn systems thinking very quickly.[178]

CHAPTER 7

EUREKA:
Insights into Human Energy and Weight Regulation Using a Simple – Bathtub-like – Model

It is no secret why the divide-and-conquer strategy of breaking messy problems into smaller chunks that are simpler to address was the reigning intellectual paradigm for centuries. The behavior of isolated processes is often reasonably obvious to understand, while the behavior of a complex web of interconnected processes (sometimes working in concert sometimes in opposition to one another) often is not. So, initially, the same features that made the holistic systems approach attractive—putting things back together and examining the interactions between them to better understand how the whole system works—also made the task somewhat slippery and elusive. And as inquiry extended to more complex systems (and the heightened need for answers during World War II), it became more and more apparent that a formal system of "bookkeeping" was needed to help manage the complexity.

That's where the discipline of *Systems Thinking* was helpful.

Thinking *inside* the Box

In order to understand how/why a system behaves (or mis-behaves) in a certain way in response to different environmental pressures we need to understand its *structure*. That is, we need to look "inside the box" and understand how the system is organized. How the system's variables (such as the energy consumed and expended in the case of weight regulation) are related and how they influence one another and are influenced by the system's external environment. Indeed, one of the early (core) insights to come from the young field of *Systems Thinking* was accentuating the fundamental role system structure plays in driving system behavior.

To appreciate why it is the system's internal structure—and not external environmental pressure—that is the real key to deciphering (and predicting) system behavior, consider this experiment: Imagine you are holding a slinky as shown in Figure 7.1. Then, as shown in the right panel, you remove the hand that was supporting the slinky from below. You know what happens next: the slinky will start to oscillate. The question is: *What is the cause of the oscillation?* I've asked the question many times in my lectures. The two causes most commonly cited are: gravity and removal of the hand. Both of these emphasize *external* triggers and miss a fundamental cause: the slinky's *internal* structure. To better appreciate the merits of this insight, imagine that you performed the <u>exact</u> same experiment with say, a cup. No oscillation! The outcome you'd get with the cup makes it easier to appreciate that the oscillatory behavior is latent within the *structure* of the slinky itself. In the presence of gravity, when an external stimulus (i.e., removing the supporting hand) is applied, the dynamics latent within the structure are "called forth" causing the oscillatory behavior.[179]

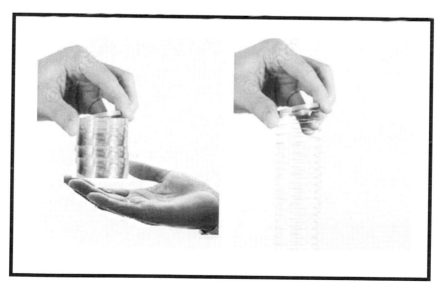

Figure 7.1: The Slinky

The example demonstrates while exogenous pressures do trigger system behavior (like displacing a slinky or pendulum), the same exogenous trigger will induce vastly different responses in different systems (slinky versus cup). It is the system's structure (e.g., a slinky's mass and its spring constant) that modulates the behavior. Hence the systems thinking tenet: to understand a system's response to environmental pressures, understand its structure.

Like X-ray (let's call it "ST-Ray"), systems thinking will help us zoom-in onto the underlying structures of systems (e.g., human energy regulation) to better understand what's generating a complex situation or problematic behavior. Let's see how.

Thinking about Structure

As systems science emerged as a serious field of study after World War II, early analyses revealed an elegant simplicity underlying the complexity of systems. One of the most important, and potentially most empowering, insights to come from the young field is that different systems—whether biological, engineering, social, or economic—shared common principles in the ways in which their components work together to perform some well-defined function. (Which, by the way, is the reason why it will be natural and useful for us to use analogy and metaphor from simpler and every-day systems to explain and explore the workings of human bioenergetics.) Furthermore—and even more surprising—that the rich variety of the systems does *not* rise from an enormous variety of "building blocks." Rather the richness we observe around us arises from the mixing-and-matching of a few (three) basic and relatively simple building blocks that make up the DNA of all systems. Just as in biology, where the mixing and matching of only four DNA molecules produce the enormous variety of living things from daisies to dinosaurs, these building blocks are common to a very large variety of systems and phenomena revealing an elegant simplicity underlying the complexity of systems.

Understanding and learning to recognize these generic "building blocks"— our goal in this chapter—is a powerful leverage that will allow you to see through complexity to the deeper structures and patterns that drive (and thus help explicate) seemingly complex events and phenomena. Specifically, we'll see that all dynamic systems—the human body being a perfect example—are made up of three fundamental building blocks: *stocks* and *rates* of flow threaded together by information *feedback* loops.

Simple–Bathtub-like–Analogy

Like all systems—both technological and biological—the human body obeys the laws of thermodynamics that define the immutable principle of energy conservation—changes in stored energy equals energy intake minus energy expenditure. If we eat too many calories or are too inactive relative to the calories we eat, the excess energy is stored—primarily in the form of body fat.

Thermodynamics notwithstanding, most people intuitively understand that while human energy regulation involves complex energy transformations (such as from the chemical energy within the food's nutrients to mechanical/heat energy or to fat tissue), at some basic level the process resembles that of filling and draining a bathtub. That is, the level of energy stored in the human body changes as a function of the rates of energy *flowing in* (ingested) and *flowing out* (expended) (Figure 7.2). And that is essentially true… *at some basic level.* (We'll see later, additional elements will need to be added.)

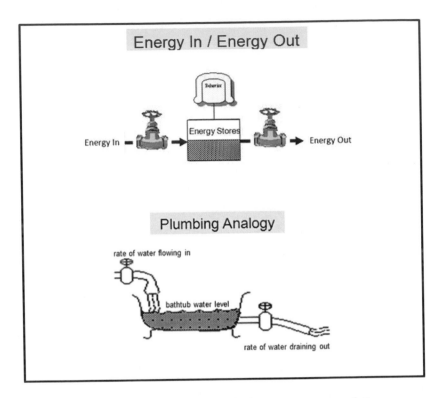

Figure 7.2: Plumbing analogy for human energy regulation

The bathtub analogy provides the perfect construct to introduce two of the three building blocks that all systems are made of: the stocks (tubs) and the rates (faucets/drains). (The third building block—feedback—will be introduced a little bit later.) Both the bathtub and the fat compartment in the human body can be thought of as "containers" (or *stocks* in systems thinking lingo) that accumulate the difference between stuff flowing in and stuff flowing out. In the case of the bathtub that "stuff" is the water flowing in/out while in the case of human energy regulation it is the energy (calories) ingested by eating and expended through physical activity.

This simple stock-and-flow structure—a single stock of "stuff" with an inflow that replenishes it and an outflow that drains it—is by no means unique to human energy regulation… or to "plumbing." Rather, it characterizes many types of real-life systems and everyday tasks—such as managing a checking account or a company's inventory. Indeed, such stock-and-flow structures are so ubiquitous in our lives that system thinkers (including this author) have long argued that a better understanding of the relationship between stocks and the flows that alter them—that is, resources that accumulate or deplete and the flows that alter them—is fundamental to understanding and managing a wide range of real-life systems.

In this book, however, our focus is squarely on the system of human energy and weight regulation. And what we will soon learn is that: (1) Understanding the underlying stock-and-flow structure of human energy regulation will provide us tremendous insight into the workings of the system (its behavior and misbehavior); and (2) By understanding few simple book-keeping rules (that govern how a stock is affected by its flows) we can better predict the system's behavior.

To simplify the schematics (and hence the discussion), I will adhere to the formal (more compact) representation of stock-and-flow structures commonly used in the *Systems Thinking* literature. All such structures are represented more generically as shown in Figure 7.3. The stock (whether a bathtub or fat reserves) is be represented by a rectangle (suggesting a container holding the contents of the stock). The inflows/outflows are represented by pipes with arrows pointing into (adding to) or pointing out of (subtracting from or draining) the stock. And the faucets on the pipes regulate the speeds (rates) of the inflows and outflows.

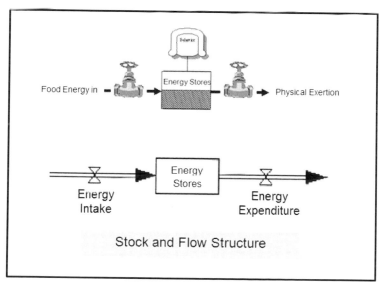

Figure 7.3: Stock-and-Flow Structure of Human Energy Regulation

Understanding your Body's Stock-and-Flow Dynamics

Stocks and flows constitute the two fundamental (and complementary) processes, accumulation and flow respectively, that characterize how reality works and how systems change—whether it is the energy regulation of our bodies, water in a bathtub or money in the bank. (For the mathematically inclined readers: stocks and flows correspond to the two key operations in calculus... integration and differentiation.) To effectively manage such stock-and-flow systems requires (as was argued earlier) two skills: understanding (in this case, what is a stock and what is a flow) and prediction (how changes in the inflows and outflows affect the level of the stock... and vice versa).

Given the importance and ubiquity of stock-and-flow structures in everyday tasks (including filling a bathtub, managing a checking account, or controlling an inventory), you would think that people should be able to infer their dynamics quickly and reliably. Yet, there is considerable evidence of a fundamental lack in the human understanding of stock accumulation and rates of change: a difficulty (unimaginatively) called the stock–flow (SF) failure.[180] (Indeed, the evidence keeps mounting that many real-world individual, organizational, and social problems are rooted in the misunderstanding of the basic processes of stock and flow dynamics.) The stock–flow failure appears to be rooted in failure to understand and/or properly apply basic (bookkeeping) principles of accumulation and are often exacerbated by the application of inappropriate seat-of-the-pants type heuristics.[181]

Which naturally brings up an important question: Do these "challenges" also apply to human judgment about personal weight and energy regulation—an activity that most people are intimately experienced with? The question is *not* an academic one. If such stock-and-flow failures do indeed apply to human judgment about weight/energy regulation, they could potentially undermine obesity prevention and management efforts. It is, thus, a question that is important to investigate.

To find answers, we conducted a study to assess people's understanding (or misunderstanding) of stock-and-flow relationships that underlie the dynamics of weight gain/loss. The study (conducted in 2012 / 2013) was called the SIGOS study—an acronym for the Systems Inspired Global Obesity Study. Below I provide an overview of the study and its major findings. (The study results were published in the premier systems thinking journal the *System Dynamics Review* [January 2014, Volume 30, Number 1].)

Systems Inspired Global Obesity Study

The SIGOS study is a worldwide study that was conducted in 2012 to assess public and health-professionals' understanding (or misunderstanding) of stock-and-flow relationships that underlie the dynamics of weight gain/loss. For that, we created an experimental task to assess the degree to which people correctly infer the dynamics—and thus their risk—of weight gain/loss during the holiday season.

Overeating during the holiday season is an annual "ritual" undoubtedly familiar to (and, I suspect, dreaded by) most people and has been a focus of discussion and research in both the lay press and academic literature. According to some recent studies, caloric consumption during the "eating holidays" (Thanksgiving and Christmas) increases by 25 to 40 percent.[182] Such significant increases, research findings suggest, "… is a combined result of the eating environment and the food environment. The holiday eating environment directly encourages overconsumption because it involves parties (long eating durations), convenient leftovers (low eating effort), friends and relatives (eating with others), and a multitude of distractions. At the same time, the food environment—the salience, structure, size, shape, and stockpiles of food—also facilitates overconsumption."[183]

The study was conducted worldwide so as to assess performance across different populations and cultures. (Overall, twenty researchers from seven countries—US, Venezuela, Norway, France, China, India, and Sri Lanka—participated.) And to assess the extent to which professional health-training improves performance, we drew samples from two distinct populations: lay people and health care professionals (HCP).

A total of 621 subjects (seventy one percent of them from the U.S.) participated in the study. In terms of background, 59 percent of the subjects were lay and 41 percent HCP.

The Experimental Task

To assess public and health professionals' understanding of stock-and-flow relationships pertaining to the dynamics of weight gain/loss, we created a simple task that required subjects to determine how body weight (the quantity of energy in a stock) varies in response to changes in food intake (the inflow) during the holiday season. The level of daily energy expenditure (the outflow) was held constant. To make the task as concrete as possible, the subjects were provided a hypothetical overeating scenario with a graphical representation of energy intake and expenditure.

As shown on the standardized exercise sheet (Figure 7.4), Graph (a) shows the eating behavior of a hypothetical individual during the Thanksgiving/Christmas holiday season. As indicated by Graph (a), it is assumed that the hypothetical subject initially kept her weight steady at 150 lbs., with daily caloric intake (and expenditure) at 2,000 kcal. This steady-state situation changes during the holiday periods when her caloric intake increases by 25 percent. Specifically, it is assumed that her food intake rises progressively—in a linear fashion—peaking at 2,500 kcal/day on Thanksgiving, and then declines back to 2,000 kcal/day. The pattern repeats during Christmas. To simplify the task, it is assumed that her energy expenditure remains constant throughout at the 2,000 kcal/day level.

Given this scenario of energy intake/expenditure, the subjects' task was to sketch on Graph (b) at the bottom of the exercise sheet how body weight (the stock) changes over the approximately two-month period. For convenience, the initial steady state situation was pre-plotted—when body weight was in equilibrium at 150 lbs.

A note to the reader: before proceeding to the next section, I suggest you take a few minutes to sketch your own solution. It could be instructive—and maybe even fun!

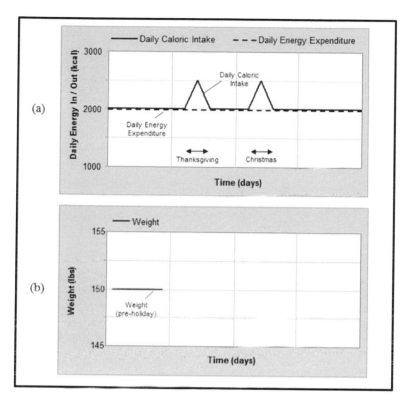

Figure 7.4: The Experimental Task

The Solution and its Characteristics

The task was designed to be simple and could be correctly handled without the use of mathematics. To tackle the task, a subject needed to apply simple rules governing the replenishment/depletion of a quantity in a stock as a function of the inflows/outflows—concepts of accumulation that should be familiar through a host of everyday tasks, including filling a bathtub, managing a checking account, or controlling an inventory.

Specifically, to solve the problem correctly (as is shown in Figure 7.5) the subject needed to apply the following two simple rules:

23) Whenever the inflow (energy intake) exceeds the outflow (energy expenditure), body weight should rise; and

24) Whenever the inflow is equal to the outflow, body weight should hold steady.

For any stock-and-flow system, the rates of flow into and out of the stock govern the rise/decline of the quantity of the stock. And the above simple rules govern *how* it would vary (qualitatively).

Note that applying these simple rules indicates that the level of the stock (body weight) depends on the relative magnitudes of the inflow and outflow—on which is larger—not whether the inflow is increasing or decreasing. And that means that a stock and its inflow may *not* necessarily move in the *same* direction (a result that many participants found counterintuitive as will be discussed below). For example, when food intake peaks at 2,500 kcal and starts decreasing towards 2,000, body weight *should still increase* because energy intake (while decreasing) still exceeds energy expenditure.

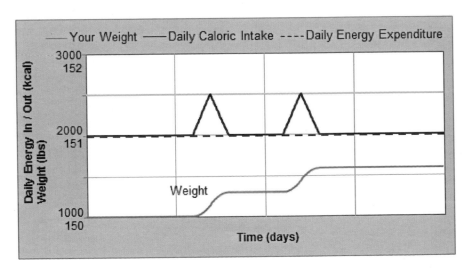

Figure 7.5: The Correct Solution

How did our Subjects Perform?

Overall, the subjects' performance was poor and their responses exhibited systematic errors. Even more disturbing, the performance of healthcare professionals was only slightly better (29 percent derived the correct weight trajectory versus 24 of lay subjects). Too many drew trajectories that violated even basic physical principles such as the conservation of energy/matter—e.g. failing to realize that the quantity in a stock <u>must</u> increase if the inflow exceeds outflow, *even if* inflow is decreasing. And there was a widespread tendency among both lay and HCP subjects to match the trajectory of body weight to energy intake.

Common Difficulties

Two aspects of the experimental task that many participants found particularly counterintuitive deserve some discussion. First, there was a widespread tendency among experimental subjects (both lay and HCP) to match the trajectories of body weight to the energy intake pattern. The majority of those who failed to provide the correct trajectory sketched a weight trajectory that matched the (incorrect) pattern shown at the bottom of Figure 7.6 below (in which the rise and fall in body weight *matches* the rise and fall in food intake). Did you?

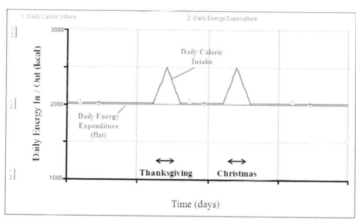

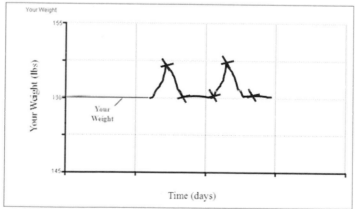

Figure 7.6: (Erroneous) Pattern-Matching Response

This tendency to pattern-match illustrates a basic misunderstanding of the difference between what causes *a flow* to move in a certain direction (increasing/decreasing) and what causes the associated *stock* to rise or fall.

The key to whether a stock's level increases or decreases is not whether its inflow rate increases or declines, but rather whether the inflow's magnitude is greater or less than that of the outflow rate. Period! If it is greater, then that would mean more "stuff" is being added to the stock than is being drained out. For example, when food intake peaks at 2,500 kcal and starts decreasing to 2,000, body weight should still increase because energy intake (while decreasing) still exceeds energy expenditure.

That means that a stock and its inflow may *not* necessarily move in the *same* direction (a result that many participants found counterintuitive as was discussed above).

Research studies indicate that employing this (erroneous) pattern-matching heuristic (Figure 7.6) is by no means unique to our SIGOS subjects. Rather, it has been a robust finding in stock-flow experimental studies covering a wide variety of task settings.

It appears that many people have difficulty applying the principles of accumulation correctly, failing to grasp that the quantity of any stock, such as the level of water in a tub, rises (falls) when the inflow exceeds (is less than) the outflow. Rather, it appears that people often use intuitively appealing but erroneous heuristics such as assuming that the output of a system is positively correlated with its inputs. That is, people assume that the output (the stock) should "look like" the input.[184]

Second, many subjects failed to appreciate that the process of stock accumulation provides systems with *inertia* and *memory*. Notice (in Figure 7.5) that after the Christmas feast body weight does not drop to its original level—even as food intake drops back to its pre-holiday level. Instead, body weight remains "stuck" at its maximum level! And that is because, at any point in time, the amount of energy in the body (the stock) reflects the *cumulative* effect of the net inflows over outflows, not merely what is going on at that very moment.

Stocks are, therefore, said to provide systems with inertia because they provide a "memory" of all past events in the system (Figure 7.7)—in this case, a memory of the fact that in the preceding two months the inflow equaled or exceeded the outflow (and was never below it). Failure to recognize the stock-related inertia in personal health may be a "self-serving" (and I suspect pervasive) misconception that have potentially serious implications in judging/managing health risks. It may explain, for example, why many people fail to adequately compensate for their overeating during the holidays.

Such a failure to compensate was demonstrated in a recent two-phase study in which scientists at the National Institutes of Health tracked the amount of weight gained by 195 adults between Thanksgiving and New Year's Day, and then, in phase two, checked on them a year later. Not surprisingly, the research team found that most of their experimental subjects did gain weight over the holidays. What was of greater concern, however, was the "striking" lack of after-holidays compensation by most of the participants. (To lose the holiday pounds, energy intake must decrease to a level *below* energy expenditure. In the SIGOS experiment that would be dropping below 2,000 kcal/day—i.e., below the system's outflow rate.) The inevitable result: the amount of weight gained during the holidays never came off for most subjects (for 165 out of the 195, or 85 percent).[185,186]

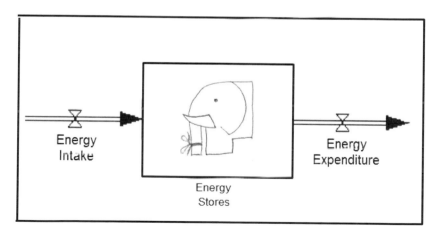

Figure 7.7: Stocks—like elephants—never forget

Our findings raise some serious concerns. Most fundamentally: that people can't effectively manage what they don't understand. If people misunderstand the basics of stock-flow dynamics that underlie human energy regulation, they are likely to draw erroneous inferences about their risk. And this, in turn, could seriously undermine obesity prevention and management efforts.

The sooner *lay* people understand the basic stock and flow concepts underlying human bioenergetics, the sooner they will reject wait-and-see strategies and learn to turn down the "tap"—before the tub overflows! Even the few simple "rules" governing the replenishment/depletion of a stock as a function of its inflows/outflows (such as those discussed earlier) can help clear up significant muddles in public thinking about the dynamics of weight gain/loss.

Beyond Fat Reserves and Bathtubs

The difficulties people have with this exercise often surprise them. They are surprised because the system is rather simple: there is only one stock; the outflow is constant; and the inflow follows a simple pattern. The key underlying process in the task—a process of replenishment/depletion regulating the quantity in a stock—is a familiar one, and the task requires only little calculation and no knowledge of higher mathematics.

Surprise notwithstanding, the results do provide some very useful insights. They suggest that inferring the dynamic behavior of even a simple system (a single stock with two flows) is perhaps not as intuitive as we think. They also suggest that poor performance arises not from a faulty understanding of system structure (in the SIGOS experiment the participants had *perfect* knowledge about the system's pieces and their relationships), but from the apparently innate inability to use their knowledge to properly infer system behavior. That is, from an inability to mentally "run" our mental model of some system or situation to figure out how it behaves over time.

Behavior-decision scientists and cognitive psychologists have long sought to explain why this is so. Why haven't we evolved an innate "simulation" capacity to "run" the complex mental models we hold of our world? And how do we manage without it? Now, they think they know why.

MIT's Sterman and Booth Sweeney provide a very plausible evolutionary explanation for the apparently innate limitation to reason dynamically, and they use the bathtub exercise as the context for their point:

> [As in many real life situations,] it is not necessary to understand the relationship between flows and stocks to fill a bathtub—nature accumulates the water 'automatically.' It is far more efficient to simply monitor the level of water in a tub and shut off the tap when the water reaches the desired level—a simple, effectively [goal-seeking] process, which, experiments . . . show, people can do well. Thus for a wide range of everyday tasks, decision makers have no need to infer how the flows relate to the stocks—it is better to simply wait and see how the state of the system changes, and then take corrective action. In such settings [dynamic reasoning about] stocks and flows offers no survival value and is unlikely to evolve.[187]

Unfortunately, the wait-and-see strategy can fail spectacularly in systems with long time delays and where effects are irreversible—as in the case of human health and disease.[188] When it comes to our bodies, many processes can be hard, if not impossible, to reverse, and even when self-repair is possible the often long delays mean that there is little opportunity for corrective action through outcome *feedback*.

In managing personal health we need to manage by *feedforward*—which involves choosing actions and designing plans on the basis of expectations about the future state of the system. To manage by feedforward we need to be able to *predict*.

Luckily, that's precisely where computer modeling can help. Unlike a mental model, a computer simulator can reliably and efficiently trace through time the implications of a messy maze of interactions. And it can do so without stumbling over phraseology, cognitive bias, or gaps in intuition.[189] Furthermore, by tailoring model parameters, computer-based tools (as we will see in Part III) can be easily customized to fit the precise specifications of different individuals.

Systems Thinking Building Block #3... A Peek Ahead

The simple bathtub model of human energy regulation, though simplistic, provided us with some useful insights into the dynamics of human energy regulation. For example, helped us better understand the risks of weight gain that persists after overeating during the holiday season—even as we revert to pre-holiday food intake levels.

The model, however, is far from complete. For example, it does *not* show us how/what regulates the two faucets that regulate the energy in and energy out flows—obviously important determinants of the system's performance. It turns out; the body's *stock* of fat plays a big role in regulating its two rates (the *in* faucet and the *out* drain)!

Because of the importance of ensuring sufficient energy reserves for survival and reproduction, our bodies cannot leave energy regulation to chance. And so it has evolved a multitude of *involuntary* homeostatic mechanisms to regulate *both* sides of energy flow—energy intake and expenditure. These important homeostatic mechanisms in the system are examples of *feedback* ... the third building block... and the focus of the next chapter.

Extending our bathtub model by incorporating the feedback processes in human energy regulation will help us appreciate why dieting to lose those extra pounds (after the holiday season) is often not as straightforward as people hope—why people tend to lose less weight than they expect... much less. Understanding *feedback*—the third building block—will also help you understand the *how*.

CHAPTER 8

Feedback:
The Third Building Block

As I explained earlier, all systems—whether simple or complex, whether biologic, technologic or economic—are made up of surprisingly few fundamental building blocks. We already learned about two of them, namely, (1) Stocks (or bathtubs) and (2) Rates (or faucets). In this chapter I introduce you to the third: feedback. The goal is twofold: (1) Elucidate what feedback is and what it does—which is to provide channels of communication so the stocks and rates can coordinate their respective values; and (2) Understand the crucial role feedback plays specifically in human energy regulation.

Understanding the myriad feedback processes that underlie energy regulation will help you in two ways: as you look back to explain (and properly diagnose) what has happened (e.g., to understand why losing weight has not proven to be as straightforward as advertised) as well as when you look forward (e.g., to devise personalized weight-loss strategies that work). Indeed, feedback plays such an important role in human physiology that misperceiving feedback may be hazardous to your health!

Feedback is all Around Us

To introduce the important concept of feedback, I will use examples of feedback processes from three familiar (everyday) systems. The three examples I picked are deliberately quite different to underscore a point I made earlier, namely, that different systems—whether biological, engineering, social, or economic—shared common principles in the ways in which their components work together to perform some well-defined function. For example, we will see that the same feedback mechanisms that govern how the components in engineering systems (such as in an autopilot say) work together to perform some goal-seeking function also govern the goal-oriented behavior of human and other living systems.

I'll start with our "running" bathtub example introduced in the previous chapter. Because of the obvious parallels between the filling and draining of water in a bathtub and the intake, storage and expenditure of energy, I will continue to tap this bathtub metaphor to clarify many concepts in human energy regulation in this and subsequent chapters. An added bonus: because water, unlike energy, is something we can see and touch, the filling/storing/draining processes will be easier to visualize.

So, let's assume you are observing someone filling the bathtub with water— say in preparation for taking a bath. If you observe the process, what you'll see is this: faucet opening → water flowing → water level rising (Figure 8.1). (Assume the outflow or draining rate is constant or zero.)

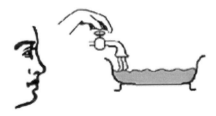

Figure 8.1: Filling the bathtub

But wait! These observed processes do not tell the whole "tub-filling story." Most notably, they miss the essence of what regulates the tub-filling process, namely, the person's tub- filling <u>goal</u>.

When we fill a bathtub to take a bath, we'll have a "desired water level" in mind—that's our goal. We plug the drain, turn on the faucet, and watch the water level rise. As the water level rises, we adjust the faucet position to slow the flow of water and then turn it off when the water reaches our desired level. Thus, the more complete, and more accurate, representation (or model) for what is happening looks like this:

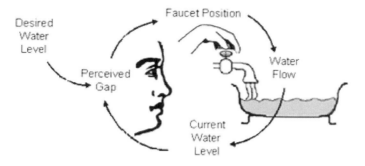

Figure 8.2: Filling the bathtub… what *really* is going on

Notice that the goal—our "desired water level" –and the arrow-like connections (which are cause-and-effect connections) are not visible in the *physical*
system. If an intelligent extraterrestrial was watching and trying to figure out how
the tub fills, it might take a while to figure out that there's an invisible goal and a
discrepancy-measuring process going on in the head of the creature manipulating
the faucets. But if it watched long enough (assuming it is an intelligent extraterrestrial), it would figure that out.[190]

When we observe a process like this in daily life, we see the picture of
Figure 8.1 (without the connections), and we naturally think of the faucet controlling the amount of water in the tub. Period! That is, we think of unidirectional
cause-and-effect:

Faucet opening → Water flowing → Water level rising

We do not mentally close the loop and realize that not only do our actions
affect the water level *but* the water level in turn affects our actions:

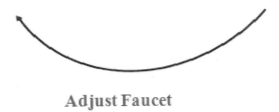

Faucet opening→ Water flowing → Water level rising

Adjust Faucet

Figure 8.3: Closing the loop

The cause-and-effect relationships, in other words, are mutual rather than one-way: the faucet's opening affects the water level <u>and</u> the water in the bathtub, through our sight and action, controls how long the faucet is opened and when it is turned off. And this applies to many things we do—not just tub-filling. In daily language we refer to these circular effects with references such as: What goes around comes around; Closing the loop; and Boomerang. All these are references about *feedback* effects.

In all such examples, an action taken by a person or thing comes back—directly or possibly through a chain of causes and effects—to eventually affect that person or thing. That's what feedback is... the closing of the loop: the situation of X affecting Y and Y in turn affecting X, perhaps through a chain of causes and effects.

Without feedback it would be almost impossible for a system (or for us) to achieve some desired goal. Think about the bathtub example. If the system was simply as depicted in Figure 8.1—with no feedback from the bathtub to the decision maker—how would we know when to stop filling? We won't.

Understanding the fundamental role that feedback plays in regulating most systems—whether biologic, mechanical or social—was an important breakthrough to come from the young field of systems thinking. In the remainder of this chapter you will learn that we humans rely on feedback—both consciously and subconsciously—to control many processes in daily life. Indeed, feedback processes underlie all goal-oriented behavior—and that's a lot of behavior! Anytime you seek to accomplish some goal you rely on feedback about the results of your actions in order to decide whether you should intensify your efforts or terminate them.

More Feedback Examples

Our bathtub filling example nicely demonstrates all three building blocks and the interactions between them (see Figure 8.4). These are: (1) Stocks (or bathtubs); (2) Rates (or faucets); and (3) Feedback (the information/causal links between them). And it demonstrates why in real systems (even familiar ones), the causal links that form the feedback are not as visible as the bathtub and the faucets and, thus, are usually a little harder to discern. To see them takes some training and requires more effort—we have to squint *with our mind* to see causal relationships. That's what you will learn to do in this book.

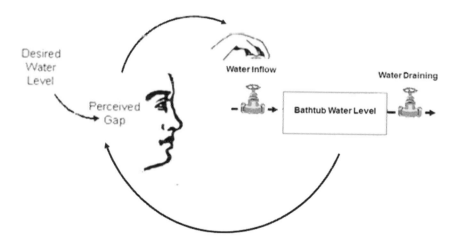

Figure 8.4: The three building blocks and the interactions between them

The bathtub filling scenario demonstrates how feedback drives conscious goal-seeking behavior by a human. Interestingly, similar feedback structures also drive goal seeking processes that are involuntary (and unconscious) in human physiology as well as in non-human goal-seeking processes (such as in mechanical systems).

Let's see two examples.

We will stick with our bathing friend and the bathtub, but shift attention to the bathroom's thermostat—an electromechanical devise that aims to maintain the bathroom at a desired temperature say a comfortable 65 degrees Fahrenheit.

A thermostat is a device that is used to control a room's heating or cooling system so that it maintains a certain temperature or keeps the temperature within a certain range. The thermostat does this by switching heating or cooling devices on or off. To do its work, the thermostat relies on feedback. For example, on a cold wintery day the thermostat would initially turn on the heating system to raise room temperature. When the temperature in the bathroom reaches a certain upper limit, the heating is switched off so that the temperature begins to fall. When the temperature drops to a lower limit, the heating is switched on again. Provided the limits are close to each other, a steady room temperature is maintained.

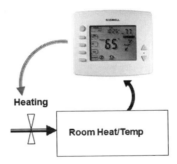

Figure 8.5: Thermostat regulating room temperature

That the system works almost exactly like the bathtub filling process discussed earlier can be seen in Figure 8.6 below. The figure depicts the two loops side by side: on the left is our familiar bathtub filling loop and on the right the feedback loop for regulating room temperature. Both work exactly the same way: where the state of some system we aim to control (water level in a tub or room temperature) is compared to our goal for the system, and if a discrepancy is detected, corrective action is taken to close the gap and bring the system back in line with the goal. Indeed, such a feedback process underlies all goal-oriented behavior. Nature evolves such goal-seeking feedback mechanisms and humans invent them as controls to keep system states within desired bounds.

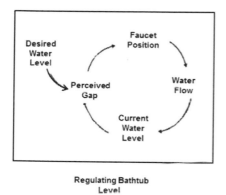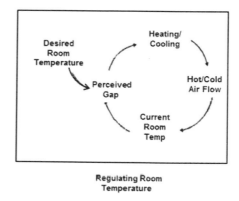

Figure 8.6: Bathtub filling loop and feedback loop for
regulating room temperature

The two examples demonstrate how we rely on feedback to achieve our
goals both by directly regulating our own behavior (opening/closing a faucet) and
indirectly by incorporating it into mechanical controls we invent (thermostats).
Just like humans, nature evolves such goal-seeking feedback mechanisms to keep
system states within desired bounds. The human body is the perfect example.

Our physiology relies on feedback… lots of it in fact. Essentially all organs
and tissues of the body rely on feedback to perform regulatory functions that help
maintain the body's internal stability, even under extremes in our natural environment. More than a century ago, the French physician Claude Bernard correctly
attributed this internal stability to ". . . the exquisite capacity of the body to monitor its internal state and to make adjustments to compensate for any perturbation
of that stability."[191] In 1939, Walter Cannon, an American physiologist, coined the
term "homeostasis" to characterize this remarkable ability that is key to the survival of humans and most other living organisms. Indeed,

> [I]f one had to describe, with a single word, what physiology is
> all about, that word would be *homeostasis*. . . . [I]t refers to [feed-
> back] mechanisms by which biologic systems tend to maintain the
> internal stability necessary for survival while adjusting to internal

or external threats to that stability. If homeostasis is successful, life continues; if it is unsuccessful, disease and, perhaps, death ensue.[192]

My third feedback example demonstrates the parallels between the mechanical and the physiologic (Figure 8.7). Consider how our core body temperature is regulated: If body temperature should rise—on a hot day or after a burst of physical activity—it creates a "gap" between "desired body temperature" and "actual body temperature." When this is sensed by the brain, the command is issued to the sweat glands to induce sweating. And it is the evaporation of the sweat—rather than the sweating per se—that would eventually cool the body down. Furthermore, in a manner very much analogous to the bathtub above—where the rise of the water level causes us to adjust the faucet position and ultimately turn it off when the water reaches our desired level—the brain relies on feedback from the body (sensory information) to determine that the goal is achieved (core temperature back down to 98.6 degrees Fahrenheit) to stop the sweating. (The same loop works to *raise* body temperature if it drops below the desired 98.6 degrees Fahrenheit say on a chilly night—in this case by inducing shivering.)

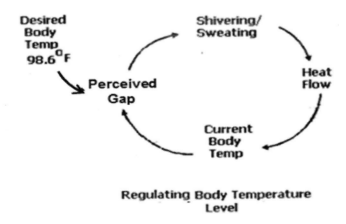

Figure 8.7: Regulation of body temperature

So, as you can see whether in regulating conscious human behavior (filling a tub), controlling a mechanical system (thermostat) or regulating a biologic system's internal state (body temperature), different systems—whether biological, engineering, social—share common principles in the ways in which system components work together to achieve their desired goals.

Understanding (and learning to recognize) these circular feedback processes and how they regulate behavior can be very helpful in understanding how and why systems behave the way they do—e.g., how systems seek to achieve and then maintain some desired goal (like a person filling a bathtub or a thermostat that's set to maintain a room's temperature) and why systems "fight back" and resist intervention (when a snowballing-type feedback dominates).

In the next chapter, we will apply all this to human energy regulation. We'll see that human weight/energy is indeed regulated by feedback process—but with a twist. In the case of the body's feedback process that regulates core body temperature, the system serves us well because in this case the system's goal (maintaining body core temperature at 98.6 degrees Fahrenheit 98.6) works just fine for us. Dieting is different. When individuals reduce food intake to diet, they do so not because their physiology requests it. They do it for personal reasons usually at variance with physiological drives—reasons that are cognitive and deliberate rather than physiological and automatic. Indeed, successful dieting entails overriding the body's built-in homeostatic physiologic controls (e.g., to eat when hungry) with cognitive controls aimed at achieving an individual's personal aesthetic or health aspirations for what his or her weight should be.[193] So what can we expect when we try to override a system's built-in goal? "Resistance!" That's exactly what happens when we go on a diet. The system's feedback processes "fight back."

Understanding feedback will help us clarify all this and that, in turn, will help you become a better (more informed) *manager* of your body.

CHAPTER 9

Human Energy Regulation:
The "Complete Package"

Our well-being—indeed our life—literally depends on feedback. As we started to see in the previous chapter, the human body relies on a multitude of hormonal-based homeostatic mechanisms that act to maintain the body's internal stability in the face of changes in its external or internal environment. Examples include regulation of the body's temperature, the stomach's pH level, the blood glucose level, regulation of arterial pressure, regulation of oxygen and carbon dioxide concentrations in the extracellular fluid, etc. Although not directly visible to us, these (among many other) feedback processes are key governing mechanisms by which many of the body's systems are controlled and regulated. Human energy and weight regulation is no exception. Which is why, I believe, understanding the role of feedback in human weight/energy regulation is crucial for effectively managing our weights and our bodies. As we shall see in this chapter, not only is the system profuse with homeostatic processes, but these feedback processes operate at multiple levels—homeostatic processes at the physiologic level, between the physiologic and the behavioral, and between people and their external environment. Furthermore (as I hinted), they have interesting "twists" in how they operate.

The Simplistic Feedback-less Model

To appreciate the utility of "feedback understanding," (and the pitfalls of feedback-less thinking), I'll start with the public's widely shared feedback-less (and incorrect) mental model of energy regulation, expose its limitations, and then correct it.

Figure 9.1 depicts what can be described as the reigning mental model by which most dieters explain weight gain and predict treatment outcomes.[194] It is a simplistic ("feedback-less") model of the human energy regulation system. Body weight is viewed as being dependent on the balance between energy intake (EI) and energy expenditure (EE), both of which are assumed to be under voluntary control. From this, the caloric calculus for weight loss becomes pretty straightforward: reduce daily caloric intake below the daily energy requirements, increase energy expenditure (through increased physical activity for example), or do both and observe your weight drop proportionally and steadily.

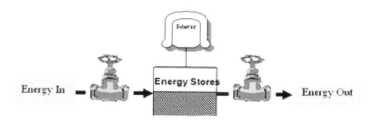

Figure 9.1: Simplistic ("feedback-less") mental model of
human energy regulation

Unfortunately, it is *not* that simple.

In reality, unbalancing the energy balance equation in the direction of weight loss has proven *not* to be that straightforward. Because of the importance of ensuring sufficient energy for survival and reproduction, the human body has evolved a multitude of *involuntary* homeostatic mechanisms to regulate *both* sides of the energy balance equation.

... our bodies cannot leave energy metabolism to chance; lack of energy means failure to thrive, and often, failure to survive. Thus it is an oversimplification to say that fat balance is just a matter of the difference between what is consumed and stored, versus what is mobilized and oxidized. This is true, but it shall turn out that one must also consider the body's ability to regulate the rate at which all energy-yielding nutrients are oxidized, and to alter the proportions according to a logic that is part of our ancestral heritage.[195]

Furthermore, the two limbs of energy balance are not independent, but instead are physiologically linked—interacting in complex ways, and often compensating for each other.[196] This means we cannot voluntarily change one, say decrease energy input, and expect that the other (energy expenditure) will hold steady.

Let's see how... and why all of this matters a great deal.

On the Energy-Input Side

Because eating is under conscious control, food intake has always been seen as a matter of an individual's decisions—or, rather, of a failure to make decisions.[197] (That is perhaps why obese people are stereotyped as lacking in self-control, and why being obese elicits scorn as often as sympathy.[198]) And, obviously, there is some truth in that. It is, however, far from the whole story. Metabolic and physiologic feedback mechanisms play a major, albeit less visible, role in regulating our energy intake (Figure 9.2).

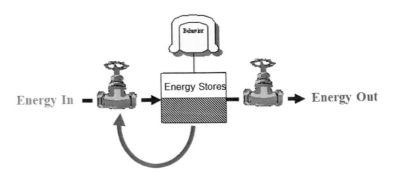

Figure 9.2: Adding the feedback link

During the past half-century, scientific research into human feeding regulation have shown that the initiation and termination of feeding are very complex processes that are part reflective part reflexive. They also have shown that, like other forms of human behavior, food intake is an activity that is mediated by the brain.[199] Specifically, a small region at the base of the brain, the hypothalamus, has been shown to play a major role in controlling food intake and energy homeostasis. (In animal studies, for example, placing tiny lesions in this area causes obesity or leanness, depending on where the lesions are placed.[200])

The emerging conception of the biological drivers of human food intake (which themselves, as we shall see, are not the sole drivers) is that they are controlled by two regulatory subsystems, one short-term and the other long-term. The aim of the short-term component is to provide energy substrate to meet the immediate and short-term metabolic needs of the body by controlling the onset and cessation of feeding on a meal-to-meal basis. After a large meal, the unused portion of ingested food energy (remaining after immediate metabolic needs are satisfied) is stored—primarily in the body's depot of fat reserves. The function of the second long-term regulatory component is to monitor the depletion/repletion of these (longer term) reserves.

The brain plays critical roles in both the short term (regulating appetite) and the long term (monitoring the body's energy reserves). In recent years, considerable research has focused on decoding the signals that continually shuttle between the brain and the stomach. Now, scientists believe that they have a pretty good understanding of how (1) incoming signals from diverse sources within the body are integrated in the brain to produce a real-time picture of the body's energy status, and (2) how the brain, in response, orchestrates output messages to trigger or suppress appetite.[201]

The *short-term* component of the system controls the onset and cessation of feeding on a meal-related basis. As a meal is consumed, the ingested food interacts with an extensive array of chemo- and mechanoreceptors along the gastrointestinal (GI) tract that relay information about the ingested food to the hypothalamus (mainly via the vagus nerve).[202]

From personal experience we know that,

[A] full belly is a simple but sure sign that the body has recently taken in energy as food, and [is often cause] to reduce appetite. One way that this physical state is communicated to the brain is via distension-sensitive nerve fibers that carry signals from the stomach and intestine, ultimately reaching appetite-control centers.[203]

In addition to gastric distension, gut peptides—such as cholecystokinin (CCK) and ghrelin—provide added signals to the brain about the amount of food eaten and the kinds of nutrients received.

In a part of the hypothalamus called the arcuate nucleus (ARC), indicators of energy and feeding status that are coming from these diverse sources act upon groups of neurons associated with appetite regulation. And it is the stimulation of these neurons that induces in us feelings of hunger or fullness and, ultimately, causes us to start or stop eating. For example, when the appetite-related neurons are stimulated by an empty stomach, the ARC cells release appetite-stimulating peptides (such as the neuropeptide Y or NPY), which act to induce appetite and promote eating.[204] Conversely, following food consumption, signals from the stomach and intestine to the brain activate a second type of neurons (the satiety-related group), producing the opposite, anorexigenic effect—or loss of appetite.[205]

Note the similarity between the body's feedback/homeostatic process to maintain body temperature at 98.6 degrees Fahrenheit and the body feedback/homeostatic process to maintain energy reserves. In the case of body temperature: if body temperature should rise—on a hot day or after a burst of physical activity—command is issued to the sweat glands to induce sweating. And the evaporation of the sweat—rather than the sweating per se—would eventually cool the body down. Similarly, when our energy reserves drop, we feel hunger, this induces us to eat until hunger is gone. Both are examples of the archetypical goal-seeking feedback strategy we rely on—both consciously and subconsciously—to control many processes in daily life: where the state of the system is compared to some goal, and if a discrepancy is detected, corrective action is taken to close the gap and bring the system back in line with the goal.

It is not enough that our bodies muster enough energy resources to fuel our immediate metabolic and physical activities. To enhance survival in a food-scarce environment and inevitable periods of energy deprivation, the human energy regulation system—like that of the many other species that do not have constant access to food—evolved to maintain the body's *long-term* energy reserves. In this two-tier system, energy-yielding nutrients in a meal are used to fuel the body's immediate metabolic and physical activities, and any excess is rearranged into long-term storage—primarily in the form of fat reserves—to be used between meals and overnight, when fresh energy supplies run low. The long-term regulatory component monitors the depletion/repletion of these fat reserves.

To be able to maintain the body's energy reserves long-term, the regulatory system must be able to sense the status of the body's energy stores and adjust feeding accordingly—i.e., adjust the frequency and/or size of meals. The system's two key components to accomplish this are: 1) the adiposity signals that "report" the status of the body's fat stores to the brain; and 2) the brain centers that receive and decode the signals to influence feeding behavior.[206]

The system's first limb, the adiposity signaling mechanism, consists of hormones (such as leptin) that are secreted by the body in proportion to the size of its aggregate fat mass. For the leptin adiposity signals to influence energy balance, they must somehow be transduced within the brain into hunger/satiety signals, thereby influencing the frequency and/or size of meals. Recent leptin-related discoveries have helped reveal just how elegantly this is accomplished. As the adipocyte's hormonal signals cross into the brain's hypothalamus—the area of the brain that plays a major role in controlling food intake and energy homeostasis—stimulation of the brain's leptin receptors serves to enhance or decrease the potency of the brain's endogenous hunger/satiety signals. That is, the sensitivity of the brain to the (short-term) meal-initiating and meal-terminating signals is modulated, in part, by the size of the adipose mass, so that

> [An] individual who has recently eaten insufficient food to maintain its weight will be less sensitive to meal-ending signals and, given the opportunity, will consume larger meals on the average. Analogously, an individual who has recently overeaten and gained excess weight will, over time, become more sensitive to gastrointestinal meal-terminating signals [and tend to eat smaller meals over time].[207]

In this way, the brain's short-term signals that control the size and/or frequency of individual meals are adjusted in proportion to changes in body adiposity[208,209]

The functions of the long- and short-term sub-systems, thus, overlap, with clear cross-talk between the adiposity-regulatory centers in the brain and the brain regions that produce the basic drive to eat. Any change in short-term energy balance sufficient enough to alter fuel stores (e.g., during prolonged dieting) elicits compensatory changes in the long-term regulatory system. These changes, in turn, induce pressures (via the short-term sub-system) to reverse the under-feeding and replenish the depleted energy stores.[210]

Fighting the Feedback

The eating behavior of humans is unique because it is, on the one hand, controlled by biological states of need and, on the other hand, cognitively mediated—one can always decide not to put fork to mouth. We are the only species on the planet ". . . in which hungry individuals will voluntarily refuse to consume readily available, appealing food"211 in order to meet some particular objective—from achieving aesthetic or health goals to demonstrating a moral conviction (e.g., as in a political hunger strike).212

Overriding the body's wired-in feedback link from energy stores to appetite is in fact what dieting is all about. Successful dieting entails overriding the body's built-in homeostatic controls with cognitive controls aimed at achieving an individual's personal aesthetic and/or healthy aspirations (hence the "X" in Figure 9.3 below).

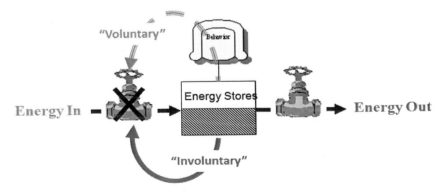

Figure 9.3: Voluntary and involuntary feedback on EI side

Notice that dieting constitutes a type of situation we have not encountered before: it aims to override an operating feedback process. That makes it fundamentally different from say body temperature regulation. There is no inherent conflict in the case of the body's feedback process that regulates core body temperature because in this case the system's goal (maintaining body core temperature at 98.6 degrees Fahrenheit 98.6) works just fine for us. On the other hand, when individuals reduce food intake when on a diet, they do so for personal reasons usually at variance with physiological drives—reasons that are cognitive and deliberate rather than physiological and automatic. In essence, they are seeking to block a goal-seeking system from achieving its goal. So, what can we expect? A "fight."

When we go on a diet, the feeling is that we are engaged in an inner conflict in which we are pulled in opposite directions. That conflict is between the cognitive and the biologic, between one's desire to keep to a strict diet and the urge to ". . . gobble down that doughnut that someone has placed on the table in front of you."[213]

Not unlike resisting temptations, persevering to finish tiring tasks, breaking bad habits and the like, dieting to lose weight or trying to keep it off is an act of self-control.[214] In all such cases, self-control is the process of the self-exerting control over the self. We do it any time we inhibit immediate desires or gratification, and when we prevent ourselves from carrying out a strong but undesirable impulse.[215] In exercising self-control, people exert cognitive control over their bodies' impulses rather than allowing them to proceed automatically, often because they see that to be in their best long-term interest.

And, as we all know, self-control is no leisurely stroll in the park. It can be (and often is) a challenge and people are often frustrated by their failures to keep promises and resolutions and to resist temptations. Controlling one's diet and maintaining a desired weight is no exception. All too often, we give in and indulge in the "forbidden" behaviors because we lack the self-control to restrain ourselves.[216]

In Part III, we will revisit this fight. We'll discuss how the act of self-regulation is an effortful process that requires not only strength to override impulses and resist temptations—but also *skill*. And I will offer strategies to help you win.

On the Energy-Expenditure Side

The homeostatic process to regulate feeding on the energy intake (EI) side is one of the body's mechanisms to maintain energy reserves during caloric deprivation. It is not the sole mechanism.

Because of the importance of ensuring sufficient energy for survival and reproduction, the human body has evolved a multitude of *involuntary* homeostatic mechanisms to regulate *both* sides of the energy balance equation. That is, as with appetite, energy expenditure both consumes (drains) the body's energy stores and is simultaneously regulated by them (Figure 9.4). This overlapping regulation of/by energy reserves effectively links the two limbs of energy balance. The result: energy intake and expenditure in humans are not independent, but instead are physiologically linked—interacting in complex ways, and often compensating for each other.[217] And this means we cannot voluntarily change one, say decrease energy input, and expect that the other (energy expenditure) will hold steady.

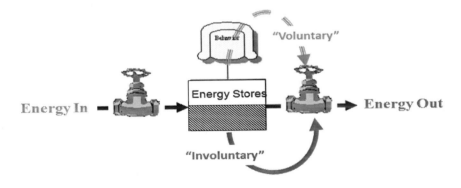

Figure 9.4: Feedback on the EE side

For example, when significant weight is lost on a diet, the loss is interpreted by the body as a deprivation "crisis" that needs to be contained… and is. To restrain the rate of tissue depletion, the body compensates by slowing its metabolism (akin to the body changing its light bulbs to fluorescent lights to save energy). Only now scientists are starting to better understand the multitude of ways this is accomplished. One possible mechanism is through transformations in muscle fibers.

Muscle biopsies taken before, during and after weight loss show that once a person drops weight, their muscle fibers undergo a transformation, making them more like highly efficient "slow twitch" muscle fibers. A result is that after losing weight, your muscles burn 20 to 25 percent fewer calories during everyday activity and moderate aerobic exercise than those of a person who is naturally at the same weight. That means a dieter who thinks she is burning 200 calories during a brisk half-hour walk is probably using closer to 150 to 160 calories. [218]

These adaptations (which may seem diabolical and frustrating to dieters) are neither capricious nor mysterious, and have a lot to do with the body's *homeostatic* processes—its adaptive (and defensive) mechanisms that continuously aim to maintain the body's internal stability in the face of internal or external threats to that stability.

Transformations in muscle fibers are not the body's only adaptation. Additionally, as both fat and fat-free tissue are shed, maintenance energy requirements—that's the amount of energy the body requires to maintain the cells and sustain the body's essential physiological functions—drop, since there is simply less "stuff" to maintain.[219]

For a person on a diet, the combined effect of these two energy conservation measures is to effectively shrink the diet's energy deficit, which in turn (and unfortunately for the dieter) dampens the rate of weight loss. For example, if a female dieter who expends a total of 2,000 calories per day cuts daily dietary intake to 1,500 calories, she would initially induce a daily caloric deficit of 500 calories. But (days or weeks later) as some weight is lost, the body's energy requirements also drop. The total energy expenditure level thus falls from 2,000 down to, say, 1,800 calories. As a result, the daily energy deficit effectively shrinks from 500 to 300 calories—a 40-percent decrease.

(Interestingly, all this is consistent with the simple "bathtub analogy" to human energy regulation. As with the body's maintenance energy expenditure, water flowing out of a drain at the bottom of a bathtub will *not* flow out at a constant rate. As the bathtub empties ["loses weight"] and the water level falls, water pressure at the drain decreases causing the outflow rate to drop.[220])

Our bodies' wired-in feedback processes to regulate (protect) its energy reserves are the reason why weight-loss strategies are rarely as straightforward as advertised. It is why weight lost tends to decline with time—even if the prescribed diet *is* maintained—and why people tend to lose less weight than they expect... much less. Ignoring the body's *involuntary* homeostatic mechanisms may sell more diet books but will inevitably lead to spurious predictions of treatment outcomes. Which should be of concern, since patients' expectations about treatment outcomes and the degree to which they are met—or not met—affect self-efficacy and in turn long-term motivation and commitment.

A *Multi*-Feedback System... with Several Twists

From the above we can see that the body's energy regulatory system is somewhat more complex and nuanced than the goal-seeking feedback systems we've examined—such as filling the bathtub, setting a thermostat to maintain room temperature, and regulating body temperature. In at least two ways: 1) It is regulated by *multiple* loops—on both the energy input and expenditure sides; and 2) It combines both voluntary and involuntary elements.

But that's not all. The body's energy regulatory system is also different in that its goal is not fixed... rather, it ratchets up. I explore the implications of that next.

"A Moving Target"

The essence of any homeostatic system is the control mechanism that acts to bring the state of the system being controlled in line with some goal or target. This is true whether the target is the speed of an automobile, the temperature of a room, or the body's core temperature. If the controller—the car's cruise control, the room's thermostat, or the brain—senses a discrepancy between the desired and actual states, it initiates corrective action to bring the state of the system back in line with the goal. In the human body, a multitude of hormonal-based control processes maintain the body's internal stability in just this fashion. In most cases, the homeostatic process strives to maintain some body variable within a set (and invariant) normal level. For example, the human body seeks to maintain core temperature at around 98.6 degrees Fahrenheit in the face of variable (sometimes

108

extreme) ambient temperatures and/or activity levels. If the body's state deviates from normal, the body initiates corrective actions (such as sweating or shivering) to return itself to the desired state.

The regulation of the body's energy stores is different in a very significant way: its target is not static (like desired body temperature). Instead, the set point in energy store regulation is a moving target that can ratchet up over time. In this case, a dynamic (or moving) control scheme was obviously necessary to allow for the natural growth in body weight from childhood through adulthood. In addition, such an adaptive control scheme would have conferred a survival advantage throughout human prehistory, allowing for the buildup of energy reserves in times of plenty. A key regulator in setting and resetting this moving target is fat-cell size.[221]

Recall that the primary form in which excess food energy is stored in the body is fat in the fat tissue. The amount of fat in a person's body reflects both the number and the size of the fat cells. Through childhood and adolescence, the number of fat cells increases gradually and continuously as the body naturally grows in size (their number increasing approximately fivefold between the ages of one and 20 for a non-obese individual).[222,223] After reaching adulthood, a person's fat cell number may continue to increase as a result of weight gain.

When a person experiences a positive energy balance and starts to gain weight, initially the excess energy gets stored in the body's existing stock of fat cells, increasing them in size. Fat cells can expand in size a long ways, but not forever—they have a biologic limit (about 1.0 μg of fat).[224,225] When the cells approach maximal or "peak" size, a process of adipocyte proliferation is initiated, increasing the body's fat cell count. Thus, obesity develops when a person's fat cells increase in number, in size, or, quite often, both. *Once fat cells are formed, however, the number seems to remain fixed even if weight is lost.*[226]

Because the body strives to maintain normal fat-cell size, the increased number of fat cells that invariably accompanies excessive weight gain results not only in an elevation of body weight but in the defense of that body weight.[227] Thus, unlike a typical goal-seeking regulatory process, the target of the body's energy storage regulatory system is not static—say like desired body temperature. Instead, the set point in energy-store regulation is a moving target that ratchets up over time.

Here is a hypothetical example to explain how this adaptive scheme works.

Consider the case of an average male, "Mr. Average," or "Mr. A" for short. He is six feet tall and weighs 180 pounds—which would translate into a body mass index (BMI) of 24. A fat-tissue analysis indicates that fat cells in his body number 25 billion and are of an average size, 0.5 µg. Mr. A's weight has remained relatively steady over the last few years. Like most of us, he has experienced occasional, modest fluctuations, sometimes gaining, sometimes losing a few pounds, but always managing to revert back to what he justifiably considered his "normal" weight. But then some change in lifestyle—perhaps a move to the city, or a change of jobs or family status—embarks him on an extended period of positive energy balance (e.g., persisting nutritional excess and/or diminished physical activity). When we revisit him a year later, we find that he has gained 40 pounds.

To accommodate his expanded fat mass, his fat cells would have grown in size and increased in number. This would not occur uniformly throughout his body because newly acquired fat is never deposited uniformly among the body's distributed fat stores. Fat deposits are modulated by body enzymes, such as the enzyme lipoprotein lipase (LPL), which is mounted on fat cell membranes, and whose activity is partially regulated by sex-specific hormones—estrogen in women and testosterone in men. In men, for example, fat cells in the abdomen produce abundant LPL, and, as a result, men tend to store fat there and develop central obesity.[228]

Unhappy with his new state of affairs, Mr. A decides to go on a diet to lose weight—and he does. His target, not surprisingly, is to drop back down to 180 pounds, the weight he considered "normal" before his recent (temporary, he hopes) weight gain. Unfortunately for Mr. A, the escalation in his weight and the changes to his body (at the cellular level) that accompanied it are neither completely "passing" nor completely reversible. As some of his fat cells grew and divided (particularly in those areas that experience larger increases), his fat cell number would have increased, say, to 28 billion. As a result, as he starts losing the weight, the "I am at target level" signal from the body's energy stores to the brain will come at an elevated body weight—the one associated with 28 billion cells at an average size of 0.5 µg. This will happen at a body weight around 200 pounds. A drop in weight below this newly elevated target level, say to his original 180 pounds, will necessarily cause his 28 billion fat cells to shrink to an average size that's below 0.5 µg. This will be interpreted as a depletion of energy reserves below "desired," and so would trigger his hormones to scream to the hypothalamus, "Eat, eat, eat!"[229]

Gaining a significant amount of weight, thus, produces some irreversible anatomic and physiological changes that cause body energy reserves to be regulated at a higher set point. Specifically, *fat cell theory* maintains that the body's dynamic set point for energy regulation may be determined by the size of fat cells, and the weight at which this occurs depends on the number of cells. Weight loss beyond the point at which cells reach normal size would signal a depletion of energy reserves below "desired," and so induce overeating to refill fat cells.[230,231]

Research in fat-tissue cellularity is also starting to shed light on precisely how fat cells signal the brain the status of their size. The mechanism is believed to be analogous to how mechanoreceptors lining the gastrointestinal tract sense gastric distension and relay information about the stomach's nutrient content to the brain. As fat cells fill with fat and increase in size, the stretching of the fat-cell membrane (and the associated increase in the cell-membrane tension) signals the brain as to the size of fat cells. Both hormonal and enzymic mechanisms mounted on fat-cell membranes appear to be involved in this signaling process.[232,233]

Thus, fat-cell size and number, together, modulate eating so as to maintain aggregate fat stores while striving to maintain fat-cell size at some normal level. This creates a dynamic mechanism that sets (and resets) the set point for the human energy regulation system. And because the body strives to achieve and maintain normal fat-cell size, the increased number of fat cells that invariably accompanies excessive weight gain will result not only in an elevation of body weight, but in the *defense* of that body weight.

The significance of this for obesity treatment and prevention is clear: It is crucial to intervene before excessive weight is gained and fat-cell proliferation sets in. Otherwise we risk being caught in a "biological trap:" Becoming fat from eating too much and then continue to eat too much because we are fat—because our bodies are seeking to maintain the higher weight associated with the elevated number of fat cells. Appetite, in other words, not only shapes body weight, but (a growing) body weight also influences appetite!

CHAPTER 10

Misperceiving Feedback May be Hazardous to your Health

Reality is made of circles but we see straight lines.

Peter Senge

"Feedback-Challenged"

Most people, experiments consistent show, are predisposed to thinking in straight lines (linear thinking).[234] That is, to view the world in terms of unilateral causation, independent and dependent variables, origins and terminations. Examples of open-loop thinking are everywhere, as when thinking: appetite affects weight; exercise affects body composition; stimuli affect responses; ends affect means; desires affect actions. All those assertions are incomplete, however, because each of them demonstrably also operates in the opposite direction: weight affects appetite; body composition affects exercise; responses affect stimuli; means affect ends; actions affect desires. In every one of these examples causation is circular, not linear.[235] But we do not see that.

There are two primary reasons for why we tend to see straight lines even when reality works in circles. The first is visibility: what we see when we open our eyes.

When we look at some system, we (naturally) see the physical "stuff." We see material things like bathtubs, water, dollar bills, food, etc. What we do not see are the cause-and-effect interrelationships between objects. Going back to our bathtub example: the physical actions of tub filling such as faucet opening → water flowing → water level rising are readily observable (left picture below). Less so are the information (causal) links that actually regulate the tub filling process: the bather's "desired water level"—his/her goal—and the information about the level of water in the tub that causes him/her to adjust the inflow rate and ultimately turn off the water when the level in the tub reaches the desired level. The cause-and-effect links, are more difficult to see because they are not physical objects, they are *relationships* between objects.

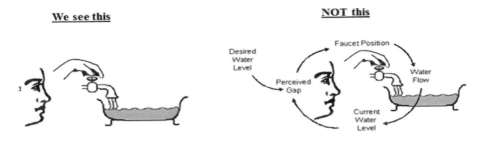

Figure 10.1: What we see… and don't

In the case of human energy and weight regulation, the feedback relationships are even harder to see. The rise and fall of our energy stores, for example, are not as visible as the rising and falling water level in a bathroom tub.

In addition to the lack of visibility, a second important reason why we often fail to close the loops is *delay*. There is often asymmetry in the delays associated with cause and effect. By that I mean that the effect of some action by an object X on another Y may be immediate and directly apparent, but the feedback effect of Y on X may be delayed by days or months (see Figure 10.2). In our daily lives, it is not at all uncommon for the consequences of actions we take to be delayed and thus not evident to us in the moment an action is being taken (as when smoking today leads to lung cancer many years in the future). And because when judging causal relationships we are conditioned to using cues such as the temporal and spatial-proximity of cause and effect when there is delay, we often fail to "close the causal loop."[236]

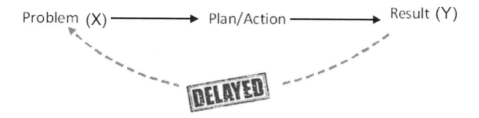

Figure 10.2: Delays in feedback systems

Whether as a result of invisibility or delay, the misperception of feedback comes at a price: vulnerability to unanticipated (often undesired) surprises. And when we are unpleasantly surprised, we are quick to claim these to be unfortunate side effects. But do not fool yourself, side effects are *not* an inescapable feature of reality; rather, they are a sign that our "feedback challenged" understanding of the system is narrow and flawed.[237]

Weight-loss is a good case in point.

Surprise, Surprise... Our Body Fights Back when Dieting

The ubiquitous weight-loss rule (also known as the 3500 kcal per pound rule) is the basis for the "standard" prescriptions you'll find in most self-help diet and weight-loss books (as well as official recommendations from institutions such as the National Institutes of Health and the American Dietetic Association in the USA). These go something like this:

> Your weight is determined by your energy balance. . . . If you burn the same amount of calories as you eat, your weight stays the same. . . . If your goal is weight loss, subtracting 500 calories a day from this figure should promote losing about a pound a week, because 3,500 calories equal a pound [and 7 days x 500 calories per day = 3,500 calories per week].[238]

This simplistic open-loop model (see depiction below) is the staple mental model by which most dieters explain weight gain and predict treatment outcomes.[239]

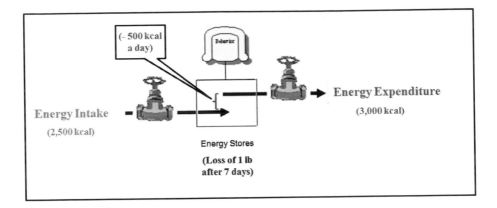

Figure 10.3: Simplistic open-loop model

It is a linear model (with body weight dropping in direct proportion to the size and duration of the diet's energy deficit as depicted in Figure 10.4), it is unbounded... and it is wrong.[240] For example, it takes weight loss projections to absurd values—a negative energy balance of 1,000 calories per day would shed about 8 lbs. in a month and an unlikely 100 pounds in a year!

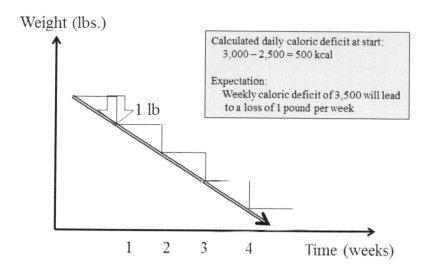

Figure 10.4: Body weight dropping in a linear (straight-line) fashion

In reality, losing weight has proven not to be that *straight*-forward. Weight loss tends to decline with time—even if the prescribed diet *is* maintained—and people tend to lose less weight than they expect... much less. That's primarily because of physiological *feedback* adaptations to the loss of body tissue.

Specifically, the drop in body weight leads to involuntary changes in both the resting metabolic rate (and does that using two pathways) as well as the energy cost of physical activity.[241] (As explained in Chapter 9), when any significant weight is lost on a diet, the loss is interpreted by the body as a deprivation "crisis." To restrain the rate of tissue depletion, the body compensates by slowing its metabolism. This metabolic adaptation (captured by link 1 in Figure 10.5) is achieved chiefly through hormonal mechanisms that enhance the tissues' metabolic efficiency—a process I likened earlier to changing one's "light bulbs" to fluorescent lights to save energy. Additionally, as weight is lost (and both fat and fat-free tissue are shed) maintenance energy expenditures (MEE)—that's the amount of energy the body requires to maintain the cells and sustain the body's essential physiological functions—drop, since there is simply less "stuff" to maintain (link 2). Finally, as body mass declines, the energy expended in weight-bearing physical activity (referred to as the thermic effect of activity or TEA) also declines since less energy would be needed to move a lighter body (link 3). The size of the drop in TEA will naturally depend on the types of activities. As an example, consider what happens in walking: In a mile of walking, a 90-kg person (198 lbs.) burns about 105 kcal, but a 70-kg person (154 lbs.) walking the same distance will burn only 80 kcal.[242] That's almost a 25-percent difference.

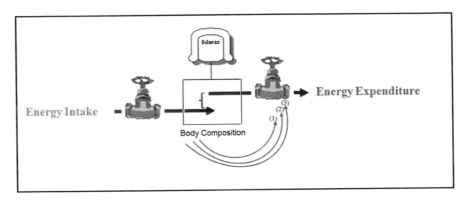

Figure 10.5: Change in body weight & composition
affect energy expenditure

For any dieter, these energy-sparing adaptations cause the diet to become progressively less effective. The result? Weight-loss plateaus at a level that's significantly higher than the ubiquitous 3,500 kcal per pound rule would predict.

That the body appears to have a mind of its own may seem diabolical to frustrated dieters, but in truth, the body's resistance is neither mysterious nor capricious. Let's not forget that, throughout human history, food deprivation has ordinarily been the result of ecological scarcity. Hence, our built-in physiologic defenses in response to food deprivation are the body's attempt to survive in the face of food scarcity—nothing diabolical there. There was simply no evolutionary reason for our bodies to anticipate (or be designed for) self-imposed deprivation in an ecology of plenty—aka "dieting."

Unfortunately for the dieter, additional homeostatic adaptations occur during food restriction that create even more protection against tissue loss. The thermic effect of food (TEF) drops. TEF constitutes the various metabolic costs associated with processing a meal, which include the costs of digestion, absorption, transport, and storage of nutrients within the body. (It is referred to as the thermic effect of food because the acceleration of activity that occurs when we eat—as the GI-tract muscles speed up their rhythmic contractions, and the cells that manufacture and secrete digestive juices begin their tasks—produces heat). The TEF accounts for approximately ten percent of total daily energy expenditure in moderately active individuals, but obviously can increase or decrease depending on the amount and the composition of a person's diet. Since TEF constitutes the metabolic costs of processing a meal, eating less while on a diet would naturally lower the thermic effect of food (link 4 in Figure 10.6 below).

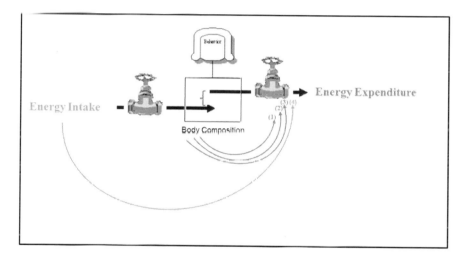

Figure 10.6: Link from EI to EE

The combined effect of these energy conservation adaptations is to progressively dampen the diet's energy deficit. As a result, a given decrease in energy intake causes a negative energy balance—and weight loss—of ever-decreasing magnitude. It is why weight lost tends to decline with time—even if the prescribed diet *is* maintained—and why people tend to lose less weight than they expect... much less (Figure 10.7).

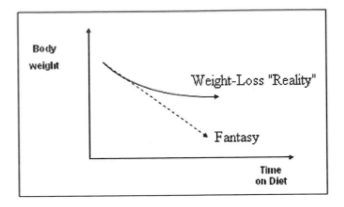

Figure 10.7: Weight loss during prolonged underfeeding is
curvilinear not linear

It is precisely these homeostatic (feedback) adaptations that can help us both understand as well as anticipate the curvilinear-type pattern of weight loss that has frustrated many a dieter: the (brief) initial phase of gratifying loss in weight that invariably tapers off with time, ultimately leveling-off at a new steady-state weight that's substantially higher than expected or hoped for.

Ignoring the body's energy-sparing mechanisms that aim to limit tissue loss during caloric deprivation (as does the ubiquitous 3,500 kcal per pound rule) may sell more diet books, but will inevitably lead to spurious predictions of treatment outcomes. Which should be of concern, because people's expectations about treatment outcomes and the degree to which they are met—or not met—are likely to affect self-efficacy—the belief in one's ability to accomplish one's goals— and in turn their long-term motivation and commitment.[243]

Feedback Operates at Multiple Levels

Feedback is not limited to homeostasis in our physiology.

The human energy regulation process, it is becoming increasingly clear, does not operate as an isolated physiologic/biologic system. Rather, it is a complex biopsychological phenomenon with interactions between the physiologic and the behavioral, and between people and their external environment.

The human species is different from all others in that psychological, cultural and social conventions can be major determinants of food intake and can significantly modulate the impact of metabolic and physiologic signals.[244] One characteristic of humans is that we not only eat food, but we also think about it. In humans, unlike, say, bears or oysters, eating behavior is not only controlled in accordance with biological states of need, but it is also a cognitively mediated activity. To us, in other words, food is both a nutritional entity and a cognitive construct.

In the next chapter we will extend our analysis beyond physiology and explore the behavioral dimension, and in Chapter 12 extend the circle even more to look at the environmental/socio-economic.

Moving beyond biologic does not imply denying biology. Rather,

[It] involves viewing biologic phenomena within their social contexts and examining the tight interrelations between the social and the biologic at multiple levels. Neither does it imply denying individual-level explanations, but rather entails integrating them into broader models incorporating interactions between individuals, as well as group-level or society-level determinants.[245]

That's the strength (and promise) of the systems approach. It allows us (even nudges us) to expand our boundaries and to integrate variables that otherwise would be isolated from each other. This allows us to integrate our knowledge of the multiple dimensions, and to examine the interactions between them, such as between the physiologic and the behavioral, and between people and their external environment.

CHAPTER 11

Beyond Physiology... The *Reward* of Food

We might like to believe that we eat only if hungry and stop eating when full... but, it doesn't work that way. Everyday experience confirms the superficially trivial fact that "... people often eat more of better-liked foods when offered an ad libitum choice, and that the experience or anticipation of highly liked food can stimulate its consumption *in the absence of an energy deficit or perceived state of hunger* (italics added)."[246] Human appetite, it turns out, is not only asymmetric but is also elastic, a design that served us well over the eons of human existence. In an environment in which food resources were unpredictable and starvation was a major cause of death it behooved our hunter-gatherer ancestors to overeat voraciously whenever the opportunity presented itself, allowing them to build up reserves of fat against future famine.[247]

Overly exploitative behavior when palatable food resources become abundant is not just unique to humans. Most mammals will eat beyond their needs when presented with foods that are highly appetizing.[248] For example, when wild primates—the mammalian taxon humans belong to—are placed in environments where palatable food is always abundant overeat their way to obesity. (In one study, wild baboon females averaged 50% greater body mass, and had 23% body fat compared with 2% for their wild-feeding counterpart.[249])

What drives humans and other animals to ignore satiety signals and eat more than is needed (or optimal)?

In one word: *reward.*

The *Reward* of Food

Three decades into the obesity epidemic, the powerful modulating effects of reward on feeding behavior can no longer be argued (Cornier et al., 2007). In our modern food-replete environment, food consumption—not to mention *overcon-sumption*—is rarely induced by acute energy deprivation.[250] The evidence—sub-stantial, mounting and summarized below—suggests that among well-nourished populations the primary stimulus for eating is more and more the gratification of food rather than energy deficit.

The human energy regulation system, it is becoming increasingly clear, is not operating as an isolated physiologic system. Rather, it is a complex biopsy-chological phenomenon with interactions between the homeostatic (physiologic) processes of energy regulation and the reward- (or hedonic-) effects of food. This is not to say that food deprivation is not a powerful motivator of feeding in humans (and animals). It is... and probably always will be. But in our modern environment of abundance, the hunger-induced physiologic drive to seek food is becoming increasingly secondary.

According to the emerging positive-incentive theory, people in modern industrialized societies are not driven to eat by declines of their energy resources below set points. Rather, people are drawn to eat by the anticipated pleasure of eating (i.e., by food's positive-incentive value):

> [P]eople will consume highly palatable foods when such foods are available because they have evolved to find pleasure in this behav-ior. Positive-incentive theorists do not deny that major reductions in the body's energy resources below homeostatic levels increase hunger, as well as eating, if food is available. They do, however, view this relation differently than do set-point theorists. According to set-point theory, reduction of the body's energy resources below energy set points is the main motivating factor in food consump-tion; according to positive-incentive theory, humans and other ani-mals living in food-replete environments rarely, if ever, experience an energy deficit. This is because they find the consumption of high positive-incentive value foods so rewarding that when such foods are readily available, they consume far more than they need to meet their energy requirements.[251]

Humans (and animals) will work for food—the quintessential definition of a reward i.e., the willingness to engage in otherwise unrelated behaviors that extinguish in the absence of the reward. "If feeding were controlled solely by homeostatic mechanisms, most of us would be at our ideal body weight, and people would consider feeding like breathing or elimination, a necessary but unexciting part of existence."[252] However, humans will pay large sums of money for an excellent meal and almost any mammal will eat beyond its homeostatic needs if presented with highly palatable food.[253]

Many factors interact to influence a food's positive incentive value, and individual differences exist, but for most people anticipated taste is among the most important:

> [People develop] a relish for particular tastes that are in nature associated with foods that promote human survival. For example, humans normally develop a liking for sweet, fatty, and salty tastes— tastes that in nature are usually characteristic of foods that are rich in energy and essential vitamins and minerals... Superimposed on these species-characteristic taste preferences and aversions are individual preferences and aversions that each person develops through interactions with other members of the species and through experiencing the health-promoting and health-disrupting effects of the foods he or she eats.[254]

But would reward-driven eating over-ride the drive for balance and promote overeating in a food-replete environment? The evidence suggests the answer is yes—the drive for reward can indeed assert dominance over the drive for balance.[255] Sometimes, aggressively so. In a recent study, for example, "81% of respondents reported that in situations in which they have access to a large supply of preferred foods, they frequently (overeat) until they feel ill."[256]

In a major new research thrust, scientists are seeking to understand how the liking and wanting of food work together to affect the reinforcing value of food and ultimately overeating behavior. Central to this effort is work in neuroscience which is shedding light on the brain's neurotransmitter systems that orchestrate the workings of this feeding-related reward system.

Already several studies have revealed that food rewards and drug rewards share some common neural substrates (e.g., opioid receptors were found to play key roles in both). Apparently, it is more than a linguistic accident that the same term, craving, is used to describe intense desires for palatable foods and for a variety of drugs of abuse.[257] By comparing diets rich in sugar with diets rich in artificial sweeteners, neuroscientists have demonstrated that it is the palatability of the food rather than its energy content that activates the opioid system.[258] Furthermore, there is evidence that the brain's endogenous opioid systems regulate the hedonic value of food intake *independently* from the ongoing metabolic needs of the individual.[259] This suggests that, given the high priority of feeding, mammalian brains have evolved several overlapping neuronal systems that potentiate eating behavior.[260]

Typical of the behavior induced by stimulating the reward circuitry of the brain—represented by endogenous opioids, dopamine and serotonin—is to "come back for more."

> Whether the opioid circuits are activated by highly palatable foods or by drugs, they enable the body to perceive a rewarding experience... A highly palatable food tells the brain, 'This is a desirable object, get more'...

> [Case in point:] Martin Yeomans at the University of Sussex, in England, has done experiments in which he keeps interrupting people as they eat to ask them how hungry they are. Halfway through their meals some people rate their hunger levels higher than before they started to eat.[261]

Another explanation for over-consumption of palatable food is evidence (from animal studies) that eating food rich in fat and sugar blunts the brain's satiety signals. In experiments on mice, it was found that satiety signals (e.g. cholecystokinin and leptin) were suppressed on diets rich in fat and sugar leading to a prolongation of the meal and ultimately to overeating and adiposity.[262] See sidebar.

A new study suggests that (Oreos)"America's favorite cookie" is just as addictive as cocaine or morphine -- at least in lab rats.
Researchers found that in lab rats, eating Oreos activated more neurons in the brain's "pleasure center" than exposure to drugs like cocaine and morphine. / Bob MacDonnell, courtesy of Connecticut College.
A new study suggests that high-fat/high-sugar foods stimulate the brain in the same way that drugs do.
Researchers also looked in the nucleus accumbens, or the brain's pleasure center, and measured how much c-Fos, a protein marker that signals brain neuron activation, was expressed. In simple terms, they were looking at how many cells were turned on in response to the drugs or Oreos.
The researchers saw that Oreos activated significantly more neurons than cocaine or morphine.
This correlated well with previous studies. Previous studies have shown that highly-processed carbohydrates like cakes, cookies and chips could affect this same pleasure center in the brain by triggering the release of dopamine, a neurotransmitter that is released when the brain senses something that is a reward.
This could explain why people have a hard time turning junk food down. It may explain why some people can't resist these foods despite the fact that they know they are bad for them.
Overall, it lent support to the hypothesis that high-fat/high-sugar foods can be viewed in the same way as drugs of abuse and have addictive potential.

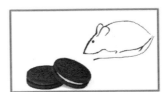

In summary, the following may be deduced about human appetite regulation: The reward of food is a powerful modulator of feeding behavior and in a palatable-food-replete environment drives us to eat beyond our needs. Which, as Pine et al. argue, makes perfect evolutionary sense:

> From the perspective of our evolutionary analysis, the reason humans living in modern industrialized societies tend to overeat is that the presence, the expectation, or even the thought of food with a high positive-incentive value promotes hunger. Because in nature high positive-incentive value foods are rich sources of vitamins, minerals, and energy, it is important that such foods be consumed each time the opportunity presents itself so that the nutrients they provide can be banked as protection against potential future food scarcity.[263]

Rewards Galore in our Current Food Environment

From the above, we see that overeating cannot be simplistically attributed to an absence of willpower or a sudden upsurge in moral failure. It is a psychobiological challenge—one that's apt to become more difficult in a modern environment in which highly palatable foods are increasingly omnipresent.[264,265] Foods rich in sugar and fat were relatively scarce in most natural habitats, but today they are cheap and easy for the food industry to deploy. By combining fats, sugar and salt in innumerable ways, food industry scientists, not being malicious but seeking to increase profits, are successfully creating foods that push our evolutionary buttons to get us to buy and eat more.

> Foods high in sugar, fat, and salt, and the cues that signal them, promote more of everything: more thoughts of food... more urge to pursue food... more consumption... more opioid-driven reward... more overeating to feel better... more delay in feeling full... and ultimately, more and more weight gain... Hyper-palatable foods are hyper-stimulants. And when a stimulant produces reward, we want more of it.[266]

So, does this mean we can safely hop on the "food industry is the real culprit for the obesity epidemic" bandwagon?

Not so fast.

While much discussion of the people-environment interactions, whether in academic or public discourse, continues to cast such interactions in terms of one-way causal connections (hence the finger pointing between obesity researchers and the food industry), the reciprocal influence of individual and environment shouldn't be ignored. People influence their settings, and their settings then act to influence their behaviors (including health behavior). As Winston Churchill once observed (while commenting on the design of The House of Commons), "We shape our environment, and then our environment shapes us."

So perhaps we should look at the issue from both sides.

What's Cause... What's Effect?

Food and beverage companies argue that they create new products in response to consumer demand (e.g., for convenience foods) and that offering choice is what a free society is all about (Figure 11.1).

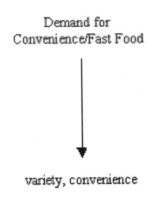

Demand for
Convenience/Fast Food

variety, convenience

Figure 11.1: Food industry view

That's a "crock" in the view of the health industry! For it is more than a misnomer, many health experts argue, to suggest that it's simply a person's free-ly-chosen "lifestyle" to eat non-nutritious, high-fat energy-dense fast foods when healthier foods are much more expensive or all-together unavailable. Our choice of foods, they argue, is not only a matter of personal preferences, but is also very much a function of what food is available in the variety of food outlets we have access to in our communities—the restaurants, supermarkets, and vending machines. The unavailability of certain healthful foods in the environment (home or school or neighborhood) obviously precludes their consumption. Thus, it is erroneous to imply that it is simply a person's freely-chosen "lifestyle" to eat poorly when the food supply is characterized by an abundance of palatable, energy-dense fatty foods or when supermarkets have fled the neighborhood and been replaced by fast food restaurants. As shown in Figure 11.2, this points the "finger" in the other (upward) direction.

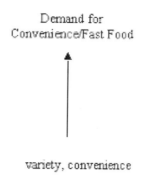

Figure 11.2: Counter view

This view is probably more in tune with what most people think—because it is more comforting. When trying to explain the causes of some bad behavior, it is an all-too-common human tendency to blame it on some convenient scapegoat. The "enemy is out there" syndrome is actually "a propensity (in each of us) to find someone or something outside ourselves to blame when things go wrong... When (our actions) have consequences that come back to hurt us, we misperceive these new problems as externally caused."[267] The "enemy is out there," however, is almost always but a self-serving cop out.

In the case of the mutual finger pointing between the food industry and health advocates, both assertions are equally incomplete. The more complete statement of causality is that influence is mutual rather than one-way. The two linear relationships interact to create a closed-loop in which the variables mutually influence one another. *And that's what exacerbates the problem.* The consumer responds to availability, lower prices, convenience, and variety by increasing consumption of those foods. Increasing demand for fast food draws more players into the market to share the spoils increasing competition and innovation which ultimately increases productive attractiveness (better quality, more variety, lower prices). With more attractive products, that are attractively priced, and that are offered at more locations demand increases even more. And so on (Figure 11.3).

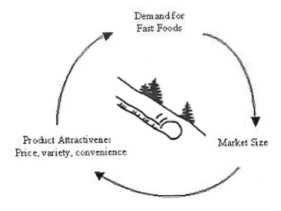

Figure 11.3: The more complete statement of causality

Which raises an interesting question: In such cycles of cause-and-effect what is the cause and what is the effect?

When any two events are related interdependently, designating one of those two as cause and the other effect is an arbitrary designation. If you examine any causal loop you will see why.

> In any causal loop no variable is any more or less important than any other variable. No variable in a loop controls other variables without itself being controlled by them. You can start the sequence anywhere you want by changing any variable. That change initially looks like a cause that triggers subsequent events in the loop. But the changes within the loop keep happening and eventually come back and modify the initial change which you had intentionally made. And that cycling back means that what was originally a cause is now suddenly an effect. This is a prominent feature of any structure of causal circuits. It should be kept in mind when you are tempted to argue that some changes are more important than other ones. If you have a genuine causal circuit, then any change made anywhere will eventually itself be changed by the consequences it triggers.[268]

When we are caught in such a reinforcing cycle we rarely make the trip around the loop just once. Rather—and that's what makes these types of reinforcing loops particularly potent—they are self-reinforcing dynamic processes that keep feeding on themselves. Seeing this is terribly important. For it is the self-reinforcing (snowballing) dynamic that can escalate a problem or trend—like fast food—into troublesome levels. With each trip around the loop, the phenomenon strengthens as the process feeds on itself, and given enough time an initial small "event" can morph into a major development. That's essentially how all epidemic scenarios arise.

The systems thinking discipline of closing the loops helps us see such escalation structures—structures in which we may be "trapped." Many times (as in this case) such structures are of our own creation. Only when we recognize such self-inflicted structures, can we begin the process of freeing ourselves.[269]

The Two Flavors of Feedback

Notice that the behavior of the feedback loop of Figure 11.3 is *different* from the many goal-seeking examples we discussed in Chapter 8—those that regulated the filling of a bathtub or maintained room/body temperature. In all such goal-seeking systems the feedback processes act to counteract and oppose any deviation from the goal. Such balancing (also called self-correcting and negative) loops counteract and oppose change. For example in the case of body temperature, if it should rise above 98.6 degrees Fahrenheit → instructions from the brain are issued to induce sweating → the evaporation of the sweat cools the body, causing body temperature to drop back down.

The feedback loop of Figure 11.3 is not, however, goal-seeking. It is a different type of loop known as a positive or reinforcing or deviation-amplifying loop. Positive feedback loops are different in that they amplify and reinforce change. That is, a deviation or perturbation in one of its variables is not suppressed rather it is amplified. You can experience this self-reinforcing process by walking yourself around the fast-food loop (Figure 11.3): More demand for fast food increases the size of the market, with more players innovating and competing productive attractiveness improves (better quality, more variety, lower prices) which further increases demand, and so on.

Positive feedback processes can be mighty "engines" of change because with sufficient cycling, small deviations can be amplified into major escalations. In folk wisdom, we speak of them in terms such as "snow-ball effect," "bandwagon effect," or "vicious circle," and in phrases such as "the rich get richer and the poor get poorer."[270]

In summary, the important distinctions between the two types (and there only two) of feedback are as follows: If the tendency in the loop is to reinforce the initial action, the loop is called a positive or reinforcing feedback loop; if the tendency is to oppose the initial action, the loop is called a negative or balancing feedback loop. Positive feedback is a process in which the effects of a small disturbance on a system include an increase in the magnitude of the perturbation. That is, A produces more of B which in turn produces more of A. In contrast, a system in which the results of a perturbation act to reduce or counteract the perturbation is a negative feedback system. Understanding (and learning to recognize) the two flavors of feedback can be very helpful in understanding how and why systems behave the way they do—e.g., why systems "fight back" and resist intervention (when negative feedback dominates) and/or escalate to troublesome levels (when positive feedback dominates).

The Figure below best illustrates the difference between the two feedback effects. A system dominated by deviation-balancing or negative feedback is like a marble placed at the lowest point of smooth-sided bowl—pushing the marble off the equilibrium creates a force opposing the displacement.[271] A system dominated by deviation-amplifying or positive feedback, on the other hand, is like falling off a cliff—the slightest disturbance causes the ball to fall off the peak and keep going.

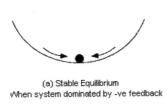

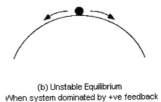

(a) Stable Equilibrium
When system dominated by -ve feedback

(b) Unstable Equilibrium
When system dominated by +ve feedback

Figure 11.4

(Reproduced from: Sterman, J.D. (2000), *Business Dynamics: Systems Thinking and Modeling for a Complex World*, Boston, Massachusetts: Irwin McGraw-Hill., and by permission of the McGraw-Hill Companies.)

Two Flavors of Feedback Operating at Multiple Levels

The reinforcing fast-food loop (Figure 11.3) example serves to underscore another important insight: feedback processes can operate at a *macro* scale. A very macro scale! In this case, the feedback process characterizes people-environment interactions at a societal-level. An interesting characteristic of such macro level feedback effects is that they rarely operate as simple isolated phenomena. Rather, they are often part in a dense web of socio-economic interrelationships.

In the next chapter we see that first hand as we explore the confluence of multiple socioeconomic and technological feedback effects that came together and fed on each other in the second half of the last century to fuel the obesity epidemic in America. Figure 11.5 below— which portrays nested feedback processes operating at the physiologic level, between the physiologic and the behavioral, and between people and their external environment—will provide a roadmap for our discussion.

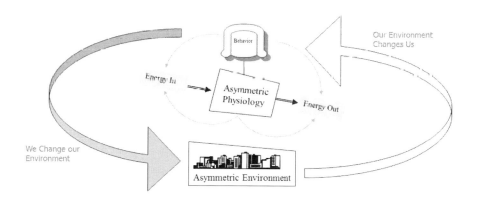

Figure 11.5 Feedback processes operate at multiple levels

CHAPTER 12

America's Obesity Epidemic:
A Case Study

One of the few reasonably reliable facts about the obesity epidemic is that it started around the early 1980s. According to the National Center for Health Statistics, the percentage of obese Americans had been relatively stable at around 13-14 percent, but then unexpectedly and quite dramatically shot up in the 1980s. By the end of that decade, nearly one in four Americans was obese. Any theory that tries to explain obesity in America has to account for this singular feature of the epidemic.

Starting with the obvious: The human body, like all systems—whether technological or biological—obeys the laws of thermodynamics, which define the immutable principle of energy conservation. Body weight can increase only if energy intake exceeds expenditure. And so, the upward trend in the population's weight itself constitutes evidence that the amount of calories consumed was exceeding those burned off by a growing proportion of the American population.[272] However, this explains neither what started the trend nor why it has persisted. It also does not explain whether the imbalance is caused by eating too much food, not expending enough energy, or both.

These are the important questions that I aim to answer in this chapter.

Tilting the Energy Balance: More Energy In

There is growing evidence to confirm what many of us don't want to admit: "We're fat because we eat a lot—a whole lot more than we used to."[273]

Caloric consumption data compiled by the U.S. Department of Agriculture (USDA) indicate that per capita food consumption in the U.S. remained relatively steady between 1900 and 1965, albeit with occasional moderate declines—for example, during World War I and the Great Depression. Since 1965, however, the food/caloric consumption of Americans markedly increased, and particularly so between 1980 and 2,000. USDA data indicate that over the two decades, the number of calories consumed per person per day in the United States increased by 20 percent, from 2,200 to slightly more than 2,700 calories—a 500 calories increase that's the equivalent of one Big Mac per person per day. (Recent data from the U.S. Department of Agriculture, the Centers for Disease Control and Prevention and the University of North Carolina food research program, suggest that calorie consumption may be starting to decline—slightly. Daily food diaries tracked by government researchers and estimates of food production suggest that calories consumed daily by the typical American adult may have peaked in 2003 and over the last decade declined by 1.5 to 2.5 percent. While the reduction is small and represents just a fraction of that change required to reverse the obesity epidemic, it is good news nevertheless.[274])

The U.S. Department of Agriculture (USDA) data on the growth in America's appetite point to two things: (1) after remaining roughly constant, the number of calories consumed has risen markedly and in lockstep with the recent escalation in obesity; and (2) the growth in energy intake is substantial enough to account for a significant chunk of the inflation we are witnessing in our aggregate "fat reserves."

What drove this increase in food consumption?

An often mentioned driver is food abundance—the result of significant improvements made in the last half century in the production and processing of food. While food abundance— not only in the United States but in many other industrialized countries—has undoubtedly afforded their populations an opportunity that humans had not previously had, "to eat food merely for pleasure and to consume more than the body needed to survive," having such an opportunity is not, however, a *sufficient* condition for over-consumption.[275]

More abundant food supplies, in other words, may have facilitated increased caloric intake, but it does not, by itself, provide a satisfying explanation for it. Obesity and abundance are sort of analogous to lightning and thunder. Though related, lightning is not what causes thunder. Rather, both lightning and thunder are caused by an electric discharge (the fundamental cause) that we perceive first visually and then aurally. To find the "cause behind the causes" of obesity, we, thus, need to dig a little deeper.

Researchers in epidemiology and public health, as well as in economics and systems science, have mined almost a century's worth of nutritional data in search of answers. And the emerging "perfect storm" theory is that the trigger that induced obesity's escalation (and energy intake) was not a single factor, but, rather, the confluence of multiple interacting factors.

Perfect storms arise rarely but violently when a number of (necessary and sufficient) weather elements come together at the right time. In a similar sense, the escalation of obesity (and energy intake) in America was not triggered by a single factor, but, rather, was induced by the confluence of multiple socioeconomic and technological factors that came together and fed on each other in the second half of the last century.

Let's see how.

How America's Eating Habits Changed

As late as the 1960s, the primary cost of food (as much as 60 percent of its total cost) was the time spent in the household preparing it. Back then, most Americans cooked their own food at home using mainly raw agricultural products. That consumed a significant amount of time, with the typical American housewife spending more than two hours per day cooking and cleaning up.[276]

America's eating habits started to change in the second half of the last century, when a growing number of women began to enter the labor force. According to David Cutler, Edward Glaeser and Jesse Shapiro of the Institute of Economic Research at Harvard University, the resultant evolution of new roles for women turned out to be one of the most important developments affecting America's eating habits in the past 50 years.

What started drawing women into the labor force? In the decades after World War II, the United States' economy experienced an important shift from an emphasis on the production of goods to the provision of services. Many of the new service-oriented jobs were white-collar jobs requiring little demanding physical effort; they were far removed from the dirty factory setting and, for these reasons, seemed more "appropriate" for women. Service industries such as banking, insurance, health, and education, which were growing rapidly, were more than happy to open their doors for more women to enter the labor force in order to sustain their rates of growth.

A number of other factors were also helping nudge more and more women through those doors. For example, the civil rights movement helped improve opportunities for and the treatment of women and minorities in the workplace, making paid work more attractive. Women's educational attainments were also, and at long last, catching up with those of men, allowing women more access to interesting and lucrative employment. And, last but not least, the women's movement helped accelerate the influx of married women into paid employment by making paid work appear more desirable to them.

As with many other social trends that escalate, the process fed on itself. For example, in this case, women's increased employment opportunities led to a decline in the birthrate, which meant that women spent fewer of their adult years raising preschool-age children and, thus, had more years available to spend in paid employment.[277] By the end of the twentieth century, women accounted for more than 60 percent of the labor force, up from 29 percent in 1950.

As more household time was diverted to outside employment, there was correspondingly less time and energy available for home activities such as food preparation and cleanup.[278] One important economic consequence of the growth of women's participation in the labor force was the increase in the economic value of their time—that is, their time spent in the household was more scarce and, thus, more valuable.

With less time to prepare meals, consumers would place a premium on fast and convenient food.

A confluence of technological innovations helped "grease" these socioeconomic trends and reinforce the changes in women's lives and the structure of the American family. Comparable to the mass-production revolution in manufactured goods that happened a century earlier, technological innovations in the preparation, packaging and distribution of food were making it increasingly possible for firms to mass-prepare food, preserve it, and distribute it to consumers in convenient locations for ready consumption.[279,280]

As in many fields (in engineering, business, or medicine), revolutionary change rarely arises out of a single great innovation or invention. Rather, it often comes about when a diverse set of "ripe" technologies fit like pieces of a jigsaw puzzle to form new "ensembles" of technologies that allow us to do things we couldn't do before or to do them in a much better way.[281]

By the 1950s and 60s, there had already been many important technological innovations in food processing, distribution, and home preparation. But most were developed separately and applied in isolation, offering marginal improvements. By the 1970s and 80s many of the pieces were in place and when finally *integrated* they would make the modern convenience foods possible and revolutionize the food environment. For example, even after deep-freezing technology had been available for some time, frozen foods still were not widely used (except, perhaps, in the military, where they played an important role for the military during the war). But when integrated with technologies for vacuum packing, improved preservatives, and artificial flavors, they made modern convenience foods possible because they made them more available and tastier. And in the home, microwave ovens (another "component" technology) allowed for rapid heating of those frozen and pre-prepared foods.[282]

Similarly, technological innovation was also revolutionizing the distribution of food.

> In order to produce food in one location that will be nearly ready for consumption in another location, [it was necessary to] surmount five main technological obstacles: controlling the atmosphere; preventing spoilage due to microorganisms; preserving flavor; preserving moisture; and controlling temperature. Innovations in food processing and packaging over the last three decades have improved food manufacturers ability to address each of these issues.[283]

As technology made it increasingly possible for firms to mass-prepare, preserve, and distribute food to consumers for rapid consumption, market production of food increasingly became a substitute for household production of food.[284] By lowering the time price of food (i.e., the time needed for preparation and clean-up), the switch from individual to mass preparation was a godsend to the growing number of time-strapped two-earner American households.[285]

Never had food been easier to prepare. Rising incomes allowed families to buy the latest appliances, from microwave ovens (in 83 percent of American homes by 1999) to nonstick pans and automatic dishwashers, which cut cleanup time.[286] By 1999, thanks to the abundance of processed foods and better kitchen appliances, the amount of time involved in meal preparation and cleanup was cut in half—from two hours per day in the 1950s to less than one.[287,288]

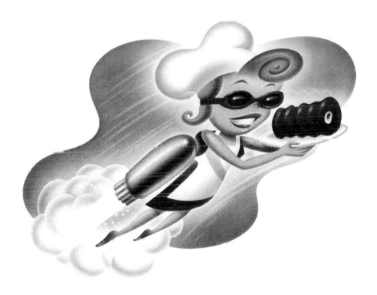

Figure 12.1
(Illustration courtesy of Dan Picasso.)

Postwar prosperity and technology were, thus, working together to create a climate that accelerated the reallocation of time from housework to outside work. With fewer hours needed to prepare food, women were freed up to do more wealth-generating activities outside the home. This, in turn, brought even more demand for convenience in food preparation and spurred the long-term trend toward eating out.[289] The two trends, in other words, fed on each other: The increased labor-force participation of women and the greater number of hours they worked stimulated the demand for inexpensive convenience and fast food, and vice versa.

All this had a Profound Impact on *How we Eat*

The socioeconomic-technological factors that changed family structures were also shaping *how* we eat. With both heads of the household working and the time available to prepare meals in short supply, fast and convenient foods were at a premium.

> Convenience [became] part of the unconscious cost-benefit analysis people make when choosing where and what to eat. Eating out increases, and with it comes deterioration in diet. What is eaten at home is also likely to be convenience foods.[290]

The public, thus, appears to have made an unconscious decision to accept the deterioration of their diet as a tradeoff for convenience and time. Instead of the wife staying at home and having time to prepare healthy meals, couples opted to both work, gaining financial benefits, "even though they now may get their dinners at drive-through restaurants."[291] To students of behavioral decision making, this tradeoff is neither surprising nor irrational.

Health is only one of many factors people consider as they make lifestyle choices—what to eat, where to work, and how to play. The incentives of economics, convenience, and the value of time (to name a few) can be more important than health in influencing individual choices. Because health consequences are often delayed and/or may be perceived as low risk, they very often have less of an impact on our choices than factors with immediate influence, such as short-term financial reward and convenience.[292]

The issue here is not information or the lack of it (e.g., about the consequences of unhealthy eating), but *incentives*. Even when people know that eating home-prepared food is healthier, rational couples may elect to eat more convenient but less healthy food because they value their high-paying, two-career lifestyles and because they may not be willing to pay the price—in effort, expense, or time—for a traditionally cooked meal.[293]

Still, what this effectively does is push the puzzle back a step. What we now need to explain is how the demand for and consumption of convenience and fast food induced an *increase in calories consumed.*

The increase in food/caloric consumption was induced through two mechanisms that relate to the *time* and *space* dimensions of how we eat.

1) The *time* mechanism relates to *when we eat.* And because time is money… at what cost. It is about how convenience food provided affordability and convenience of eating anytime, all the time.

2) The *space* (or place) mechanism relates to *where we eat.* It is about how fast food provided the opportunity to eat anywhere, everywhere.

The First Mechanism: The *Time* We Eat

The switch from individual to mass preparation lowered both the time *and* monetary costs of food consumption. The decrease in the *time cost* of food was, however, the bigger deal.

As with any product or service, when thinking about the cost of food consumption, one tends to think in terms of monetary costs. But with food consumption, cost includes both time and money. Both of these cost components have declined over the last several decades, albeit at dramatically different rates. Consider first the monetary cost of food. According to the Bureau of Labor Statistics, with the exception of a spike during the oil shock in the 1970s, food prices have been dropping by an average of 0.2 percent a year since World War II.[294] Such a drop in food prices, while welcome, is too modest to have played a significant role in the upward jump in the population's caloric intake.[295] By contrast, the drop in the *time cost* of food has been quite dramatic—and, so, of greater significance.

As already mentioned, back in the 1950s-60s, the primary cost of food for the average American household was the time spent in food preparation and cleanup. But that was before those technological innovations in convenience-food production and distribution had kicked in. As technology made it increasingly possible for firms to package and distribute mass-prepared foods, market production of food increasingly became a preferred substitute for household production of food.[296] Professional labor and capital in the supermarket and the factory replaced labor in the home, reducing food-preparation time. Time savings translate into cost savings—a translation that economists Cutler, Glaeser and Shapiro estimate amounted to a 29-percent reduction between 1965 and 1995 in the per-calorie cost of food.[297]

Reductions in the time cost of food preparation led to an increase in the amount of food consumed through a standard price mechanism, just as reductions in any good's cost should lead to increased consumption of that good. When a meal takes two to three minutes to prepare, it is neither difficult nor expensive to eat anytime and all the time. A person on a diet is less likely to have a mid-afternoon snack if it requires a ten-minute walk to the corner store for ingredients and an hour of meal preparation and cleanup. That same person, though, is much more likely to have a snack if the vending machine is ten yards away.[298]

And so, while the dazzling array of new food technologies and the widespread availability of microwave ovens and vending machines have been a boon to the time-strapped American family, they have come at a cost. The increased convenience and reduced time between when we want a meal and when we can eat it would create a new and fattening pattern of eating.[299]

In a hunt for insights into exactly *how* Americans were consuming more convenience foods, Cutler, Glaeser and Shapiro had to mine decades-worth of nutritional data, but, in the end, did find their answer: The escalation in caloric consumption has been most evident in America's growing *snacking* habit. The increased convenience (and variety) in our diet had provoked a shift in our eating patterns toward frequent "grazing"—small but cumulatively hefty snacks, as opposed to regular meals. In the last thirty years, the amount of energy we consume through snacks nearly doubled. Americans are eating more, in other words, because they are eating more frequently.[300]

Americans, across all age groups, are snacking more often and deriving more energy from snacks than ever before. Oliver[301] provides some revealing statistics on America's escalating snacking habit:

> In the mid-1970s. . . . Americans only got about 13 percent of their
> calories from snacking, a relatively small percentage. Today, men

and women are getting almost 25 percent of their daily calories from snacking, the caloric equivalent of a full meal a generation ago. The average American male consumes more than 500 calories a day from snacks, the average female more than 346 calories a day. . . Americans spend more than 38 billion dollars a year on snack foods, more than what they spend on higher education.

In the past 30 years, an enormous number of tasty snacks have been introduced into the U.S. food market, many falling into the nutrient-poor, high energy-dense categories.[302] These are distributed through vending machines that dot our workplaces, ensuring that cheap, high-fat, high-calorie snacks are no more than a few yards away.[303]

Snacking increases food consumption not only because people eat more times during the day—and on food that is often energy-dense—but also because snackers do not compensate for the snacks they eat by eating less at their regular meal times.[304,305] In one recent study that's typical of the many that have been conducted, researchers examined the impact of a snack consumed after a standard lunch on subsequent food consumption. "The researchers fed subjects a snack (400 kcal) at various times after a 1300-kcal lunch. [The Result:] the snack neither reduced the amount of food consumed at the dinner meal nor increased the time before the subjects requested their dinner meal."[306]

Studies that track longer-term energy intake are consistent with these findings. They show that total daily energy intake of adult snackers is, on average, 25-percent higher than that of non-snackers.[307] The average adult snacker, in other words, is eating the equivalent of four full meals a day—not three.[308]

Soft Drinks: The Liquid Snack

When we quench our thirst, we don't just drink water anymore, a zero-calorie affair. We grab a soft drink instead. Each 12-oz serving of a carbonated, sweetened soft drink provides about 150 kcal, all from sugars, and contains no other nutrients of significance.[309] A soft drink is the prototypical (junk) snack.

The upward trend in per capita consumption of sweetened beverages correlates closely with the rising rates of obesity. Market research data show that since the 1970s, soft-drink consumption increased by more than 130 percent (or 200 calories)—more quickly, in fact, than the consumption of any other food group.[310,311] Today, soft-drink consumption accounts for approximately seven percent of the energy in our diet, with the average American drinking soda at an annual rate of about fifty-six gallons per person—that's nearly six hundred twelve-ounce cans of soda per person per year.[312,313,314] (I alluded earlier to encouraging recent findings showing a slight decline in the calories consumed by the average American since the early 2000s. An encouraging component of that trend—if sustained—is a commensurate decline in the amount of full-calorie soda drunk. Given the very high peak we "scaled" and now need to decline from, however, soda consumption still remains at a level that's too high in absolute terms.[315])

One reason the growth in soft-drink consumption is of concern to those in public health is that the intake rates are even higher among adolescents and children.

> [In the 1970s,] . . . the typical teenage boy in the United States drank about seven ounces of soda every day; today he drinks nearly three times that amount, deriving 9 percent of his daily caloric intake from soft drinks. Soda consumption among teenage girls has doubled within the same period, reaching an average of twelve ounces a day. . . . Soft-drink consumption has also become commonplace among American toddlers. About one-fifth of the nation's one- and two-year-olds now drink soda.[316]

In 2001, a group of researchers from the Department of Medicine at Children's Hospital in Boston who were studying childhood obesity and its causes singled out childhood consumption of soda as their target.[317] The researchers tracked 548 ethnically diverse Massachusetts schoolchildren (average age, eleven) for nineteen months, looking at the association between their weight at the beginning of the study, intake of soda, and weight at the end of the study period. The results were quite revealing. For one thing, 57 percent of the kids increased their intake over the study's nineteen-month period. The association between soda consumption and weight gain was so clear-cut that the researchers could even link specific amounts of soda to specific amounts of weight gain. Each daily drink, they calculated, added 0.18 points to a child's body mass index (BMI), regardless of what else they ate or how much they exercised.

But perhaps the most interesting finding was that ". . . the kids were doing something with the soda that few people initially understood: . . . [T]hey were not compensating for those extra empty calories when they sat down for regular meals."[318] In other words, as with solid snacks, consumption of energy-containing beverages elicits little dietary compensation. The obvious implication: Because sugar-sweetened drinks represent energy added to, not displacing, other dietary intake, they must induce an increase in total energy consumption.[319]

Additional studies on adults confirmed that soft-drink consumers tend to have a higher daily energy intake than non-consumers.[320] For example, one researcher "examined 7-day food diaries of 323 adults and found that energy from drinks added to total energy intake and did not displace energy ingested in [meals]."[321] And in a Danish study, results showed not only a lack of compensation, but also how rapidly increased soft-drink consumption can affect weight.

> [The Danish] scientists studied overweight volunteers who were given soft drinks sweetened with either sugar or artificial sweeteners but were allowed to eat freely otherwise. During [the] ten-week study the people having sugared drinks consumed an extra 500-700 calories per day from the soft drinks. Those receiving the sugared drinks did not compensate for the extra calories and gained 3.5 pounds during the ten weeks.[322]

What particularly troubled the Danish researchers was that these results could occur in such a short time.

In a recent *Scientific American* article, Barry Popkin explained how evolutionary history may account for our imprecise and incomplete compensation for energy consumed in liquid form.

> For most of our evolutionary history, the only beverages humans consumed were breast milk after birth and water after weaning. Because water has no calories, the human body did not evolve to reduce food intake to compensate for beverage consumption. As

a result, when people drink any beverage except water their total calorie consumption rises, because they usually continue to eat the same amount of food.[323]

Several other researchers postulated the specific physiological mechanisms that may account for this phenomenon.[324] It goes like this: Because liquid "meals" are of larger volume, lower energy density and lower osmotic potential,[325] they are emptied from the stomach at a more rapid rate. The more rapid transit of fluids causes nutrient sensors in the gut to have a shorter exposure time to their nutrients and, as result, the signals influencing meal termination are weaker.

The Second Mechanism: *Where* we Eat

The forces that drove demand for convenience in food preparation—namely, the increasing scarcity and increasing value of household time—have also spurred the long-term trend toward eating out.

As moderately priced fast-food chains such as McDonald's and Burger King began spreading across the country in the postwar era, and with their new and increasingly popular credit cards in hand, many more Americans started dining out. Eating out, once done mainly by travelers and office workers, became another popular option for families to save time in the kitchen.[326] Consider these stats:

- Today, Americans spend about half of their food budget and consume about one-third of their daily calories on meals and drinks consumed outside the home—mainly at fast-food restaurants. That's nearly double the percentages in the 1970s.[327]
- "The average American eats out more than four times a week."[328]
- "On any given day in the United States about one-quarter of the adult population visits a fast food restaurant."[329]
- "The time spent by an average customer in a fast food restaurant is a blistering eleven minutes"[330]

Between 1970 and 2014, the number of fast-food restaurants grew from some 70,000 to close to 240,000, ensuring that Americans are not more than a few steps from immediate sources of a rich variety of fast foods. Today, fast food pervades virtually all segments of society, including local communities, hospitals, and—what to many is a troubling development—public schools. According to a survey by the Center for Disease Control (C.D.C.), about 20 percent of the nation's schools offer brand-name fast food in their cafeterias.[331,332] Fast-food companies such as McDonald's and Pizza Hut have, for years, been offering schools financial incentives for allowing them to set up shop on school grounds. With many schools chronically short on funds for supporting academic programs and other activities, the financial incentive is understandably irresistible.[333]

The introduction of the drive-through window some forty years ago made it possible to pick up fast food and eat on the run or take it home, which offered more time savings and quickly caught on.[334] Capitalizing on the trend, fast-food companies introduced menus and packaging to make it convenient for us to nosh on the road. Chips, candy and soup are packaged in containers that snuggle neatly into car cup holders. And, in the newest wrinkle (and thanks to "cooperation" from the car manufacturers), those cup holders can heat and cool our meals or beverages to keep them at the right temperature.[335] Today, 60 percent of fast food sold in the United States is purchased at the drive-through.[336]

Fast Food: Eat Anywhere, Everywhere

The increasing frequency of fast food use has undeniably increased Americans' total energy intake.

One of the most in-depth studies on the association between fast-food use and increased caloric intake was conducted by a group of epidemiologists from the University of Minnesota in 2001. The study involved almost 5000 adolescent students in thirty-one secondary schools and tracked their use of fast-food restaurants through daily dietary diaries. The results were striking:

Fast food restaurant use was positively associated with intake of total energy, percent energy from fat, daily servings of soft drinks .

. . and was inversely associated with daily servings of fruit, vegetables, and milk. . . .

A boy who never ate at a fast-food restaurant during the school week averaged a daily calorie count of 1952; one who ate fast food one to two times a week (as did more than half of all the children in the study) consumed an average of 2192 calories a day (12% more); while those who ate fast food three times or more a week (one fifth of the studied) consumed an amazing 2752 calories a day (40% higher).[337]

For additional proof that these results were due to a causal relationship between fast food and energy intake and were not the consequence of some other unrecognized or incompletely controlled socioeconomic or demographic factors, additional studies were conducted in which subjects were used as their own controls—that is, comparing the energy inputs of the *same* subject on days with versus days without fast food. The earlier results held. For example, in one of these studies, the child-subjects were found, on average, to eat 126 kcal/day more on days with fast food compared to days without fast food.[338]

Comparable findings of a strong association between frequency of fast-food restaurant use and total energy intake were observed for adults. In one representative study, total energy intake was 40-percent higher among males and 37-percent higher among females who reported three or more visits to a fast food restaurant during the past week, compared to those who reported never eating at a fast food restaurant during the past week.[339]

All of which raises the question: What is there about fast food that induces an increase in caloric consumption?

Several factors inherent to fast food seem to contribute to increased energy intake. Below, I categorize these factors along two broad dimensions: *qualitative* and *quantitative*.

The *Qualitative* Dimension

The first obvious mechanism is taste. (As discussed in Chapter 11), studies in humans demonstrate that taste is an important reason individuals choose the foods they do—*often more important than healthfulness*[340]—and that food consumption significantly increases with food palatability.[341]

Like any consumer product, fast food is "designed" for consumer appeal—specifically, to appeal to our primordial taste preferences for fats, sugar, and salt.[342] Fast food is designed to give us the tastes that generations of evolution have caused us to crave.

> We are hardwired to love the taste of fat, salt, and sugar. Fatty foods gave our ancestors the calorie reserves to weather food shortages. Salt helped them retain water and avoid dehydration. Sugar helped them distinguish sweet edible berries from the sour poisonous ones. Through our taste for fat, salt, and sugar, we learned to prefer the foods that were most likely to keep us alive. Almost everything we love about fast food are things that our hunter-gatherer forefathers would, well, kill for.[343]

The industry's pursuit of allure is extremely sophisticated, and it leaves nothing to chance. To determine the precise amount of sugar or fat or salt that will send consumers over the moon, some of the largest companies are now using brain scans to study how we react neurologically to certain foods. The world's biggest ice cream maker, Unilever, for instance, parlayed its brain research into a brilliant marketing campaign that sells the eating of ice cream as a "scientifically proven" way to make ourselves happy."[344]

According to data gathered by the United States Department of Agriculture, fast foods contain on average 20-percent more fat than home-cooked meals.[345] That's a big jump for an average measure, and because it's an *average*, there are apt to be many fast-food items with an even higher fat content. For example, a Big Mac with a medium order of French fries has 1,020 kcal and 54 g of fat—that amounts to half the total recommended daily energy requirement, but as much as 83% of recommended daily fat intake.[346] Besides the fat, fast foods—the Big Mac with

French fries and a soda remains a good example—are also higher in salt and sugar and much lower in fiber than home-cooked food.[347]

Food containing larger and more condensed amounts of fats and sugars is not only tastier, but is also more stable—meaning that it has longer shelf life and can better retain good "mouth-feel" after an hour under the fast-food heat lamp.[348] All of this helps explain why the most popular fast-food items are generally high in fat, and why many of the lower-fat, so-called "light" fast-food options that some fast food restaurants have recently introduced have not been popular with customers.[349]

Inducing *active* over-consumption of food through appetite stimulation may be the simplest explanation for why tasty fast food appears to promote excess energy intake and weight gain, but it is not the only mechanism.[350] Recent research on human appetite control and feeding regulation has revealed two additional mechanisms. The higher energy density of high-fat foods induces *passive* over-consumption, and the low thermic effect of fat allows us to retain more of it.

When people eat fat-enriched foods, they unawares tend to consume more energy as a result of the higher energy density of fat. Because this does not appear to be consciously intended—that is, it occurs passively, without any apparent effort on the part of the eater—the phenomenon has been referred to as passive over-consumption.[351]

Perhaps the most illuminating work on this phenomenon has been the pioneering studies by Dr. Barbara Rolls and her team at Pennsylvania State University. Over the last two decades, Dr. Rolls' studies on human satiety have demonstrated that the number of calories in a given volume of food—i.e., its caloric or energy density—makes a big difference in how many total calories people consume at a given meal, as well as throughout the day. And that's primarily because people tend to consume a *constant volume* of food at a given meal, irrespective of its energy content.[352]

In a series of experimental studies, Dr. Rolls and her team have demonstrated that food volume has "the overriding influence" on satiety—on what makes us feel full. Food bulk, not energy content, in other words, is the key to what makes our bodies say we've eaten enough. The corollary of that, of course, is that if people consume a constant volume of food at a given meal, then more total energy is consumed when the diets are high in energy density—as more calories are packed into a given weight or volume of food—than when they are low in energy density.[353,354]

Why would our system evolve to monitor weight and volume rather than energy or nutrient content? Blundell and King, two scientists at the Biopsychology Group at the University of Leeds in England, have a very plausible theory. They argue that because weight (before the advent of processed foods) was very often a good predictor of energy value and nutrient content, our system has "learned" to rely on weight as a reliable "cue"—i.e., to associate the weight and volume of food consumed with its energy value and nutrient composition. Given the inability to sense visually the energy or nutrient content of food, it makes perfect sense that food weights and volumes become the important variables that we monitor subconsciously.[355,356]

> [This] . . . does not mean that weight is fundamentally more important than energy content. . . . [I]t does mean [however] that humans [and animals] have learned during the course of their lives (and long-term exposure to food) that weight is very often a good predictor of energy value or nutrient content.[357]

Dietary fat is the most energy-dense macronutrient, containing more than twice as much energy per unit weight than either protein or carbohydrate (nine calories per gram for fat versus four calories per gram for both proteins and carbohydrates). Thus, a small quantity of food rich in fat has very high energy content.[358] In contrast, because water increases food volume without adding calories, foods such as vegetables and fruit, which have a high water content, cause us to feel full on fewer calories and lead to reduced energy intake.[359] After water, which has zero calories, fiber contributes the most to food volume for the fewest number of calories, supplying 1.5 to 2.5 calories per gram.[360]

A telling statistic that underscores the association between fast-food composition and caloric intake comes from the USDA. They calculate that if fast food had the same average nutritional composition (and so the same energy and fat density) as food prepared and cooked at home, Americans would consume approximately 200 fewer calories per day. That's an extra pound's worth of energy *every twenty days.*[361]

The fact that fast food is eaten . . . well, fast, further contributes to *passive* over-consumption. Like any regulatory feedback process, the body's physiologic system that regulates appetite takes time to kick in—it takes time for the body to sense that food has reached the stomach and to shut off the feeling of hunger.[362] After eating a full meal, the satiety signals that tell us we've had enough may not kick in for a full half-hour—that's long after the blistering eleven minutes the average customer spends eating a fast-food meal.[363,364] Speeding-eating fast food, we tend to stuff ourselves before our brains have the chance to slow us down. And, of course, the higher the energy density of the food we overeat, the higher the number of calories we ingest.

Active and passive over-consumption are the two primary mechanisms by which fatty fast food induces more energy consumption—in both cases, through inducing *intake*. Fast-food consumption contributes to the expansion of our fat stores in a third way: *When we eat fat-enriched foods, we tend to retain more of it.* And that's because of the low thermic effect of fat.

When we overeat, the body needs to work—expend some energy—to store those extra calories (whether ingested in the form of fat, carbohydrates or proteins) as body fat. Because, compared to the other two macronutrients, the pathway from dietary fat to body fat requires fewer metabolic steps, fat is the one that's stored most efficiently—i.e., with the least amount of "losses." For example, storing excess energy from dietary carbohydrate or protein into body fat requires an expenditure of approximately 25 percent of ingested energy. By comparison, storing excess energy from dietary fat into body fat stores uses less than five percent of the ingested energy intake.[365] And so, when the excess food we eat comes from fat-enriched fast food, we will tend to retain more of it.

The *Quantity* Dimension

The fast food quality "issues" are further compounded by a growing trend in the United States toward larger portion sizes. The explosive expansion we're witnessing in menu items with labels such as *Big, Mega,* and *Super* is not some ploy by food companies to make us think we are getting more—we really *are* getting more.[366,367]

The portions of fast food we are now getting dwarf those of past generations—in some cases, the portions are two to five times larger than the portions our parents were served in the 1950s and 60s.[368] Consider:

- A typical hamburger in the 1950s weighed 2.8 ounces and contained 200 calories. The typical hamburger today weighs 6 ounces and packs 600 calories.[369,370]
- A serving of McDonald's French fries ballooned from 200 calories in the 1960s to 450 calories in the mid-1990s to the present 610 calories.[371]
- Beverage sizes have also increased dramatically. "Soft drink containers morphed from eight ounces to twelve ounces to sixteen ounces and then to twenty ounces as the standard serving size."[372]
- Even our cookies are getting supersized—with some "monster" cookies today up to 700 percent larger.[373]

Interestingly, this massive super-sizing trend appears to be mainly a U.S. phenomenon. When a group of University of Pennsylvania researchers compared restaurant and supermarket meals in the U.S. and France, they found the French portion sizes to be significantly less hefty. A soft drink in France was a third smaller, a hotdog 40 per cent smaller, and a carton of yoghurt almost half as big. Even the croissant—perhaps the most iconic French food item—was smaller. A Parisian croissant is a one-ounce affair, while in Pittsburgh it's two.[374,375] (It is probably no coincidence that the French people are seriously leaner, and France's obesity rate is 7.4 percent, one fourth that of the U.S.)

What underlies this American-Gallic disparity? Perhaps it's the cultural compulsion of Americans to get the most bang for the buck.[376] "More is better" seems to be a mantra for most Americans. We wanted bigger cars, bigger houses, bigger portions—and more is what we got: "Portions big enough to feed a horse."[377]

And how did it all start?

The late David Wallerstein, a theater manager from Chicago and a longtime director of McDonald's, is sometimes credited with the super-sizing trend.

> In the mid-1960s, Mr. Wallerstein realized that customers were reluctant to buy two bags of popcorn because they felt gluttonous, but would happily buy one jumbo bag. He later persuaded Ray Kroc, McDonald's legendary leader, to use the same strategy with French fries, and the race for ever-larger portions was on.[378]

It was a brilliant marketing strategy, one of those rare propositions that were win-win for both consumers and food sellers. From the consumer's point of view, large portions not only *seem* like bargains—they actually are. For a relatively small increase in price, super-sizing greatly increases the number of calories we get.[379] For example: A 16-oz soft drink at 7-Eleven runs you just under five cents per ounce, while a 32-oz Big Gulp costs just 2.7 cents per ounce.[380] And at McDonald's, it costs only 60-percent more to upgrade from a Quarter Pounder to a Medium Value Meal, which includes fries and a soda, for 125-percent more calories,[381] and an additional 87 cents buys almost three times as many French fries.[382]

From the restaurants' point of view, larger portions also proved a profitable option. Compared to the costs of marketing, packaging and labor, the cost of the added ingredients to super-size a menu item is small.[383] On average, food accounts for about a third of the total cost of running a restaurant; such things as labor, equipment, advertising, rent and electricity make up the rest. So, while it may cost a restaurant a few pennies to offer 25-percent more French fries, it can raise its prices much more than a few cents and still offer the consumer a good deal. Smaller portions, by contrast, translate into lower profit margins—it's half the food, but it still requires all the labor. The result is that larger portions proved a reliable way to bolster the average check at restaurants.[384]

As the U.S. market size grew and as raw materials for food became even more abundant and cheap, food companies started competing for the consumer's dollar by increasing portion sizes rather than by lowering prices (which, of course, would have lowered revenues). Consumers responded predictably. They started favoring restaurants on the basis of portion size, which helped sustain and fuel the trend.[385]

With all this going for it, it is no wonder that the super-sizing trend that began in the late 1970s has increased steadily ever since.[386] "As of 1996 some 25 percent of the $97 billion spent on fast food came from items promoted on the basis of either larger size or extra portions."[387]

Obviously, larger portions provide another "opportunity" for more caloric consumption, but could human appetite be *expanded* by merely offering more and bigger portions? The answer appears to be yes. Experimental studies on humans have established that there is, indeed, a significant positive association between portion size and energy intake, indicating that we eat more when served larger portions.[388] "Super-sized" and "monster" meals, in other words, do encourage consumption of larger portions.[389]

In a 2001 study, nutritional researchers with Barbara Rolls' group at Penn State University demonstrated that the presence of larger portions *in themselves* "nudged" people toward eating more.

> Men and women volunteers, all reporting the same level of hunger, were served lunch on four separate occasions. In each session, the size of the main entree was increased, from 500 to 625 to 750 and finally to 1000 grams. After four weeks, the pattern became clear: As portions increased, all participants ate increasingly larger amounts, despite their stable hunger levels.[390]

In the experiment, food intake was 30-percent higher when people were given the largest compared to the smallest serving—a significant increase—prompting the researchers to confidently conclude that, "human hunger could [indeed] be expanded by merely offering more and bigger options."[391]

But the researchers didn't stop there. Additional studies that investigated the underlying mechanisms helped reveal something both interesting and hopeful for the future. They revealed strong cultural underpinnings to our apparent "compulsion" to eat more when served larger portions. The insights into the role of culture emerged from the work the Rolls group did with children. The experiments showed that before the age of three, portion size does not influence a child's energy intake. However, that begins to change sometime between the ages of three and five years as children develop and learn social and cultural conventions regarding food and eating.[392]

In a series of experiments, Dr. Rolls and her colleagues examined the eating habits of two groups of children, one of three-year-olds, another of five-year-olds:

> Both groups reported equal levels of energy expenditure and hunger. The children were then presented with a series of plates of macaroni and cheese. The first plate was a normal serving built around age-appropriate baseline nutritional needs; the second plate was slightly larger; the third was what we might now call "supersized." The results were both revealing and worrisome. The younger children consistently ate the same baseline amount, leaving more and more food on the plate as the servings grew in size. The five-year-olds acted as if they were from another planet, devouring whatever was put on their plates. Something had happened. As was the case with their adult counterparts . . . the mere presence of larger portions had induced increased eating.[393]

These results suggest that, as children grow and develop socially, they shift from eating primarily in response to physiologic signals of hunger and satiety—essentially, trusting their gut—to eating that depends more on environmental influences, such as the amount of food served, time of day, and social context. The older children had learned that cleaning the plate is what is expected and that they will be rewarded for doing so.[394]

As children grow into adulthood, they retain the expectations that the amount of food that others serve them is appropriate. As a result, many of us decide how much food to eat at a single sitting on the basis of how much food we are served. Indeed, in a survey conducted by the American Institute for Cancer Research, "67% of those polled said that, when dining out, they finish their entrees most or all of the time."[395] This is why experts tend to believe that it is no coincidence that Americans became fatter at the same time that they began eating out more and as restaurants began super-sizing their portions.[396]

And so, while we might like to believe that people will stop eating as soon as they feel full, it doesn't work that way. Human appetite, it turns out, is surprisingly elastic, a fact that—as with the asymmetric design of the system—also makes excellent evolutionary sense since our survival over the eons of human existence was more acutely threatened by starvation than by obesity. Unfortunately, while the system represents a useful adaptation in an environment of food scarcity and unpredictability, it's problematic ". . . in an environment of fast-food abundance, when the opportunity to feast presents itself 24/7. Our bodies are storing reserves of fat against a famine that never comes."[397]

Tilting the Energy Balance: Less Energy Out

The recent rise in the U.S. population's caloric intake could very well have been stifled had there been a balancing increase in energy expenditure. However, the population's increased energy intake has been accompanied by a decline in energy output. This energy "depression" is adding to our collective energy surplus.

For our hunter-gatherer ancestors, there was a natural coupling between the input and output of energy. They could feast on more food, for example, only if they expended more muscular energy to hunt and gather additional foodstuffs. Conversely, a decrease in food availability meant death for some and, consequently, less energy consumption by the collective tribe. Long-term, the caloric intake and output of those early humans tended to balance out, despite seasonal fluctuations in food availability and the ongoing need for high-energy output.[398]

This balance has now been disturbed.

Today, in the United States, as well as in most other affluent nations, energy expenditure and energy intake have been largely decoupled. Unlike the hunter (whether man or beast), humans no longer need to exert themselves so much to obtain food energy. And in terms of the calorie-to-effort return ratio (i.e., the human effort necessary to obtain a given amount of food energy), calories, from childhood on, are available at the lowest cost in human experience.[399]

In the remainder of this section, we'll explore how (and why) caloric expenditure has been dropping in the United States. We will see how the socioeconomic and technological changes that lowered the time and monetary costs of consuming calories (effectively reducing the real price of food and inducing an increase in food consumption) have contributed to the rise in obesity in a second way: by simultaneously raising the cost of expending calories and inducing a decrease in energy expenditure.[400] We also will look at how the time pressures that fueled the demand for convenient and fast food have increased our " . . . need to get places faster, which causes us to drive rather than walk, to take the elevators instead of the stairs, and to look to technology for ways to engineer inefficient physical activity out of our lives."[401]

Work: Engineering Energy Expenditure out of the Workplace

As the U.S. economy continues to shift from an emphasis on the production of goods to the provision of services, fewer and fewer Americans are working at jobs that are "sweat-friendly."[402] Recent census data show that the proportion of the workforce employed in occupations requiring heavy manual labor, such as farming, masonry, carpentry, and heavy manual factory work, continue to decline, while the proportion of the workforce employed in more sedentary white-collar jobs is rising. Many of these new service-oriented jobs—in industries such as banking, insurance, health, and education— require little energy expenditure, often nothing more active than pressing keys on a computer.[403,404]

Meanwhile, even on the farm and on the factory floor, places that traditionally required high energy expenditure, we find that modern labor-saving technology is increasingly performing the tasks once performed by our bodies.[405] It is estimated that a hundred years ago, as much as 30 percent of the energy used in farm and factory work came from muscle power; today, only one percent does.[406]

In gradual, often subtle ways, physical exertion continues to be technologically engineered out of the American lifestyle. Even small savings add up over a year, a decade, and a lifetime. French et al,[407] worked out an interesting calculation to demonstrate how, in an office setting, the cumulative effects of small decreases in energy expenditure that occur by substituting e-mail for walking to a nearby office could be significant over long time periods.

A 145-lb person expends 3.9 kcals/min walking and only1.8 kcal/ min sitting. Energy expenditure thus doubles by walking versus sitting. If one spends 5 min/day, 5 days/week, walking to cowork- ers' offices to interact, it would result in approximately 5000 kcals/ year expended, compared with only 2500 kcals/year for the same

amount of time spent sitting at the computer sending those cowork-
ers e-mails. Walking versus sending e-mail could expend about a
pound more energy per year.

Although the example is hypothetical, as the authors remind us, "[T]he
point is that small but consistent reductions in energy expenditure due to increased
computer use could have a significant cumulative impact over time."

The drivers underlying these trends are not just technological; they are economic as well. As is often said, "Economics craft institutions into energy-saving
enterprises."[408] In many industries, minimizing physical labor and replacing it with
technology has certainly been an effective strategy to save cost. While (on balance)
this has been good for our pocketbooks, it has had profound (and unintended)
consequences on the economic incentives that drive us to burn calories (Figure
12.2)

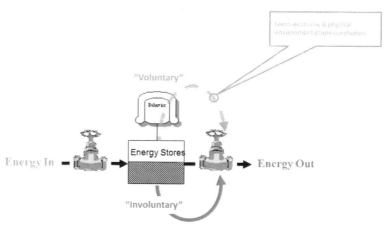

Figure 12.2: Socioeconomic incentives shape our choices

Simply put, when work was strenuous, we were, in effect, being *paid* to
exercise. Today, as more and more jobs become increasingly sedentary, we must
pay for physical activity[409]—not only in the money we pay to get into the gym, but
in foregone leisure time.[410] To expend serious calories in our society today often
involves a choice between going to the gym and spending time with our spouse
or kids.[411]

In the home, increasing reliance on prepared foods and the proliferation of labor-saving appliances—such as washing machines, dishwashers, microwave ovens, self-propelled lawn mowers, and automatic garage door openers—have caused household-related work to also markedly decline, further compounding the problem.[412]

Here, too, the small savings from devices such as electric toothbrushes and TV remote controls become sizable when added up over a year, a decade, and a lifetime.[413] For example, Professor Andrew Prentice, head of the International Nutrition Group at the London School of Hygiene and Tropical Medicine, calculates that the seemingly insignificant switch to using a cordless phone robs us of the equivalent of a ten-kilometer walk each year (because it relieves us from finding a stationary phone). Using a television remote rather than getting up to change channels, he reckons, saves enough energy to add up to as much as an extra pound a year.[414]

Whether in the farm, factory, office, or home, technology is increasingly performing the tasks our bodies once performed. It is all adding up to an environment where fewer of us are expending the energy necessary to maintain a grip on our growing appetites.[415]

Moving About: Transport and Urban Design

As we've already seen, culture and economics shape people's preferences relating to food and, in turn, energy intake. Similarly, human behavior relating to physical activity and energy expenditure is a function of both lifestyle preferences and the characteristics of our physical environment. How our neighborhoods are built—for example, with/without cycle and foot paths, street lighting, and public transport—influences the use of active transport (walking, cycling) over motorized transport. Participation in active recreational activities is similarly affected by community services, such as the availability of recreational facilities, parks, sports grounds, and community clubs.[416]

Our modern urban environment is increasingly one of our own making.[417] And what we have created are neighborhoods and communities that stifle—dis-incentivize—rather than promote physical exertion. Nowhere is that more true than in how we get from place to place.

For decades, planners have designed our cities, towns and suburbs on the assumption that every trip will be made by car. In many neighborhoods (including my own), sidewalks are a rare curiosity—and what would be the point, since most also lack stores and entertainment destinations within walking distance?[418]

> Even those willing to risk it are put off by the growing distance we have put between ourselves both from others, and from the places and things we need and desire. . . . Shopping centers are concrete islands surrounded by highways too treacherous to access by foot. Workplaces are inaccessible by public transportation. . . . Libraries, parks, and playgrounds are surrounded by acres of parking lot, making their access by anything but car if not out of the question, then at best unappealing.[419]

The pervasive availability of automobiles, combined with urban and suburban designs that make the automobile the most convenient transportation mode, has had a huge influence on how we "choose" to move around.[420] More than ever, the private vehicle is the dominant mode of transport for commuting, shopping and other activities. In 2010, almost 90 percent of us drove to work.[421] Federal studies show that three out of four trips as short as a mile or less are made by car.[422] It seems as though we are conducting many aspects of everyday business without ever having to step out of our cars including eating our—you guessed it—fast food.[423] As stated earlier, it is estimated that up to 60 percent of fast food sold in the United States passes through the drive-through.[424]

There are now more American households that own at least two vehicles—60 percent—than those that own one (30 percent).[425] (As of 2014, only ten percent did not own a private vehicle.[426]) As cars proliferate their production costs and selling prices drop, this increases affordability and ultimately sales. In often subtle and indirect ways, this maintains the pressure to keep molding our communities for the convenience of automobile transport.

Moving around less is not just a "grown-up" problem; children are not moving much either. A recent study, for example, found that fewer than 13 percent of students walk to school. That was partly because the schools were built on large sites at the edge of communities, beyond walking distance for most students.[427]

But, studies also show, even when schools are within walking distance, many school districts *prohibit* the children from walking to school because of safety and litigation concerns. With many communities lacking sidewalks for safe walking, who can blame them?[428]

You get the picture?

Everywhere, it seems, there are obstacles to human exertion. And so, even those of us who try to sweat a little often find it difficult to expend the energy. The net result is a push toward collective positive energy balance and obesity (Figure 12.3).

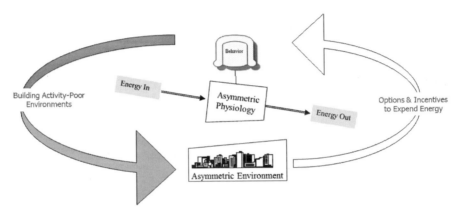

Figure 12.3: We changed our environment, and our
environment is changing us

That's precisely what researchers at San Diego State University's Active Living Program found when they conducted a large-scale field study to assess the impact of neighborhood characteristics on energy expenditure and the prevalence of obesity.

[The] researchers . . . surveyed residents in two neighborhoods in San Diego—one that was close to retail and public buildings and one that was far removed from those amenities. They found that people in the more 'walkable' neighborhood took one to two more walking or biking trips a week on average than those in the less walkable neighborhood. . . . [And, surprise, surprise] . . . about

60% of the respondents in the less walkable neighborhood reported being overweight, compared with 35% in the walkable area.[429]

Play and Leisure

When it comes to our leisure-time activities, the U.S. can rightfully claim to be the "passive-entertainment" capital of the world[430]—an "honor" we'd rather do without.

In the twenty-first century electronic frontier, Americans are spending most of their leisure time watching television, using computers and video games, e-mailing others, searching the Internet, and enjoying other electronic activities— all highly sedentary activities that require nothing more active than sitting for extended periods and pressing keys on a keyboard.[431]

Data from the *American's Use of Time Study* show that as the obesity epidemic was picking speed in the 1980s, people were spending six times more time watching television than they did exercising or doing sports (close to four hours a day, every day).[432] Hardly anyone believes this to be just a coincidence. The typical American child now spends more time watching television than doing any other activity except sleeping.[433] The sad statistic for an educator like myself is that "[by] the time American children finish high school, they have spent nearly twice as many hours in front of the television set as in the classroom."[434]

Television has been present in virtually every household in the United States for some time, but what is new (and of concern to some) is the dramatic increase in recent years of the percentage of households with two or more television sets. In the 1960s, for example, ". . . only 12% of US households had more than one television set, by 2000, 76% of US households had more than one television set (and more than half of those, or 41% of all households, had three or more sets)."[435] Many of those extra sets are going into children's bedrooms—along with computers and video game consoles. In many homes, children's bedrooms are changing into little media arcades. A recent survey of children in grades three through 12 found that a record 68 percent have TVs in their rooms.[436] "Even the nation's youngest children are watching a great deal of television. About one quarter of American children between the ages of two and five have a TV in their room."[437]

A large number of studies (forty at last count) have demonstrated that TV time correlates with weight gain, and that the relationship is linear: the more hours of television viewed per day, the higher the prevalence of obesity.[438,439] Television watching contributes to weight gain, research findings suggest, through at least three mechanisms. First, television viewing is a completely sedentary activity that requires the viewer to expend very little energy—not much more, in fact, than the energy expended sleeping (the so-called resting/maintenance metabolic energy rate).[440] Second, television watching is often associated with increased food consumption. That's because people like to snack while watching TV.[441] Worse still, what they eat is often the high-calorie, high-fat foods heavily peddled in TV commercials.[442] And third, television-viewing replaces the time that could be spent on more vigorous physical activities. As Professor Norman Nie, Director the Stanford Institute for the Quantitative Study of Society, likes to say, "[T]ime is hydraulic," meaning that time spent watching television is time taken away from other activities.[443] Quite simply, people who spend more time watching TV tend to exercise less.[444,445]

A recent report by the U.S. Surgeon General revealed that only 22 percent of adults in America engage in physical activity on a regular basis, while more than half of the adult population maintains an almost totally sedentary lifestyle. These are troubling findings, but not particularly surprising given the American public's persistent addiction to their "electronic tube."[446]

With the advent of the Internet and the availability of broadband connections, television viewing among children has started to decline (some estimate by as much as 18 percent from the 1980s levels). Unfortunately, the drop in television viewing is not translating into more calories burned. On the contrary, kids are more than compensating for TV viewing time by using computers for surfing the Internet, instant messaging, or playing video games. It is estimated that the average child aged 2-18 now spends close to 40 hours per week on these sedentary visual activities—the equivalent of an adult's full-time job.[447]

As after-school outdoor activities yield to computers, video games and television, parents are not fighting back; rather, many are embracing these modern-day baby sitters.[448] Beyond the usual concerns about time, money, and the need to rest, new parental concern about crime is a big reason why. Dangerous neighborhoods—or the perception of danger— discourage parents from permitting children to play outdoors.[449] Findings from a survey study suggest that close to 50 percent of all U.S. adults believe that their neighborhoods are unsafe. Such concerns only reinforce parents' inclinations to "bubble-wrap" their children, limiting childhood activity and spontaneous play. "What the surveyed parents were implying was utterly reasonable: TV-viewing may be bad, but at least my kid won't get shot, molested, kidnapped, or jumped into a gang while doing it."[450]

The Burden is Cumulative

As a result of all of this, the energy expenditure for most adults in the U.S. now rarely climbs above the *resting level*. That's a level of energy expenditure that is equivalent to between 60 and 100 watts—the energy output of an ordinary light bulb!

No wonder. U.S. citizens have all too appropriately been termed *homo sedentarius*.[451]

It is a sad irony. The environment we toiled so hard to create for ourselves, while a very comfortable one, is one that our body's energy-regulating systems were never designed for. And an increasing number of people are paying the price.[452]

It has often been said that humans are very adaptable creatures, and that is true. We can live in the Tibetan highlands, in the rain forests of Brazil, in Europe during the Ice Age, or in the Sahara Desert today. And because of this adaptability, we have always assumed that we could create almost any sort of environment for ourselves and thrive. We have also assumed that whatever environment we created for ourselves would likely be an improvement over what we had. Today, however, we have run smack into the limits of our adaptability. We have created for ourselves an environment—a food-rich, activity-poor environment—that makes a great number of us sick, and so far there has proved to be little we can do about it.

But let's not forget that, unlike a virus-induced disease, the structures underlying our obesifying environment are increasingly of our own making.[453] And, so, we can "unmake" them. However, before we can change those structures, we need to see them. For, as Peter Senge argues eloquently in *The Fifth Discipline*, "(societal) structures of which we are unaware hold us prisoner."

Exposing the societal structures underlying our obesifying environment is what I aimed to do in this chapter.

CHAPTER 13

Turning Vicious to Virtuous:
Leveraging Feedback Thinking

In previous chapters we learned how reinforcing processes (positive feedback) create a snowballing dynamic that can escalate a problem or trend—like fast food consumption—into troublesome levels (Figure 13.1 below). With each trip around the loop, the phenomenon strengthens as the process feeds on itself, and given enough time an initial small "event" can morph into a major development. That's essentially how all epidemic scenarios arise: Infectious diseases spread in a population as those who become infectious come into contact with and pass the disease to those who are susceptible, increasing the infectious population still further. As more and more people fall ill and become infectious, the number they infect starts to grow more quickly as the process feeds on itself. The same reinforcing dynamic applies to a wide variety of "social contagion" phenomena—situations in which people imitate the behavior, beliefs, or purchases of others. The key difference being that in social contagion the pathogen is an idea rather than a biological agent.

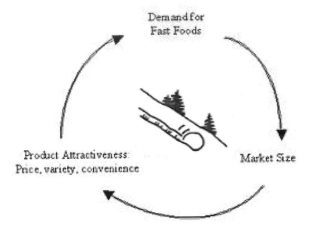

Figure 13.1: Reinforcing loop of fast food consumption

While often invoked to describe escalating problems (and characterized as vicious cycles), it is important to emphasize that positive/reinforcing feedback loops are neither inherently bad nor inherently good. Deviation-amplifying processes can be both vicious as well as virtuous (i.e., in which they reinforce in a *desired* direction). Even more interestingly… the *same* feedback process can work both for and against us. Understanding this is terribly important because it has broader implications. It's what allows us to harness the mighty power of positive/reinforcing feedback to our benefit… have it work for us rather than against us.

To demonstrate this important insight I'll use a simple example. Consider the familiar banking situation of depositing money into a savings account at, say, a ten-percent interest rate compounded annually. The feedback structure of this system is shown below.

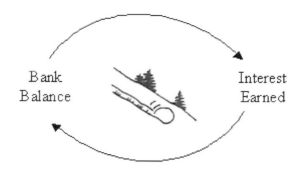

Figure 13.2: Bank savings account grows by compounding interest

Walk around the loop to convince yourself that this is a positive feedback loop—where a change made (such as a deposit that increases the account) is reinforced as we go around the loop. A larger bank balance leads to higher interest earned which when posted to the account boosts the bank balance still further which increases the interest earned even more and so on. It is a self-reinforcing process that builds on itself causing your money to grow. That's, of course, a good thing.

Now, consider what happens if the "Bank Balance" turns negative—as when taking out a bank loan at a ten-percent annual interest rate. The same compounding (reinforcing) process now works in reverse, driving the negative account more and more into the red (Figure 13.3).

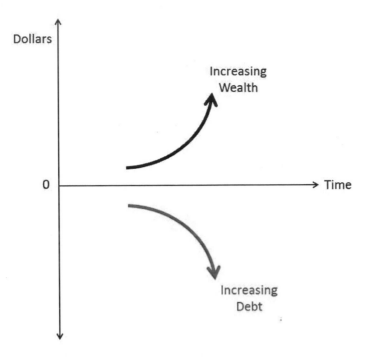

Figure 13.3: What goes up can come down

This important insight into self-reinforcing (or positive) feedback—that it can work both viciously and virtuously—is an attribute that can be exploited. At both the personal level as well as in public policy we can sometimes have an "opening" to turn a reinforcing process around so that it works for us not against us. Let's consider two examples.

My first example relates to personal behavior about exercise. In much the same way as monetary exercise in the example above (Figure 13.3), the reinforcing effect of our choices about physical exercise can work for us or against us. Let's first see how it can work against us. As already mentioned, excessive television-viewing by children replaces time spent in sports, increases food consumption and promotes weight gain.[454] The gain in weight could then push the child further in the direction of decreased activity in a self-reinforcing "vicious" spiral. It is sad, but true that "among the most prevalent consequences of obesity in children is the discrimination that overweight children suffer at the hands of their peers."[455] Chubby children, for example, are less likely to be invited to participate in sports that leaner kids play. Exclusion can also be self-inflicted, as when an obese child chooses to voluntarily withdraw because of embarrassment. Either way, lack of participation robs overweight children of the opportunity to practice and acquire skills; this accentuates their sporting ineptitude and leads to further exclusion.

Biologic mechanisms also add to this spiral of increased inactivity (Figure 13.4). As inactivity leads to weight gain, the added pounds often precipitate phys-iologic complications that hamper the child's capacity to exercise (complications such as cardiovascular problems, respiratory difficulties, and osteoarthritis).[456]

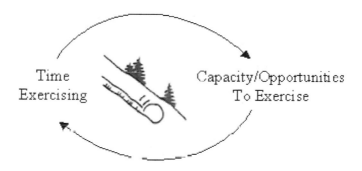

Figure 13.4: Reinforcing processes in exercising

But, as with the bank balance example, this very cycle can also virtuously work for us. Consider what happens if, in a different environment, we create the opportunity and incentives for the child to choose physical exercise—opting to play soccer, for example, over watching TV. With play and practice, skill invari-ably improves. This, of course, can be tremendously self-rewarding, as it makes the child feel better about himself or herself and about exercising. In addition, becoming a more-skilled player is apt to open up even more opportunities for future participation.

Exercising also causes physiologic capacity to expand—e.g., increasing lung, heart, and muscle capacity.[457] As the physiological capacity of the body for physical exertion expands, children can play longer and harder, leading to further expansion of physiological capacity. This, in fact, is the reinforcing mechanism that underlies the notion of "progressive training" in many sports—an intuitive "feedback" inspired practice strategy that has had a long history, beginning with the Greek Olympian Milo.

> Milo of Crotona . . . lived in Greece in the sixth century B.C. Milo is said to have hoisted a baby bull on his shoulders every day to improve his strength. As the bull grew heavier with age, Milo's strength also grew. Since that time, progressive resistance training has been an important part of the training programs of many athletes, from football players and track and field participants to swimmers and figure skaters.[458]

Bottom line: it is important to reiterate that positive feedback loops are neither inherently bad nor inherently good. Deviation-amplifying processes, in other words, can be virtuous (i.e., in which they reinforce in a desired direction) as well as vicious. It is terribly important to understand this broader implication. Learning to recognize and harness the power of positive feedback to one's advantage is a powerful conceptual leverage one gains from applying the systems approach.

Harnessing the Power of Positive Feedback in Public Policy

First rule of holes is that when you're in one, stop digging.

Will Rogers

Learning to turn feedback around—and have it work for us instead of against us—extends beyond the personal to the societal. Which is even more exciting since the dividends of a vicious-to-virtuous shift would, in this case, reach far beyond an individual's gain to the society at large. Case in point: revisiting the convenience food ←→ obesity dynamic.

Consider what happens if more and more of us shift to healthier, low-fat, higher-fiber food choices. The impact of our collective healthy behavior would ultimately re-shape our collective environment. Indeed, it *is* starting to reshape it. For example, as Americans have begun demanding healthier, low-fat, higher-fiber food choices, more and more eating establishments have changed their food preparation procedures and menus accordingly. As competition intensifies among stores, restaurants, vending- machine companies, and fast-food chains, a wider variety of choices will become available at lower costs, further encouraging healthy eating.[459] And a new *virtuous* cycle will be born.

This reinforcing process is depicted as the right-hand-side positive feed-back loop in Figure 13.5: higher demand for low-fat, high-fiber foods → market size for such foods expands → prices drop, and variety and availability increase → spurring more demand, and so on. What is of great import here is that this virtuous process will simultaneously weaken the existing vicious loop to the left. That's because, as the caricature suggests, the two loops are *coupled* via market forces—a consumer shift to low-fat, high-fiber foods will (at least in part) mean a shift away from fast foods. The two loops are, in effect, "arm wrestling" for market share.

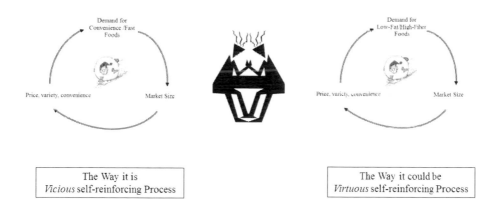

The Way it is
Vicious self-reinforcing Process

The Way it could be
Virtuous self-reinforcing Process

Figure 13.5: The *vicious* and the *virtuous*

What will that do to the fast-food loop? The potential benefit from this can be enormous since any significant shift away from fast food could potentially transform the fast food loop trajectory from accelerated growth to accelerated decline. Why? Recall that in any positive feedback process, a change in one direction sets in motion reinforcing pressures that produce further change in the *same* direction, reinforcing and amplifying the original change. The direction of change is, therefore, significant—as when, adding a deposit to an initially empty, but interest-earning, bank account will grow the account exponentially over time. If, on the other hand, the original change is downward—as when taking a loan—the value of the account will keep going south—getting more and more negative over time as the interest we owe accumulates.

This suggests that public policy can have an important role to play here, and that is to create supportive environments that make healthy choices the easy choices. In the above scenario, for example, government policy could help grease the shift to healthy eating by offering tax breaks that effectively subsidize healthy foods.[460] Similarly, public policy can do a lot of good on the energy-expenditure side by promoting active lifestyles (to help our exercising friend in the earlier example). For example, public policy levers (such as building codes and regulations, zoning ordinances, and priorities for capital investment) may be deployed so that when communities are built or rebuilt, they would be designed "to the human scale, instead of to the automotive scale."[461]

CHAPTER 14

Understanding is *NOT* Enough

Our primary focus in Part II has been on *understanding* the system of energy and weight regulation: how system variables—such as energy consumed and expended in the human system of energy and weight regulation—are related; how they influence one another; and how they are influenced by our external environment. And, along the way, this has helped us clear up some of the public's muddled thinking about human energy and weight regulation (such as the asymmetry in energy regulation and the limitations of the 3,500 kcal per pound rule).

We learned about the distinctions between stocks and flows and the feedback processes that connect them. And what emerged is a picture of human energy regulation that is far more complex and far more dynamic than the linear open-loop mental model most people have: viewing body weight as simply dependent on the balance between two voluntarily controlled processes—energy intake (EI) and energy expenditure (EE) (top of Figure 14.1). Because of the importance of ensuring sufficient energy for survival and reproduction, the human body has evolved a multitude of *involuntary* homeostatic mechanisms to regulate *both* sides of the energy balance equation (bottom of Figure 14.1). We also learned that the two limbs of energy balance are not independent, but, instead, are physiologically linked, interacting in complex ways and often compensating for each other in the face of interventions.

Not like so...

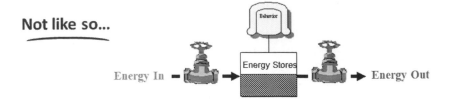

More like so...

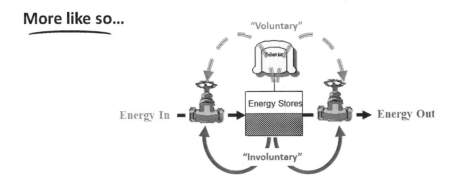

Figure 14.1: Models of human energy regulation

We learned to "mentally squint" to see that feedback processes underlie many of the interactions and mutual independences in human energy regulation. Though not directly visible to us, these circular mechanisms and their interactions account for much of what happens to our bodies over the long term—and what makes attempts at appetite control and weight reduction so difficult. As we closed the loops, the system became more realistic—but also much more complex. That is why, as is often stated, the very same traits that make the feedback-systems approach attractive—putting things back together and recognizing the feedback interactions among them—also make it somewhat slippery and elusive.[462] Or, it *used* to.

Understanding is Key—but Far from Sufficient

While understanding is an important and necessary step toward better management of any complex system it is not enough. As was argued earlier, effective control of a dynamic system—whether it is the energy regulation of our bodies or the energy regulation of an atomic reactor—requires two essential skills: understanding and prediction. Without a capability to predict the system's behavior, perfect understanding is of little practical utility. The ability to infer system behavior is essential if we are to know how our actions will influence the system. In personal health regulation, effective prediction of treatment outcomes (e.g., pounds lost from a diet) is critically important because people's expectations about treatment and the degree to which they are met (or not met) can affect their self-efficacy and long-term commitment. The two skills—understanding and prediction—are needed *together*.

Most people tend to assume that if a system's structure is well understood, predicting its behavior is a piece of cake. Unfortunately this isn't the case. When dealing with (complex feedback) systems, reliable prediction is surprisingly challenging.

Remember the SIGOS experiment? In Chapter 7, we got a taste of such prediction challenges when we tried to discern the dynamic impact of overeating during the holiday season, only to discover it was not all that obvious. The difficulty people have with this exercise is no aberration. Experiments on human subjects in many problem domains indicate that while we are generally capable of grasping the unique characteristics of systems in our environment (physical, economic, social), we are usually unable to accurately determine the dynamic behavior implied by these relationships—"running" our mental models. The human mind, experiments consistently show, is an excellent recorder of decisions, reasons, motivations, and structural relationships, but it is not that good (nor reliable) at inferring the behavioral implications of interactions over time.[463] Being able to "run" our mental model of some system or situation, in other words, is a much more difficult task for us.

And it is important to emphasize that the SIGOS exercise presented a highly simplified model of human energy regulation. For example, by holding the level of daily energy expenditure (the outflow) constant, the subjects did not have to contend and account for the homeostatic feedback adaptations from the body's energy reserves to energy expenditure. (In reality, as we learned, there are feedback effects from energy reserves to energy expenditure.)

Obviously, adding the full complement of interconnected feedback processes would make the prediction task significantly more challenging intellectually. Having to grapple with a larger number of interacting variables/processes obliges us to attend to a great many features simultaneously. So much will be going on, and some of the things that are going on will cause still other things to go on—making sense of it all quickly becomes a daunting task.[464]

To demonstrate this more concretely, let's consider the predictive task of someone designing a diet intervention. Again, as I did in Chapter 9, I'll start with the public's widely shared feedback-less (and incorrect) mental model of energy regulation, expose its limitations, and then complete it.

Figure 14.2 depicts the widely shared (feedback-less) mental model of human energy regulation in which body weight is viewed as being dependent on the balance between energy intake (EI) and energy expenditure (EE), both of which are assumed to be under voluntary control. Unbalancing the energy balance equation in the direction of weight loss would, therefore, appear to be straightforward. Using the ubiquitous 3500 kcal per pound rule it goes something like this: one pound of body fat contains 3,500 kcal. To shed a requisite number of pounds in a week or a month, one would simply use this magic number to figure out the size of the daily deficit in energy balance required. Stick with it and observe your weight drop proportionally and steadily.

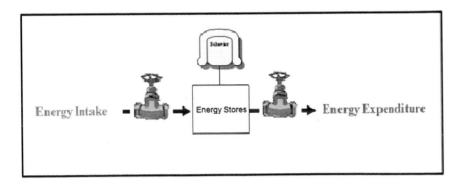

Figure 14.2 Feedback-less mental model of human energy regulation

It is an overly simplistic (and unrealistic) linear model that has proven to be too optimistic.

Missing in action: the body's homeostatic adaptations to energy deprivation that lead to changes in both the resting metabolic rate as well as the energy cost of physical activity. It is these feedback adaptations that are the reason why weight lost tends to decline with time—even if the prescribed diet *is* maintained—and why people tend to lose less weight than they expect... much less.

So let us introduce the missing feedback effects into the picture, and do it one feedback loop at a time. In Figure 14.3, loop (1) captures the metabolic adaptations to altered body weight.

- A negative energy balance à a loss in body weight → a drop in maintenance energy requirements (MEE) (as a result of the loss in lean tissue and the concomitant increase in metabolic efficiency) → a drop in daily energy expenditure → shrinking of the deficit in energy balance. (Note: this is one of three feedback effects discussed in Chapter 11, but is enough to make the point here.)

In a dieting scenario, this feedback adaptation is one of the body's wired-in defenses against tissue loss. It dampens the rate of weight loss on the diet and causes it to decline with time (even if the prescribed diet *is* maintained) until a new equilibrium body weight is reached—typically, at a level that's significantly above that expected from the 3500 kcal per pound calculation.

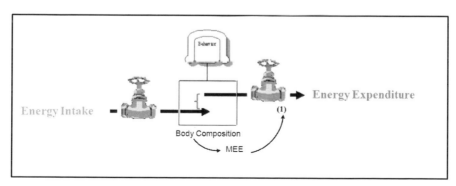

Figure 14.3: Adding Loop 1

This involuntary homeostatic adaptation complicates the predictive task for the dieter. In the figure below, the left graph shows how a simplistic linear system (without feedback compensation) would be straightforward to predict—where a pound of weight is lost at the fixed energy cost of 3,500 calories. As depicted by the graph on the right, weight loss is far more complex in reality. Not only is the weight loss achieved by food restriction invariably less than that expected from the simplistic linear model, but the feedback effects between the body's energy reserves and energy expenditure mean that the *same* energy deficit can lead to multiple possible scenarios. The outcome will depend on the many differences that exist among individual dieters, such as a dieter's initial body composition. (That's because the composition of tissue lost during weight reduction depends on the initial body fat content of the subject—obese people, for example, lose more weight as fat than do lean people, who lose more lean tissue. Because fat and non-fat tissue types have different energy densities, such differences translate into differences in the amount of weight lost.)

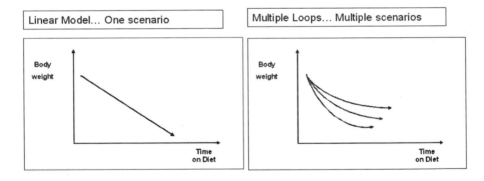

Figure 14.4: Involuntary homeostatic adaptation complicates
the predictive task

But there is more.

The outcome of a weight-loss intervention also depends on the way in which the energy deficit is engineered (e.g., dieting versus exercising). For example, if the energy deficit were to be induced by an exercise treatment rather than by dieting, such an intervention would induce an increase in muscle (FFM), which could, in turn, elevate rather than lower maintenance energy requirements (MEE). Such an adaptive response—shown in the figure below as loop 2—adds an additional wrinkle to the prediction task. In this case, the new loop counteracts rather than reinforces loop 1. By conserving and even increasing the FFM (the principal metabolically active component of total body mass), exercise partially blunts the drop in maintenance energy expenditure that accompanies diet-based weight loss.[465]

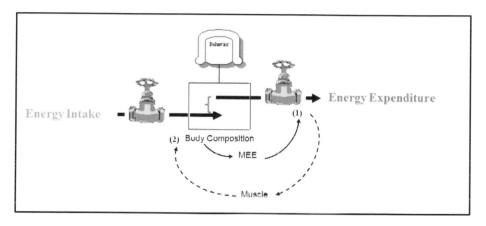

Figure 14.5: Adding Loop 2

From this simple example, we can see that even though the behavior of simple stock-flow systems may be reasonably obvious in isolation (with training in simple stock-flow rules), assessing the net *effect* of multi-loop interactions is not. Indeed, many experimental studies have shown that the ability to trace the behavior generated by a system of only two feedback loops (such as we have here) can already tax human intuition.[466]

Luckily, that's precisely where computer modeling can help. Unlike a mental model, a computer simulator can reliably and efficiently trace through time the implications of a messy maze of feedback interactions. And it can do so without stumbling over phraseology, cognitive bias, or gaps in intuition.[467] Computer modeling is thus well suited to fill the gap where human judgment is most suspect. Furthermore, by tailoring model parameters, computer-based tools can be easily customized to fit the precise specifications of different individuals.

Smarter Than We Think

A key takeaway message from the book is this: We cannot—should not—rely on intuition alone in managing our bodies. With its many interrelated subsystems and processes (some counteracting, some reinforcing) the human body is simply too complex to effectively manage by human intuition alone. The long time delays and the many interactions between many of the body's parts and processes mean that interventions (diets) can have a multitude of consequences, some obvious and many not so obvious, some immediate and others distant in time and space (as when intervention in one part of the body affects another). To effectively manage a system as complex as the human body requires a tool of "bookkeeping" that is more reliable (and efficient) than human intuition. The digital computer—a complementary innovation to systems thinking—provides us with that tool.

This is not to suggest that we all need to become model builders. What I am suggesting is that we all need to become capable model *consumers*. As computers continue to proliferate, more and more of the decisions we make—whether at home, in business, or in government—will involve the results of models. Indeed, the ability to understand and evaluate computer models is fast becoming a prerequisite for the scientist, policymaker, and citizen alike.[468]

People have already learned to rely on computer-based tools to handle the complexities of managing their portfolios and preparing their taxes. They have yet to appreciate the need to leverage computer technology to support their health-related decision-making. Yet, health is precisely the setting where complexities are the most problematic and where the stakes are the highest. Indeed, nowhere is the application of computer-based decision support more essential, and potentially more rewarding, than in managing our health and wellbeing.

In Part III, I argue for and aim to demonstrate (in layman terms) the feasibility and value of a new generation of user-friendly tools that support interaction and customization for personal health and wellness management. As we'll discuss in Part III, the quantity and quality of weight loss, whether by dieting or exercising, depends on a host of personal factors that can vary significantly among individuals. Because computer-based tools can be highly "personalized," they can provide specific, tailored solutions to dieters' individual needs.[469] We're in a position to do this because of the great advances in systems sciences, medicine, and computer technology over the last few decades. It is a truly new development.

Using today's affordable desktop computers, we can now construct silicon surrogates of human physiology that faithfully mimic our bodies' functions. And with increasingly user-friendly software, ordinary people, for the first time in history, have access to and can learn to make effective use of models of systems as complex as their own bodies. Using these tools, dieters and/or patients, like engineers, can have a laboratory in which to conduct thought experiments to test myriad sorts of what-if scenarios and learn quickly and cost-effectively answers that would seldom be obtainable through raw intuition.

PART III

"GIVE US THE TOOLS AND WE'LL FINISH THE JOB"

Churchill

CHAPTER 15

Prevention:
The Best Buy... that's still a Hard Sell

Our focus in Part III will shift to treatment and the expanding repertoire of personal information technologies that are empowering ordinary people with the data and decision-making tools they need to better manage their bodies and personal health. I will discuss several of the new generation tools that can be easily (and economically) tailored to each person's health needs, lifestyle (why they like to do or do not do) and even style of thinking.

But before getting into that, it would be remiss to overlook the important role of prevention.

The Case for Prevention

Since the onset of the obesity epidemic, treatment of the problem has received overwhelmingly more attention than prevention has. While this remains true today, interest in obesity prevention is slowly starting to attract increasing attention. That's probably because of the growing realization that it may be easier, less expensive, and more effective—at both the personal and public-policy levels—to change behavior so as to prevent weight gain, or to reverse small gains, than to treat obesity after it has fully developed.

Obesity prevention may also be the best way to address the health problems it causes. That's because many of the adverse health consequences associated with obesity result from the cumulative stress of excess weight over a long period of time and some may not fully reversible by weight loss.[470] When it comes to our body, "there are real limits to what can be done to reverse the damage caused by a lifetime of unhealthy living."[471]

As MIT's John Sterman so deliciously puts it: "You can't unscramble an egg (the second law of Thermodynamics)."[472] Analogously, many processes in health and disease can be hard, if not impossible, to reverse. For example:

- A former smoker's risk of lung cancer is always higher than that of someone who has never smoked. "The best [one] can be is a former smoker—[one] can't be a 'never smoker.'"[473]
- There is no way to repair the cancer-causing DNA damage that excessive exposure to the sun's ultraviolet radiation causes to our skin.[474]
- Repeated exposure to loud noise—from the earbuds on an iPod, a lawn mower or a Metallica concert—can destroy the inner ear's delicate sound-conducting hair cells. Dead hair cells don't grow back, and once hearing is lost, it is gone forever.[475]

Obesity is no exception. Gaining an *excessive* amount of weight can induce a wide array of irreversible anatomic and physiological changes that can lead to irreparable damage. For example, obesity is often associated with damage to blood vessels and the buildup of plaque in the arteries that no amount of exercise or diet change will reverse.[476] But perhaps the one irreversibility that annoys most dieters more than any other is the one associated with the proliferation of the body's fat cells when excessive weight is gained. As was explained earlier, the increased number of fat cells that accompanies excessive weight gain act to defend the elevation in body weight complicating the task of weight loss.

The implications of all this for obesity treatment and prevention are clear: It may be easier, less expensive, and more effective to intervene before fat-cell proliferation sets in, excessive weight is gained, and the irreversible damage incurred.

But while (in theory) there is little argument over the wisdom of prevention, to-date obesity prevention has proven to be a challenge and a hard sell in practice. Why?

Passive Strategies that often Work… Don't

In public health policy, there has been a long tradition (and a logic) to rely on so-called "passive" structural solutions—interventions that aim to "… achieve objectives for the good of society and the people in it without requiring individual behavior change and perhaps even without the knowledge of the individual."[477] Such "passive" solutions—ones that achieve change even without the knowledge of the individual—can, and have, worked for public health interventions in sanitation, air pollution, and food fortification. But they won't for obesity. Unlike the air we passively breath, personal energy balance is a product of deliberate lifestyle choices about how much and what to eat, and how much energy to expend and how. Although human body weight regulation does reflect the outcome of interactions between people and their environment (social, economic, physical), it is human *decision making* (e.g., about food, work and play) that modulates such interactions.[478]

Thus, eliminating environmental barriers to healthy food choices and active lifestyles will not, by themselves, *prevent* obesity in the population. Let's face it: no matter how many sidewalks or healthy food buffets we build, it will not be enough if people aren't motivated to use them.[479]

Fill-their-Buckets Strategies not the Answer Either

If not "passive" prevention, then the key to changing behavior and reversing obesity, many health officials and scientists continue to believe, is *information*— offering the public more and better information about healthy food choices, for example. Most (non-passive) government programs aimed at weight control are indeed based on this principle. This viewpoint relates to what the philosopher Karl Popper used to call "the bucket theory of the mind." When minds are seen as containers, and public understanding is viewed as a function of how much scientific facts are known, the focus naturally is on how much scientific facts public minds contain.[480]

That bucket-filling strategy hasn't worked either.

An irony of America's obesity epidemic is that despite the broad publicity about the obesity problem and the government's energetic mass-media-type educational campaigns (such as distributing copies of the *Dietary Guidelines for*

Americans or the many similar educational materials on nutrition and exercise), the number of obese is not declining.[481,482]

Although the notion that knowledge shapes behavior seems reasonable, the evidence to-date suggests that merely providing information does not necessarily change health behavior.[483,484] That's because, as was argued in more detail in Chapter 4, what information we choose to tune to and how we interpret that information is very much influenced by our mental models—those deeply ingrained assumptions and generalizations that form our worldview of ourselves, others, and the things with which we interact. It is through our mental models, for example, that we define the risks we face and how we act in response—e.g., whether or not to engage in prevention efforts.

While it is comforting to think (and most of us believe) that our mental models are relatively accurate and relatively objective, unfortunately that's rarely the case. Rather than serve as neutral-objective lenses, these "cognitive goggles" are more like filters"—a great deal of research on human cognition has revealed—that often get clogged and biased by our needs and emotions. In problems like obesity or drug addiction, which many believe to be caused by behavior or personality, people for example may feel they are invulnerable because they would like to believe that they do not have the weakness of character that allows it to develop in them. This mindset becomes a significant impediment to prevention. If people convince themselves that they are invulnerable to becoming obese, then they are unlikely to heed the prevention message and take the appropriate measures to reduce their risk of gaining weight. The "it won't happen to me" mindset gets in the way: Why protect yourself from an event that will not occur?

Stuffing people's "mental buckets" with nutritional guidelines and food pyramid images would not change that mindset. It's why my goal in this book (and in Part II) is *not* bucket-filling (*knowledge accretion*) but rather, *knowledge restructuring*—challenging people's deeply ingrained assumptions about health risk and wellbeing.

In that vein, our enhanced understanding of the human energy and weight regulation system—understanding the distinctions between its stocks and flows and recognizing the important homeostatic/feedback processes that connect them—helps us debunk common misconceptions about human energy regulation and about risk that, heretofore, have been shackling prevention efforts.

Let's review the *big three*.

Trust in "Wisdom of Body" to Maintain a Normal Weight?

A major driver of the obesity epidemic is that we are not only still prisoners to physiology that was vital to the survival of our Pleistocene-era ancestors; we are still prisoners to hunter-gatherer instincts that no longer apply. Most of us continue to instinctively regulate feeding behavior in accordance with the body's biological drives: to eat to our physiological limits when food is readily available and selectively focus on foods high in energy density. The practice is rooted in the mistaken belief that it is O.K. (normal?) to defer to the *body's wisdom* and "cruise" on automatic feeding control.

Given that obesity was not a common health problem throughout most of human history, it is understandable that people instinctively believe that the body's regulatory system strives to maintain stability at some "natural" body weight, defending against both weight loss and weight gain. Such a system would be symmetrical, defending against both positive and negative energy balances that threaten to cause weight change.

But, as we saw, our weight regulation system is *asymmetric*—not only in energy input (favoring over-consumption over under-consumption) but also in energy expenditure and storage. The built-in *asymmetries* in human energy regulation mean that in our current food-rich activity-poor environment "we may be all at risk." And is why it is absolutely imperative people quit cruising on "automatic feeding control" and learn to assert cognitive control in regulating feeding and energy expenditure. Not for a week, or a month, but for a lifetime.

Stock-And-Flow Misconceptions

We learned in Part II that even though stock-and-flow structures characterize many types of real-life systems and everyday tasks (such as managing a checking account or a company's inventory), people, nevertheless, have misconceptions about how such systems behave. Specifically, we learned about *two* types of mis-calculations from the SIGOS study. First, a widespread tendency to match the tra-jectory of body weight (the stock) to the food intake pattern (its inflow rate). (As I noted, the application of this intuitive but incorrect pattern-matching heuristic reflects misunderstandings about basic principles of stock accumulation and rates of change—a difficulty called the stock–flow failure.)

A second (related) book-keeping miscalculation is failure by both lay and health care professionals to appreciate that the process of stock accumulation (such as accumulation of water in a tub or fat in the human body) provides sys-tems with *inertia* and *memory*. Recall, in the SIGOS scenario (as in reality), body weight does not drop to its original level after the Christmas feast—even as food intake drops back to its pre-holiday level. Instead, body weight remains "stuck" at its maximum level! And that is because, at any point in time, the amount of energy in the body (the stock) reflects the *cumulative* effect of the net inflows over out-flows, not merely what is going on at that very moment. Stocks are, therefore, said to provide systems with inertia because they provide a "memory" of all past events in the system—in this case, a memory of the fact that in the preceding two months the inflow equaled or exceeded the outflow (and was never below it).

Failure to recognize the stock-related inertia/memory in personal health may be a "self-serving" (and I suspect pervasive) misconception that have poten-tially serious implications in managing health risks. It may explain, for example, why many people fail (post the holidays) to adequately compensate for their over-eating during the holidays. As we saw in the SIGOS study, most people—and even healthcare professionals—incorrectly assume that reverting to their pre-holiday food intake levels would return their weight to its pre-holiday level. But, as we learned, to lose the extra pounds that were gained, food intake after the holidays must decrease to a level <u>below</u> the (normal) pre-holiday level—i.e., to a level that's below the system's outflow rate.

The inevitable result of such miscalculation: the amount of weight gained during the holidays does not come off. A lack of immediate adverse consequences often mean that a gradual (and cumulative) increase in body weight is not recog-nized (or is dismissed) until people are trapped years later in an unhealthy life-style, which can ultimately result in chronic obesity.[485]

The lesson from the SIGOS study is quite clear: If people misunderstand the basics of stock-flow dynamics that underlie human energy regulation, they are likely to draw erroneous inferences about their risk. And this, in turn, could seriously undermine obesity prevention and management efforts.

Individual-Centric Fixation

Recent surveys continue to find that large segments of the population still view obesity as a "private" matter—a result of individual moral failure—rather than as a function of a changing relationship between our physiology and the environment. This mindset constitutes yet another significant impediment to prevention. If people do not understand that a fundamental driver of our obesity problem is the mismatch between our hunter-gatherer physiology and our modern (food-rich activity poor) environment—an environment surrounding all of us in modern societies—they will underestimate the risk (to themselves and their kids). And fail to heed the prevention message. Again, the "it won't happen to me" mindset (because I do not have *moral weakness*) gets in the way.

This individual-centered and simplistic view of obesity's cause is not limited to lay people. Health care professionals, it is disturbing to note, are among the chief offenders. Numerous studies of health care providers—dieticians, physicians, family doctors—reveal that many believe excess body weight simply reflects a lack of willpower, poor self-concept, and deep-seated psychological problems.[486] It is a disturbing finding because it has destructive results—including prejudice and discrimination toward the very patients for whom these professionals care.[487,488] In one study, for example, a survey of physicians found that they viewed their obese patients as weak-willed and even ugly and awkward. In another study, as many as 78 percent of the obese patients surveyed reported that they had "always, or usually, been treated disrespectfully by the medical profession because of (their) weight."[489]

While all this is certainly disturbing it is not at all surprising.

When explaining the causes of some behavior it is common for people to rely on factors that are most salient to them. The most salient thing in health behavior is the "actor" who is behaving. People are in the foreground; most everything else—situational and environmental factors—is in the background. Hence the cognitive "trap." This over-readiness to explain behavior not only in obesity, but for many dysfunctional behaviors in terms of dispositional factors such as abilities, traits, and motives is so widespread and universal that it [has been] called "the fundamental attribution error."[490]

It is a tendency that often leads to attributions that are patently wrong. An example of "Biblical" proportion is the one committed by the sailors in the Book of Jonah. When a storm hit their ship, they didn't ascribe it to a seasonal weather pattern. They attributed the cause to Jonah's sinfulness, and responded by throwing him overboard.[491] In the case of health issues, the *fundamental attribution error* creates the bias of over-attributing behavior to factors such as personal control and grossly underweighting the influence of situational factors such as the modern socioeconomic environment in which we now live.

Don't get me wrong. There is no dispute that individual-level characteristics are important determinants of individual health and that our understanding of individual-level risk factors—from choices and behaviors to unique genetic makeup—has contributed greatly (and continues to contribute) to our understanding of health in populations. (A good example is the identification of lifestyle and biological factors associated with cardiovascular disease.) However, it has also become increasingly clear that a fixation on such determinants has limited our ability to examine and understand the full spectrum of disease causation.[492,493]

In the case of obesity, one consequence of the individual-centered fixation is the field's preoccupation with why individuals are obese and how to help them, rather than with why society is obese and how to help it.[494] And this may explain why, given the current environment, approaches to weight loss that focus on the individual have been tougher than expected.[495]

One of the goals of this book is to provide a different conception of the obesity problem. In contrast to the classical, individual-centered worldview, in Part II, I advocated a systems-inspired worldview that adopts a much broader biopsychosocial perspective—one that looks beyond individuals' characteristics and behaviors for answers, to the symphony of behavior-biology-environment interactions. Moving beyond individual-based explanations does not imply denying personal responsibility or genetics, but rather involves viewing personal characteristics within their social contexts and examining the tight interrelations between the social and the biologic at multiple levels

The reason for doing this is scientific: Our object of study demands it.[496]

A 2014 study by the highly respected McKinsey Global Institute titled *Overcoming obesity: An initial economic analysis* argues that obesity is a highly complex system of countless interacting variables. And that any single intervention is likely to have only a small impact at the *aggregate level*. Only a comprehensive, systemic program of multiple interventions—what they describe as a holistic approach by the public, private, and third sectors—is likely to be effective.

I agree. In order to help the overweight lose weight we'll need to also address why society is overweight and how to help it. As I argue in upcoming chapters (and in even more detail in *Thinking in Circles about Obesity*), the challenge—and opportunity—at both the personal level (in our homes) and at the public policy level is to create supportive environments for making the healthy choices the easy choices for people (Figure 15.1).

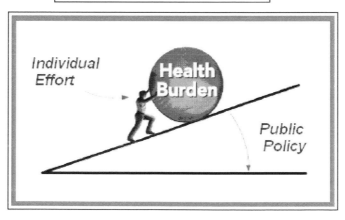

(Adopted from [Milstein, 2008])

Figure 15.1

CHAPTER 16

Treatment:
First and Foremost... Clear those Misconceptions

In the previous chapter our focus was on misconceptions that relate to the perception and management of risk—highlighting three that I argued are hampering prevention efforts. Here we shift our focus to misconceptions that may stymie treatment.

Because overweight is a complex multifactorial health issue—involving genetics, physiology, and biochemistry, as well as environmental, psychosocial, and cultural factors—it is among the most misunderstood of human conditions, and perhaps as a result among the most exploited.[497] In *The Hungry Gene*, Ellen Shell argued eloquently that "the obese and overweight are ... pummeled with bad advice and patronized with marketing campaigns. Only the marketing has paid off."

We are of course partly to blame. It is human nature, if not the American way, to seek the quick simple fix even when we look at complex problem in the face. All too often we adhere to simplified solutions, as though to a raft, because they are easier to understand... are more convenient. But beware: while quick simplistic solutions may be convenient, comfortable, and comforting—they are not necessarily effective.

Case in point: the *energy balance equation*—the staple energy calculus by which dieters (as well as many health care professionals) continue to use to explain weight gain and predict treatment outcomes.

The Energy Balance Equation... Reigning Intellectual Paradigm or Straitjacket?

Most over-weight individuals attempting to lose weight do so themselves using instructions gleaned from a book or a weight loss website. It's probably because both the nature of the problem as well as its solution seem (on the surface) to be transparent enough.

Indeed, weight-loss instructions—whether in newspaper articles, self-help books or on the Internet—cannot be simpler: a weekly caloric deficit of 3,500 calories—induced through either dieting or exercise—induces a loss of one pound in a week, ten pounds in ten weeks.

It is a simplistic one-size-fits-all calculus (also known as the 3500 kcal per pound rule) that overlooks the important fact that the overweight are *not* a homogeneous lot and that response to weight-loss intervention can vary greatly between people (Figure 16.1). It also erroneously treats energy as though it were a single currency—assumes a 1,000 kcal caloric deficit has the same effect irrespective of how it is induced through dieting (energy input) or exercising (energy expenditure). In reality, how an energy deficit is created *does* matter... and energy is *not* a single currency.

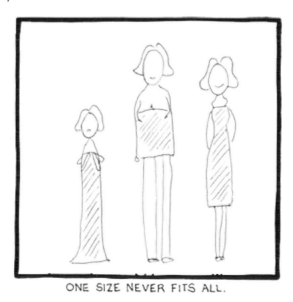

ONE SIZE NEVER FITS ALL.

Figure 16.1

As was briefly noted in Chapter 10, the simplistic energy balance equation is a crude linear approximation of what in reality is a complex non-linear system. It is also static, unbounded—and just plain wrong. For example, it takes weight-loss projections to absurd values—a negative energy balance of 1,000 calories per day would result in a loss of a whopping 100 pounds in a year!

The energy balance equation gets it wrong, in large part, because it ignores the dynamic physiological adaptations to altered body weight that lead to changes of both the resting metabolic rate as well as the energy cost of physical activity.[498] As was explained, when any significant weight is lost on a diet the loss is interpreted by the body as a deprivation "crisis" that needs to be contained. To restrain the rate of tissue depletion, the body compensates by slowing its metabolism. Additionally, as both fat and fat-free tissue is shed, the body's maintenance energy requirements drop, since there is simply less "stuff" to maintain. (These adaptations vary significantly among people, depending on initial body composition and how the caloric deficit is induced—diet or exercise.) The combined effect of these energy-conservation measures is to effectively shrink the diet's energy deficit, which in turn (and unfortunately for the dieter) dampens the rate of weight loss.

It is because of such involuntary adaptations that weight loss is almost never as straightforward as advertised. It is also why it is not linear but declines with time, even if the prescribed diet is maintained, and it is why people tend to lose less weight than they expect… much less.

Ignoring the body's energy-sparing mechanisms that aim to limit tissue loss during caloric deprivation may be easier to peddle, but will inevitably lead to spurious predictions of treatment outcomes. And that should be cause for real concern. Effective prediction of treatment outcomes is critically important in managing any aspect of personal health. In the case of weight management, effective prediction is key in setting attainable treatment goals. If one's goals are unrealistic, then failure is inevitable regardless of how hard one tries. Failure, in turn, saps motivation, undermines beliefs in self-efficacy, and drives people to give up.

Reliance on simplistic one-size-fits-all tools such as the 3500 kcal per pound rule—justifiable perhaps in the pre-Internet ages when we were computationally poor—is a bankrupt strategy that must be abandoned in favor of more intimate tools that actually fit. Today we can do better… we should do better.

People need personalized "intimate" tools that fit them and that reflect their lifestyle preferences (dieting versus exercise) not the one-size-fits-all calculation that is applied en masse. As consumers, we've come to expect customization in more and more of the things we buy, and now it needs to happen in health.

As we'll see in upcoming chapters, this is no wishful thinking. Thanks to the great advances in medicine and computational sciences over the last few decades, we *already* have the models that allow us to predict with great fidelity how the human body regulates its energy and mass. And the explosive growth of the Internet provides an economic and efficient infrastructure to deliver and *tailor* these new generation tools to large numbers of people.

But before we do that, we need to debunk a few other misconceptions that can—like speed bumps on the road—stymie our progress.

"Irrational Exuberance"

It is estimated that in any given year, 25% of US men and 43% of US women may attempt to lose weight. That's many millions of weight-loss seekers... and that's good news. The bad news: failure rates are exceedingly high.[499]

While most dieters undoubtedly understand that they would succeed more often if their weight-loss goals were more realistic (in terms of the ultimate target, the pace to achieve it or both), setting more realistic goals unfortunately rarely coincide with most dieters' personal agendas. Nor are they encouraged to. The diet industry thrives for two reasons—big promises and repeat customers. The big promises attract the customers in the first place, and the magnitude of the promises virtually guarantees that they cannot be fulfilled. It makes for a very attractive business model![500]

While in most human endeavors failure can be a powerful teacher, in the case of weight-loss, past failures, it appears, fail to engender better judgment. In one revealing study, a group of overweight women participating in a weight-loss program were asked to identify their desired weights before beginning the program. Their goal weights amounted to a whopping 32- percent reduction from their initial weight. That far exceeds the five to ten percent reduction commonly recommended by experts and reported by the most successful weight-loss studies.[501,502] Particularly interesting was the fact that the women's weight-loss targets were nearly three times the amount that they themselves had typically lost in previous efforts, suggesting that personal experience did not dampen their "irrational exuberance."

And the result? Close to a year later, the women's average weight loss was only halfway to their target weight, with almost half of the women failing to achieve even a weight loss that they stated before treatment they would consider "disappointing."[503]

Important to stress that the above study is no aberration nor is it a US-specific phenomenon. Other studies in the U.S. and elsewhere have similarly found that individuals engaging in weight loss programs have unrealistically ambitious goals and expectations. (Interestingly, the "dream" or ideal weight-loss targets consistently fall in the 25-35% range as in the above study.) And that weight-loss levels achieved in treatment mostly disappoint.[504,505]

The persistence of many dieters to shoot for unrealistic weight-loss targets—despite achieving only modest losses in previous efforts—may be rooted in the misconception that setting challenging goals can only be beneficial... and in any case is harmless. That a dieter who shoots for his/her dream body weight, no matter how unreasonable, would nevertheless always settle for what is achievable... ending up no worse than someone who had started with a more modest goal.

That's a misconception.

Research suggests that most dieters pay a hefty price for their irrational exuberance. The unrealistic goals that people set not only virtually guarantees that they cannot be fulfilled, but in fact contribute to relapse. (Not unlike a marathoner who sprints early, only to run out of gas later.) The systems thinking inspired insights we gained into the workings of the human energy regulatory system can help shed some light onto the reasons why.

The Idea of *Path Dependence*

The idea of *path dependence* is this: whether you're steering your body (body weight), or your car, taking one road towards some destination often precludes taking others and determines where you end up.[506] To explain how this applies to goal setting and weight-loss I will draw up some interesting parallels between "driving" our body weight to some target and driving a car to a destination and show how in both cases the aggressiveness of the goal often determines whether we make it or not.

In both cases, goal aggressiveness can be defined in terms of "velocity," which is the obvious metric in the case of driving a car. Analogously in the case of weight-loss: aiming to lose fifteen pounds in ten days (at a "velocity" of a pound and a half per day) is certainly more aggressive (ambitious) than aiming to lose the fifteen pounds in a month (at the slower clip of half a pound a day). Setting aggressive weight-loss targets means we aim to "drive" our body down at a high clip.

Why would velocity matter?

Consider the driving case first. Velocity matters because it affects fuel consumption—the higher the speed the higher the burn rate (and the lower the miles per gallon). For a given tank of fuel that, in turn, can determine whether we make it or not.

For a specific scenario consider driving from San Francisco to San Diego—approximately a 1,000 miles trip—on a 25 gallon tank of fuel. We'll assume our car is a modern fuel efficient car with mileage of 40 miles per gallon when travelling at 55 mph. This means if we drive at 55 mph we'll need a total of 25 gallons to complete the 1,000 mile trip (in approximately 18 hours).

Too long? We can drive faster. However, the car's gas mileage will decrease once it driven above 55 mph. For two main reasons. First, car engines do not run efficiently at all speeds. Instead they are optimized to run efficiently at speeds around 55-60 mph. Driving above this range pushes the engine's rpm, temperature, etc. outside the optimal operating parameters. In addition, driving faster increases air resistance. (The increase in air resistance is exponential, meaning wind resistance rises much more steeply between 60 and 70 mph than it does between 50 and 60.) The escalation in air resistance is highly significant since pushing the air around consumes as much as 40% of a car's energy at highway speeds.

So, assume (like most dieters) we are in a hurry... that instead of driving at 55 mph on our trip from San Francisco to San Diego we instead drive at 80 mph. At that speed (and a typical midsize car) we can expect our miles per gallon to drop from 40 to around 30 miles per gallon. This means our 25 gallon tank which would have been adequate for the trip would now only last for 750 miles.

So, does setting an unrealistic ("high velocity") weight-loss goal pose an analogous risk: the risk of running out of "self-regulatory gas? And falling shorter than what we otherwise would? Recent research findings on human self-control suggest the answer is yes.

In the remainder of this section we'll see that whether we're managing body weight or gasoline consumption, the goal we set not only defines the end to a purposeful task, but also shapes the means to achieving it. Therefore, establishing a different goal can and does create an altogether very different endeavor and, quite possibly, a very different outcome. And just as the tire-burning driver who drives fast but ends up short, dieters seeking lofty weight-loss goals are able to slash off large amounts of weight by eating very little or even starving themselves, but then run out of regulatory gas and end up, after a period of short-lived success, regaining the weight—often with "interest." For these dieters— and they are, by far, the majority—the end result leaves them worse off than if they had begun with and maintained a more modest weight-loss goal. And which often means increased frustration and other emotional costs.

Without execution, any goal—whether reasonable or unrealistic—is just wishful thinking. And the key to execution is self-control... so that's where we start.

The Self-Control Strength Model

Dieting to lose weight or trying to keep it off is an act of self-control— not unlike resisting temptations, persevering to finish tiring tasks, breaking bad habits, and the like.507 In all such cases, self-control is the process of the self-exerting control over the self. We do it any time we inhibit immediate desires or gratification, and when we prevent ourselves from carrying out a strong but undesirable impulse.508 In exercising self-control, people exert cognitive control over their bodies' impulses rather than allowing them to proceed automatically, often because they see that to be in their best long-term interest.

But, as we all know, self-control is no leisurely stroll in the park.

In dieting, as with many other cases of self-regulation, the feeling is that of an inner conflict going on in which we are pulled in opposite directions. That conflict is between the cognitive and the biologic, between one's desire to keep to a strict diet and the urge to "... gobble down that doughnut that someone has placed on the table in front of you."[509] In recent years, there has been significant advancement in our understanding of this tug-of-war like self-regulatory process and its role in weight management.

Roy F. Baumeister, Dianne Tice, Mark Muraven (all of Case Western Reserve University) together with Todd Heatherton (of Harvard), are accredited with formulating the strength model of human self-regulation.[510,511] The model helps explain self-control performance, not only statically, in terms of individual or task differences, but also dynamically, as a function of the persistence and duration of the self-control effort over time. Thanks primarily to their work, we now have a better understanding of the self-regulatory process—both its theoretical importance and great practical utility—and its role in the self-regulation of personal health.

There are three key ingredients to the model:

- The act of self-regulation is an effortful process that requires strength to override impulses and resist temptations.[512]

- The human capacity for self-regulation operates like a muscle, and is a limited resource that is partially con sumed in the process of self-control. Acts of self-control, thus, not only require the use of strength, but also reduce the amount of strength available for subsequent self-control efforts. And, as with muscular strength, after exertion self-control strength is replenished with rest.[513]

- Self-control performance is a product of an individual's level of self-control strength—availability of the resource—and his or her motivation to exert self-control—its mobilization.[514] That is, the motivation for exerting self-control and the level of self-control strength jointly determine the amount of self-control exerted.[515]

Self-control strength may, thus, be conceptualized as a reservoir or stock that is consumed and replenished over time with self-control exertion and rest respectively. Such a stock-and-flow structure (see Figure 16.2 below) would be identical to that of the plumbing analogy we used to portray the dynamics (the rise and fall) of energy reserves in the human body. That's not just a happy coincidence. It is a perfect example of the important systems thinking inspired insight that systems across diverse domains—whether biological, engineering, or social—share common patterns of structure. Sharing the same underlying structure means that for these very different types of systems—whether a physical stock like water or gasoline in a tank or a cognitive stock like self-control strength—the book-keeping arithmetic that governs the filling/depleting of the stock as a function of the filling/draining rates works the same way.

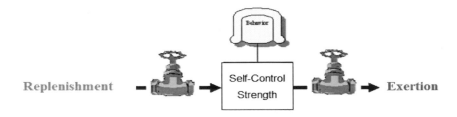

Figure 16.2: Stock-and-flow structure of self-control

The fundamental question we'll seek to answer is this: How best to use a limited resource (fuel in a tank or self-control strength) to reach some destination or goal. In the case of driving by car to some destination, this means resisting the temptation of driving too fast since this would increase the rate at which fuel will be burned, decreasing the maximum travel distance. In personal health regulation, this translates to learning to use our "tank" of self-control strength—which like a car's tank is not limitless—to sustain our dieting effort.

From personal experience we know that humans are capable of exerting modest levels of self-control and sustaining the effort day in and day out. This suggests that the amount of self-control needed for our daily social functioning—e.g., stopping at a stop sign or standing in line even when in a hurry, holding our tempers, and so forth—is low enough that normal periods of rest can compensate for the slow depletion rate. Indeed, many have proposed that the human capacity to inhibit antisocial impulses, and to do it continuously, has been a key facilitator—even a necessary condition—of civilized life.[516,517] But what about when we have to (or choose to) exert *more-than-modest* levels of self-control—such as not eating even when persistently hungry?

The conceptualization of self-control strength as a "reservoir" or stock that is consumed with self-control exertion and replenished with rest (Figure 16.2) can now be quite handy. It allows us to draw parallels between managing a physical and familiar resource (like car fuel) and a less tangible cognitive resource like self-control strength. This will help us better understand intricacies of managing this exhaustible cognitive resource, why aggressive goals can be counter-productive and ultimately learn how to maximize our self-regulatory performance.

The Very Simple Rules of Stock Replenishment and Depletion

For any stock-and-flow system, the fundamental laws of conservation and accumulation mean that the rates of flow into and out of the stock govern how the quantity of the stock varies over time. For example, if outflow is higher than the inflow, the stock level must gradually decrease and, given enough time, may completely deplete. If, and how fast, total depletion of a stock occurs will depend on the initial size of the stock and the magnitude of the imbalance between the inflow and outflow. The larger the *net* outflow and the smaller the stock's size, the faster total depletion occurs.

The key to regulating a stock's level is to manage the relative strengths of the stock's inflow and outflows rates. This is perhaps easier to see in a physical stock-and-flow system, such as that of water flowing into and draining out of a bathtub. Assume that while pouring water into the tub when filling it up in preparation for taking a bath, the drain accidentally is unplugged. Unplugging the tub's drain will not necessarily cause the tub to empty out. That will depend on whether the rate with which the water drains exceeds the rate of water flowing in—i.e., on whether the rate at which water is pouring in *compensates for* the rate at which it is being drained out.

The relative strengths of inflow-versus-outflow rates, together with the size of the stock, also explain why muscular exertion, in the case of physical activity, may or may not deplete muscular capacity and diminish physical performance. For a person living a sedentary lifestyle, for example, daily muscular exertion on daily activities such as eating, driving, working at the office, shopping, etc. is always modest, so that the drain on energy reserves (mostly the body's fat stores in this case) is slow enough that it is adequately compensated for by daily food intake. As a result, there would be no deterioration in the person's performance. Such a state of relative stability, however, changes whenever a person engages in *intense* physical activity. When a person exercises at high intensity, the muscles must draw on the body's limited glycogen reserves to obtain the glucose needed to fuel the work. The higher the intensity of physical activity, the higher the drain rate on the glycogen energy stock. Because glycogen reserves in the human body are relatively limited (a few hundred grams amounting to about 2,500 kcal), our glycogen stock can sustain only one to two hours of intense activity before it depletes.[518] Once depleted, the muscles fatigue, thus diminishing our capacity to continue exercising.

Intensity of exertion also matters when it comes to self-control. Just as humans are able to sustain low-intensity muscular exertion in daily activity, they also are capable of exerting modest levels of self-control and sustaining the effort day in and day out. This suggests that amount of self-control needed for our daily social functioning is low enough that normal periods of rest can compensate for the slow depletion rate.

The $ 64,000 question: what about when we exert *more-than-modest* levels of self-control to resist stronger impulses—not eating even when persistently hungry obviously requires more self-control than resisting the temptation to speed on the highway. Would normal rest be enough to compensate for the faster depletion rate? Or is the human capacity for self-regulation—like our glycogen stores—a limited resource that depletes relatively quickly by intense exertion?

It is an important question, and one that would require an empirical resolution. Specifically, the question to self-control researchers was whether the human capacity (stock) for self-control is large enough to sustain intense and, if necessary, extended exertion without deteriorating.

Over the last twenty years, a wide range of studies have been conducted to assess self-regulatory depletion in humans. These have included studies of human performance in controlled laboratory settings, as well as the study and analysis of people's autobiographical accounts of self-regulatory experiences—both successes and failures.[519]

Many of these studies were conducted at Case Western Reserve University by Professor Baumeister's group.[520] A major thrust of their laboratory experiments was to assess how human subjects perform when they engage *in a series* of self-regulatory tasks. In their typical experiment, the researchers had experimental subjects exert self-control on some initial task and then measured their self-control performance on a subsequent (often different) task.[521] The experiments covered a wide range of tasks, including traditional forms of self-control—such as tasks involving delayed gratification and resisting temptations (e.g., eating, smoking, and drinking alcohol)—as well as tasks involving persistence in performing frustrating mental exercises (they used anagrams) and endurance of physical discomfort (athletic or manual-labor tasks in which the subjects needed to continue performing despite physical fatigue).[522]

The results were consistent across the wide range of studies and generally point toward the following conclusions: The capacity for self-regulation, just like muscular strength, is a limited resource that is subject to temporary depletion.[523] And, as people exert self-control, subsequent self-control capability degrades over time.[524] As Baumeister et al succinctly put it, "To use it is to lose it, at least temporarily."[525]

The researchers expected and found individual differences in both innate capacity and the motivation to mobilize one's reserves. Some people, as we know from personal observation, are much better able than others to hold their tempers, maintain their diets, stop after a couple of drinks, save money, persevere at work, and so forth.[526] The experiments not only confirmed such impressions, but also empirically demonstrated that the differences in individuals' degrees of self-regulation can be substantial. In other words, when it comes to self-control strength, some people have a much larger stock than others.[527,528]

The researchers also found that *incentives* for exerting self-control influenced the degree of deterioration in self-regulatory performance. Participants who were given greater incentives to exert self-control exhibited less deterioration and performed better. In particular, tasks with more-attractive outcomes and in which success seemed more likely increased the subjects' motivation to exert self-control, and that, in turn, improved their performance. That is, self-control performance was found to be the product of individuals' motivation to exert self-control and their prior exertions of self-control.[529]

Furthermore, the experimental results also showed (again akin to muscular exertion) that self-regulation in one area reduced the subsequent ability to self-regulate in another area.[530] This suggests that different self-regulation tasks draw on the same resource. In other words, it appears that a single capacity underlies the wide variety of self-regulatory functions and that "any and all attempts at self-control require the use of this resource."[531] The good news is that the degradation in self-control strength is not permanent. With rest (sleep also plays a role, the research indicates), people normally regain their lost strength.

Since the same resource is used for many (or conceivably all) acts of self-control, we would hope that the resource were large. Apparently, it is not. The present findings reveal that (for most people) this resource is rather limited. Acts of self-regulation in many of these experiments were relatively brief, and yet performance was significantly degraded on subsequent tasks.[532]

A Challenge for the Self: How to Accomplish a Lot with a Little

An important and obvious implication of these results is that people's capacity for self-regulation needs to be managed like any other limited resource—and must not be squandered.[533]

It's a challenge not unlike managing one's energy consumption while driving a vehicle on a route where there are few refueling stops. Making the trip depends on not running out of fuel between fill-ups, and that will depend not only on how much fuel is in the tank, but also on how we manage our consumption of it (how fast we burn it). Driving at a high speed increases the rate at which fuel will be burned, decreasing the maximum travel distance. On the other hand, when driving at moderate speeds, fuel consumption would be higher, increasing our range.

To reiterate, performance in many self-control challenges is determined not only by the size of our tank (stock)—which we typically have little control over—but also, and equally importantly, on what we do with what we have—a choice we *do* control.

So, how effective are dieters at managing their limited capacity for self-regulation? On this, the record indicates some good news and a lot of bad news. First, the good news. Recent findings indicate that more and more people are getting better at losing weight, at achieving levels of weight loss that are substantial enough to improve their health, and at maintaining weight loss for extended periods. Of the estimated 55 million Americans who will go on a diet this year, we can expect that between five and 20 percent of them will succeed in losing five to ten percent of their initial body weight and will keep it off for at least a year.[534,535,536,537]

The bad news, however, is that long-term successful losers remain a minority. For the vast majority of those seeking to lose weight, long-term success remains elusive. The record continues to show that most dieters are trapped in a recurring cycle of weight loss and regain—"*Yo-Yo dieting* became the colloquial term for this process."[538] The cycle typically starts with lofty weight-loss goals, followed by short-lived losses, and invariably ending with a regain of the weight.[539,540]

Why?

The High Price of High-Velocity Dieting

When embarking on a diet, most overweight individuals tend to set weight-loss goals that reflect their image of what their ideal body weight should be—based, perhaps, on personal notions of aesthetics, advertised "poster" success stories, or standard height/weight charts read in a book or magazine article. The greater the weight-loss goal, the greater the caloric deficit must be. The greater the caloric deficit, the more acute the person's hunger and the greater the self-control needed to override the deprivation and sustain the diet—that is, the greater the drain rate on the dieter's self-control capacity (stock). That's obvious. But what is often less obvious is how much harder doing so becomes over time.

Dieters can seriously underestimate the escalation in hardship because, as psychologists have found, most people intuitively view causality in linear terms, expecting effect to be always proportional to cause. That is to say, we to tend to think that if A causes B to happen, then 2 As must cause 2 Bs to happen.

But the effort needed to accomplish a task often increases exponentially, not linearly, as the difficulty of the task increases (as when doubling to 2 As causing say 10 Bs to happen). This principle is not unique to dieting, but applies to many tasks, both cognitive and physical. Consider, for example, walking, which for most people is their major physical activity in a relatively sedentary lifestyle. "Escalating Energy Expenditure" (in Figure 16.3) portrays how energy expenditure escalates as walking speed increases, at speeds ranging from one to 10 km per hour (0.62 to 6.2 mph). It shows that as speed increases, energy expenditure rises, not in a linear fashion, but exponentially.

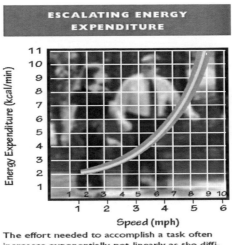

ESCALATING ENERGY EXPENDITURE

The effort needed to accomplish a task often increases exponentially, not linearly, as the difficulty of the task increases. For example, energy expenditure escalates as walking speed increases.

Figure 16.3

At low walking speeds—at the one- to two-mph pace of normal daily activities—the exertion of muscular energy (the stock's outflow rate) is modest enough that the drain on energy reserves can be adequately compensated for by daily rest and moderate food intake (the inflow rate). It is, in other words, a level of exertion that is sustainable, meaning that if we chose to, we could sustain this level of physical activity for extended periods of time without depleting our muscular energy stock. In fact, we can sustain it for extended periods, as in the case of Deborah De Williams. On Friday, October 15, 2004, De Williams arrived back in her hometown of Melbourne after having set a world record as the first woman to walk around Australia—traveling in a clockwise direction along Australia's National Highway 1. She completed the 9,715-mile walk in 343 days (which also earned her a second world record for the "longest walk in the shortest time"). Deborah De Williams had walked close to 30 miles per day, at a speed of two miles per hour. That translates into walking 15 hours a day, every day for almost a year—a sustained stock, if there ever was one.

As the speed versus energy-expenditure plot in Figure 16.3 shows, walking faster can quickly increase the rate of energy expenditure. Once our rate of energy expenditure exceeds our ability to replace it, our energy reserves deplete over time. How fast? Consider what it takes to run a marathon. The human energy "stock" (even the best stocked) is barely large enough to sustain a 26-mile marathon run (quite a bit less than De Williams' 9,715 miles.) And those resilient enough to endure that challenge will most certainly arrive with empty tanks (sidebar).

Not unlike walking or running, the self-regulatory effort in weight loss escalates not linearly, but exponentially, with the difficulty of the goal. Our body's weight set point seems to have a certain give to it, so that a person can stay a bit below it with relatively little effort. Larger weight losses, on the other hand, are difficult to tolerate. Fat-cell theory provides one possible mechanism for this physiological nonlinearity. As the enlarged fat cells of an overweight dieter (which had expanded in size during weight gain to accommodate excess energy storage) shrink back to their normal size (or slightly below it) subsequent to modest weight loss, the physiological signals to overeat and regain the weight are often easy to override. But if the weight-loss effort persists and the fat cells deplete to below-normal levels, the "volume" of the physiological message to the brain's appetite-control center increases, eventually becoming a scream: "EAT, EAT, EAT."

Experimental studies show just how "deafening" this message can become. In acute-dieting experiments, obese people who lost large amounts of weight developed a psychiatric syndrome called semi-starvation neurosis—a condition that had been noticed before in people of normal weight who had been starved. These poor experimental subjects continuously fantasized about food or about breaking their diet; they dreamed of food, and they became anxious and depressed (some even had thoughts of suicide).[541]

The bottom line: Higher goals deplete the stock faster than the speed of replenishment leading to failure. The harder we push, the harder the body pushes back. The greater the weight loss, the greater the sensation of hunger and the drive to eat and, hence, the greater the exertion of self-control and the higher the risk of self-control depletion.[542] As deprivation accumulates or escalates—many dieters would, no doubt, attest—hunger can end up consuming us, and food becomes the focal point of every thought and action.[543]

A Tale of Two Stocks

From the above we see that stock-and-flow structures underlie (at least) two important and distinct processes in the human psychobiological system for energy regulation. One is the body's energy stock, with food intake as its inflow rate and energy expenditure as its outflow rate. The other is this chapter's discussion of the stock of human self-control. And while up to this point these two sets of processes have been described separately, in reality they are not isolated phenomena. The two processes—one physiological the other behavioral—are interacting components in our multifaceted psychobiological system for feeding regulation. Indeed, it is the interaction (or *mis*-interaction) between these two stock-and-flow systems that gives rise to the dreaded weight cycling phenomenon that remains widespread among dieters.

The diagram "Dieting Regulation System" below integrates the two sets of stocks and flows: (1) the body's energy stock, with food intake as its inflow rate and energy expenditure as its outflow rate; and (2) the stock of human self-control, with its replenishment and exertion rates. And it depicts some of the interaction and cross-talk between the two processes. Specifically, you can see that in this integrated psychobiological system, "Self-Control Strength" (which we can designate as stock 1) affects adherence to the diet and, hence, the regulation of the food intake rate into stock 2, "Body Weight." This regulatory function is not a free lunch—constraining food intake to decrease and/or maintain the weight stock at a certain level requires effort which, in turn, consumes self-control strength. This means that the state of the body-weight stock (stock 2) regulates the exertion rate (the outflow rate) of the self-control stock. Stock 1 acts as a catalyst for the inflow rate to stock 2, and, likewise, stock 2 returns the favor and acts as a catalyst for the outflow from stock 1.

This two-stock feedback structure, while admittedly far too simplified to capture the full complexity and idiosyncrasies of human weight regulation, does in fact capture the essential elements that underlie human weight-cycling behavior. Let's see how.

Starting at the top stock-and-flow. From personal experience we know that humans are capable of exerting modest levels of self-control and sustaining the effort day in and day out. This suggests that if weight-loss goals are reasonable, the amount of self-control needed to restrict daily food intake would be modest enough that the drain on self-control energy reserves (stock 1) would be adequately compensated for by daily rest (the inflow rate). It is, in other words, a level of exertion that is sustainable, meaning that if we chose to, we could sustain this level of self-control for an extended period of time without depleting our self-control stock.

Unfortunately, as was noted, setting realistic goals rarely coincide with most dieters' personal agendas. When embarking on a diet, most overweight individuals tend to set weight-loss goals that reflect their image of what their ideal body weight should be—based, perhaps, on personal notions of aesthetics or advertised "poster" success stories. This comes at a price. The greater the weight-loss goal, the greater the caloric deficit must be. The greater the caloric deficit, the more acute the person's hunger and the greater the self-control needed to override the deprivation and sustain the diet—that is, the greater the drain rate on the dieter's self-control capacity (stock 1). And as we now understand (from the simple rules of stock replenishment and depletion), if our rate of self-control energy expenditure exceeds our ability to replace it, our self-control energy reserves will deplete over time. Which is what leads to the familiar weight-cycling pattern.

Dieters seeking lofty weight-loss goals are often able to slash off large amounts of weight by eating very little or even starving themselves. While initial progress towards a fanciful goal may be cause for celebration, unfortunately for most dieters it is usually a short lived one. As a dieter's futile persistence to shed an unrealistic amount of weight continues, the process ultimately depletes self-control strength. With a depleted stock 1, the dieter's grip on the feeding inflow "spigot" loosens. And with adherence to the diet progressively weakening as a result, body weight (stock 2) invariably refills. Regaining the pounds, in turn, saps motivation, undermines beliefs in self-efficacy, and drives people to give up. The result: after a period of short-lived success, the weight is regained and the effort abandoned—for a while. But weeks or months later—with rest and the replenishment of the self-control stock—the dieter may be back on the starting line for yet another trip on the weight-loss roller-coaster.

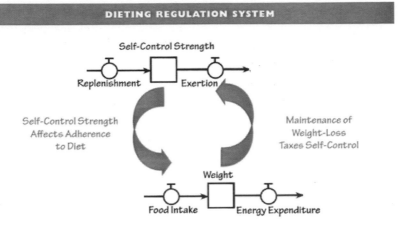

DIETING REGULATION SYSTEM

This diagram integrates two sets of stocks and flows in the human psychobiological system for feeding regulation: (1) the stock of human self-control, with its replenishment and exertion rates; and (2) the body's energy stock, with food intake as its inflow rate and energy expenditure as its outflow rate. The interaction between these two systems gives rise to the weight-cycling dynamic widespread among and dreaded by dieters.

Figure 16.4

Learning to Manage Our Stocks

Like any other limited (and exhaustible) resource, self-regulatory capacity needs to be managed and must not be squandered. But squandering it, not managing it, is what most dieters habitually do. The unrealistic goals that people set escalate self-regulatory exertion and over time induce regulatory depletion and ultimately relapse (not unlike a marathoner who sprints early, only to run out of gas later).

Thankfully, however, things may be changing.

A growing understanding of the biological factors that regulate body weight and of the cognitive difficulty of maintaining large weight losses is prompting a redefinition of the "successful" goals of obesity treatment. Slowly but surely, moderation is becoming the overriding theme in weight-loss efforts. A major impetus for this shift has been the growing evidence that moderate weight losses of only

10–15 percent of initial weight, even among substantially overweight individuals, are associated with a significant improvement in nearly all parameters of health—including blood pressure, heart morphology and functioning, lipid profile, glucose tolerance (among diabetics), sleep disorders, and respiratory functioning. And these findings are now prompting a growing number of federal agencies and health organizations to call for setting more realistic weight goals rather than striving for an "ideal" weight.

Moderating our weight-loss goals—for the target weight, the velocity to reach it or both— moderates self-control exertion and improves the prospects of reaching our goal on our "tank-full" of self-control energy. In Chapter 20, I will discuss additional strategies you can take to improve your chances of success even more. Rather than decrease caloric intake by decreasing portion sizes—which inevitably increases hunger and feelings of deprivation—we'll see how smarter food choices—specifically, about energy density—can help you stave hunger even as you cut on calories.

Ultimately, though, figuring out what works best for each individual—what weight-loss target to set, at what velocity and what meal size/composition is going to be an entirely individual matter that will require experimentation. And honest reflection. Unlike running out of gas when driving, when it comes to self-control, there's not going to be an obvious "fuel gauge" to signal depletion. Hence you need to watch yourself for subtle, easily misinterpreted signs. Baumeister offers some hints in his latest book:

> Do things seem to bother you more than they should? Has the volume somehow been turned up on your life so that things are felt more strongly than usual? Is it suddenly hard to make up your mind about even simple things? Are you more than usually reluctant to make a decision or exert yourself mentally or physically? If you notice such feelings, then reflect on the last few hours [meals?] and see if it seems likely that you have depleted your willpower.[544]

Allure of the Silver Bullet ... The Mother of all Misconceptions

Finally, we arrive at our third and final example misconception.

Americans, like those who live in the world's many other advanced economies, have grown accustomed to thinking in terms of "medical miracles" and "quick fixes" that require no effort on their part.[545] With a disease like obesity, whose causality is complex and for which treatment options are confusing, often difficult, and always prolonged, it is doubly tempting to succumb to the allure of the "silver bullet." And this may well prove to be our greatest challenge... overcoming the human tendency to seek the quick fix rather than take on the difficult demands of exercising control.

In the movies, the *silver bullet* is what slays the werewolf. It is worth noting that in the movies, Hollywood often makes the werewolf a rather innocent character transformed against his (or rarely, her) will into a monster. In many ways, that's not unlike how many of us think about our fat. (See sidebar.)

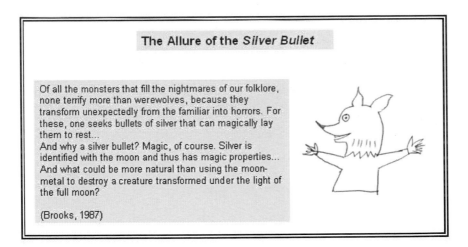

The Allure of the *Silver Bullet*

Of all the monsters that fill the nightmares of our folklore, none terrify more than werewolves, because they transform unexpectedly from the familiar into horrors. For these, one seeks bullets of silver that can magically lay them to rest...
And why a silver bullet? Magic, of course. Silver is identified with the moon and thus has magic properties... And what could be more natural than using the moon-metal to destroy a creature transformed under the light of the full moon?

(Brooks, 1987)

It has been estimated that the tens of millions of American men and women who are currently attempting to lose weight spend approximately $50 billion annually on their endeavors. Of concern is that a great chunk of the expense and the effort is wasted on ineffective, sometimes even harmful practices that extend beyond the merely unwise to the Faustian. The surging demand for a weight-loss "silver bullet" has fueled a rapid rise in fraudulent weight-loss schemes, including: slimming soaps that slough off fat in the shower; miracle pills that get rid of excess pounds without dieting or exercise; plastic earplugs that curb the appetite; and even a glittering ring called Fat-Be-Gone that, when slipped on a finger, trims hips, buttocks and thighs.[546] All dubious elixirs that divert us from the unsexy truth that basic nature and fundamental biology cannot be gamed, cheated, or transcended.[547]

But, as former HHS Secretary Tommy Thompson has bluntly declared, "There's not going to be a miracle weight-loss remedy or pill."[548]

Not only are there no silver bullets now in view, the multifactorial nature of obesity makes it unlikely that there will be any. As we look at the horizon, we see no single development—pharmacologic or surgical—that, by itself, promises a solution. The redundancy and complex compensatory interactions that characterize human energy regulation are very difficult to interrupt. When a drug blocks one mechanism or peptide, another goes into overdrive to compensate. Moreover, in the human body, energy maintenance does not operate as an isolated island, but is intertwined with other functions. The gut hormone Ghrelin is a good example of that. It not only makes us hungry, but it is also essential for tissue repair, bone strength, and muscle growth. Thus, intervening to suppress it may trigger a slew of unnerving (potentially life-threatening) consequences.[549]

Realism is not pessimism however.

While this dashes all hopes for a magical solution, our new (and enhanced) *understanding* of obesity—its multifactorial nature and biopsychosocial determinants—is, in fact, the beginning of real hope. Let's not forget that only a century ago, we took the first step toward managing infectious diseases, replacing demon theories and humours theories with germ theory. That very step, the beginning of hope, in itself dashed all hopes of magical solutions. It told us that progress would be made stepwise, with great effort.[550]

So, I believe, it is with obesity today.

CHAPTER 17

Work *with* your Body... Not *against* it:
A Judo Metaphor

Most of us approach weight loss as we would a boxing bout... seeking to knock-out a tough adversary, namely, our own body. The record to-date is pretty clear: Few can successfully land that "knockout punch." Perhaps we'd have a better shot if we approach the weight-loss "fight" differently... using the more efficient mindset of the Judo wrestler.

Judo's philosophy is to leverage an opponent's force to one's advantage, rather than confronting it directly. It has long been touted as the most efficient (and cleverest) strategy to defend oneself—if the attacker pushes, you pull and if the attacker pulls, you push.

The insights we gained from applying a systems perspective into the workings of human energy regulation suggest opportunities to deploy Judo-like tactics for weight-loss that work with (not against) our body's built-in drives. Below I present three examples. The three entry points relate to: 1) What we eat; 2) How we eat; and 3) Burning what we eat.

Judo-Inspired Move # 1: What we Eat

Hunger is the death knell of a weight-loss program.

Eric Westman, Director
Duke Lifestyle Medicine Clinic

Experimental studies demonstrate that (to our bodies) food volume has the overriding influence on satiety—that is, on what makes us feel full. Food bulk, not energy content, in other words, is the key to what makes our bodies say we've eaten enough. The meal's "bulk" that satisfies would, obviously, differ from person to person and generally tends not to be a specific number. Research by Dr. Brian Wansink and his group at Cornell University's Food and Brand Lab[551] suggests that each of us have a small weight range for the meals we eat—*a satiated or gratified margin*—where we feel content after a meal. If we eat much less, we know it. If we eat much more we also know it. But when we eat meals that fall within our *satiating margin* we are indifferent of small differences and feel fine. (In Chapter 20, I will discuss how to figure out your *satiating margin*.)

The implication (Judo move) from this is clear: If people are happy consuming a constant volume of food at a given meal, then less total energy would be automatically (and painlessly) consumed when one's diet is designed to be low in energy density.

Different types of foods can vary widely in the amount of calories they pack into a given weight or volume—in nutritional parlance, this is called the energy density (ED) of the food. It is generally presented as the number of calories per gram of food (kcal/g). Energy density values, which are influenced by the macronutrient composition and moisture content of foods and beverages, range from 0 kcal/g to 9 kcal/g. This is no typo. There is indeed something we consume a lot of that has zero calories… water. Because water increases food volume without adding calories, foods which have high water content, such as vegetables and fruit, cause us to feel full on fewer calories and lead to reduced energy intake. After water, fiber contributes the most to food volume for the fewest number of calories, supplying 1.5 to 2.5 calories per gram. In contrast, dietary fat is the most energy-dense macronutrient, containing more than twice as much energy per unit weight than either protein or carbohydrate (nine calories per gram for fat versus four calories per gram for both proteins and carbohydrates).

The "Judo move" to eat foods low in energy density is predicated on a basic fact: people like to eat. And if people are given the choice between eating more and eating less, they'll take more almost every time. Unlike diets that are based on deprivation, the Judo-inspired strategy doesn't try to fight this natural preference.

By selecting foods that are low in energy density you can eat more—probably more food than you're now eating—and weigh less because you would be ingesting fewer calories.

The good news, based on solid research, is that even modest changes in energy density can have a significant impact.

> For example, on a typical day an adult might consume 1200 g of food with an overall energy density of 1.8 kcal/g, giving an energy intake of 2160 kcal. If the average energy density of the diet was decreased by 0.1 kcal/g while the same weight of food was consumed, then the individual would ingest 2040 kcal. Thus, a relatively small change in the overall energy density of the diet would reduce energy intake by 120 kcal per day.[552]

That's a *significant* drop in daily caloric intake. Research studies suggest that most people tend to put on weight at the slow rate of two pounds a year.[553] This suggests that, in most of us, obesity results from a strikingly small—but sustained—energy imbalance. *This small energy differential is what prevention efforts need to target.* Hill et al.[554] estimate that, "most of the weight gain seen in the population could be eliminated by some combination of increasing energy expenditure and reducing energy intake by 100 kcal/day."

Hence the opportunity and reason for optimism: Energy density changes needed to close such a slight caloric gap are entirely achievable.

Several year-long clinical trials have indeed demonstrated that encouraging people to consume low-energy-dense foods does induce (long-term) weight loss. Without the deprivation! "Participants (even with) modest decreases in energy density increased the amount of food they consumed. Increasing the amount of food consumed while decreasing energy intake could contribute to the long-term acceptability of a low-energy-dense eating pattern since it could help to control hunger."[555]

As already suggested, several methods can be used to decrease the energy density of foods, including reducing the fat and sugar content and increasing the proportion of water-rich fruit and vegetables.[556] Increasing the water content of our diet should not be limited to the hard food stuffs however. When quenching one's thirst, better not to grab a soft drink and just drink water. Each 12-oz serving of a carbonated, sweetened soft drink provides about 150 kcal, all from sugars, and contains no other nutrients of significance.[557] These are not only "empty" calories… they are insidious empty calories. That's because, experimental results have shown, people do *not* compensate for whatever soft-drink calories they consume when they later sit down for regular meals. Sugar-sweetened drinks thus often represent energy added to, not displacing, other dietary intake and as a consequence invariably increase total energy consumption.[558]

"Plotting" to Incorporate Energy Density into your Dietary Plans

Incorporating energy density into your decision making about diet and nutrition helps you in two ways: in looking back and looking forward:

1) In looking back, would help you better understand what is happening e.g., why you are gaining weight or why you are hungry.

2) In looking forward, would help you design diet plans that work better for you e.g., eat more—probably more food than you're now eating—and decrease caloric intake.

In Chapter 20, I will discuss a simple tool you can use to *optimize* meal selection (when looking forward). In the remainder of this section, our focus is on task #1 above—employing energy density to help us look back. Specifically, I introduce a simple graphic tool to help you assess where you are on the energy density scale. I call it *Mi EDPP*—which stands for **Mi** **E**nergy **D**ensity **P**olar **P**lot.

To help you visualize where you are nutritionally and also chart promising directions for improvement, you need to incorporate energy density into your nutritional RADAR. However, knowing just the ratio of calories per gram (kcal/g) is not enough to assess or design a proper diet plan. You also need: total meal weight (that's the key to what makes you feel satisfied) and total calories (the key to weight loss/gain). *Mi EDPP* is a graphical tool that combines the three elements into one visual display.

Mi EDPP... Energy Density Polar Plot

A meal's weight is represented in *Mi EDPP* by the size of its circle—like for a pizza, the larger the circle the larger (heavier) the meal. Picture a set of concentric circles drawn on a page with the circles radiating out from a center (Figure 17.1). Each circle corresponds to meals with a certain weight (in grams), with the center being zero and the outer-most circle being perhaps 1,000 grams.

In the Figure below, I show two meals (pizzas). The inner smaller (red) circle is a 400 gram pizza and the outer larger (blue) circle is a 600 gram pizza. The weight of a pizza is, thus, indicated by the length of its circle's radius. The vertical axis provides a weight scale in grams (from 0 to 1,000 grams).

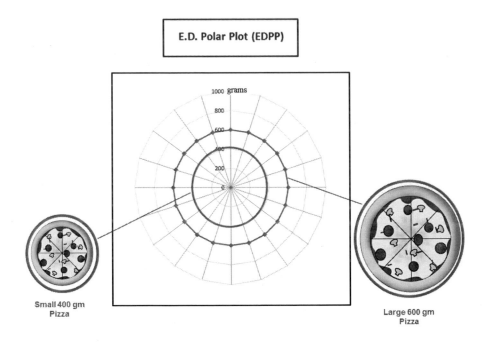

Figure 17.1 Two pizzas on Energy Density Polar Plot

Next, we add energy density to the picture.

In *Mi EDPP*, energy density is designated the same way that hours are on a clock. Starting at the top (the 12 o'clock position) is zero energy density and as we travel around the plot in a clockwise direction energy density increases. Figure 17.2 shows energy density values starting at zero at the top and increasing in increments of 0.25 kcal/g until we reach 4.75 kcal/g when we complete one rotation. Like hours on a clock, or cardinal directions on a compass, lines radiating out from the center of the circle are *constant* energy-density lines (e.g., the 1.5 kcal/g line highlighted by the arrow).

The term "polar" stems from the circular nature of the graph where all measurements start at one point—the pole or the origin. To represent a particular food item (or a meal), first move from the center (origin) of the plot vertically upwards a distance equal to its weight in grams (e.g., 600) and then rotating clockwise on that circle (shown as a dashed arc) until you reach the energy density radial (e.g., 1.5 kcal/g). Figure 17.2 shows a specific example (pizza). As indicated, the intersection of the energy density ray and the weight circle determines the food item's caloric content—in this case 600 grams X 1.5 kcal/g equals 900 calories—which is entered at the head of the arrow.

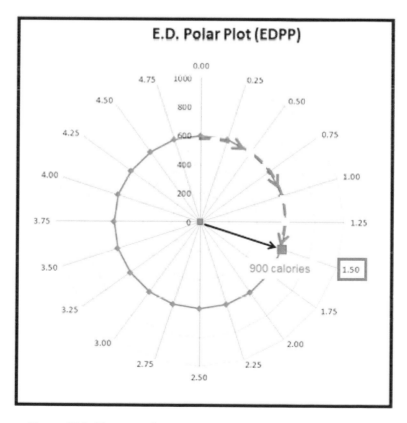

Figure 17.2: Three meal metrics: 600 grams, 1.5 kcal/gm, 900 kcal

We already saw that different pizzas come in different sizes and weights. But that does not tell the whole story. Depending on their macronutrient compositions, different pizzas can have very different energy densities. In the figure below (part "a"), I plot two pizzas with different sizes and energy densities. *Notice that they both have the same 900 calories.*

- The smaller pizza: 400 grams, 2.25 kcal/gm—say a pepperoni pizza
- The larger but lower energy density pizza: 600 grams, 1.5 kcal/gm—whole wheat crust, low-fat cheese

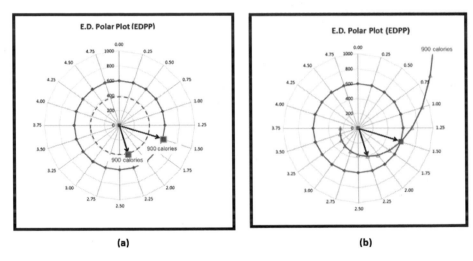

(a)	**(b)**

Figure 17.3: Different pizzas can have very different energy densities

On a *Mi EDPP*, concentric circles designate foods/meals that have the same weight while energy density radials designate foods with a particular energy density. We can also connect foods/meals with equal calories (such as the two 900 calorie pizzas in panel "b" above) to designate constant calorie foods (Figure 17.3). The resulting hook-shaped curve is called an iso-calorie curve (like the iso-bar curves you hear about in the weather forecast on your TV news) and represents foods with the same caloric level—in this case 900 calories:

- For the smaller pepperoni pizza: 400 grams x 2.25 kcal/g = 900 calories
- For the larger pizza: 600 grams x 1.5 calories/g = 900 calories.

(Note: On the book's website you will find a tool that you can use to automatically generate *your own **Mi EDPP**.*)

Now that we know how to construct the ***Mi EDPP***, let us use it.

The *Mi* in *Mi* EDPP

As I mentioned, ***Mi EDPP*** can help you better manage diet and nutrition in two ways: (1) When looking back to better diagnose what is happening e.g., why you are gaining weight or why you are hungry; and (2) looking forward to design diet plans that work better for you. In situations like personal health regulation where we often need to juggle multiple (somewhat conflicting) objectives, the trick in designing plans that work *better* for us is to try and improve whatever aspect or problem dimension we may be unhappy with (say hunger) *without* marring those aspects or decision-dimensions we are happy with (say caloric intake).

To demonstrate, let's use as an example a lunch scenario for a *hypothetical* you.

Let's assume that in order to maintain your current weight you have determined that you need to limit your lunch's caloric intake to 900 calories. (In Chapter 19, we will discuss how to determine a caloric target to lose/maintain weight.) The small 400-gram pizza (with an energy density of 2.25 kcal/g) meets that caloric target, and you decide to go for it. The problem: after eating it for lunch you remain hungry and wanting more.

The 400-gram pizza is, in other words, below *your satiating margin*. (In Chapter 20, I will discuss how to figure out your *satiating margin*.) Assume, for now, that what makes <u>you</u> happy (satiated) is a lunch weighing 600-1,000 grams. That's significantly more than the 400 gram pizza (and is why you are left hungry).

But don't despair. As promised a few pages ago, by choosing the right kinds of foods you can eat more—more food than you're now eating—without exceeding your caloric target. But how?

You can start by plotting your currently "hungry situation" on *Mi EDPP*— as point "X" in Figure 17.4. (Note that any meal that falls within the 600 gram circle—the lower threshold of *your* satiety margin—will *not* be satiating.) If we were to plot on this same figure all the food options available to you, the hundreds (even thousands) of possibilities would pretty much blanket the entire figure like a starry sky on a clear night. And the plethora of options could overwhelm (even frustrate) rather than help you. Here is where *Mi EDPP* can help. Like a road map, *Mi EDPP* helps zoom in on a narrow band of options that constitute what would be the "optimal" path for YOU. That's the path along the iso-caloric hook— depicted as a green arrow in Figure 17.4. Out of the myriad food options available, the meals that fall on this narrow band are the ones that will allow you to increase meal weight but hold calories constant at 900 kcal.

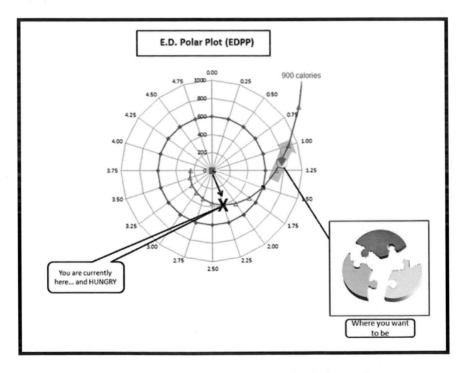

Figure 17.4: Current position… and path forward

All meal options along the iso-caloric hook between the 600 and 1,000 gram semicircles are meals that have the desirable *average* specs: all such meals are 900 calories and all are more satisfying than the current 400 gram meal. Their average energy densities will be in the 0.8 – 1.5 kcal/g range. Notice the qualifier *average* specs. That's because if you decide to design a new lunch with multiple food items and a target energy density of say 1 kcal/g (which is within the range), you are not limited to selecting individual food items with that value. You can mix and match food items—some with lower energy density others with higher—as long as the average energy density for the entire meal is 1 kcal/g. Below is one example showing a four-course lunch with components with varying energy densities that combine to produce a meal that's 900 grams, 900 calories and with an average energy density of 1 kcal/g.

Food Item	wt	calories	E.D.
Tomato soup (bowl)	500.0	350.0	0.7
Roasted chicken breast (3 oz.)	85.0	170.0	2.0
French bread (2 slices)	46.0	138.0	3.0
Red wine (4 fluid oz.)	100.3	85.0	0.8
Coffee (8 fluid oz.)	25.0	5.0	0.2
Chocolate pudding (half cup)	138.2	152.0	1.1
Totals	900	900	1.0

So, while **Mi EDPP's** iso-caloric band dramatically simplifies the search for acceptable meal options, the task of properly mixing and matching food items to compose meals with the proper weight, calories and energy density specs may still feel like a jigsaw puzzle (Figure 17.5). And if you consider that your "optimal" meal should not only satisfy the three parameters (weight, energy density, calories) but should also take into account YOUR personal preferences for certain foods (whether because of taste, availability, economics)... the challenge becomes even larger.

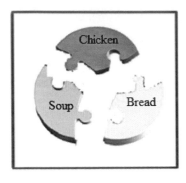 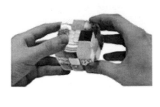

Figure 17.5: Composing a meal's jigsaw puzzle

In Chapter 20, I will provide you with a tool to help you tackle that challenge. Specifically, a tool that will help you:

1) Compose meals with different items (with different energy densities) that meet your average targets, and

2) Satisfy your personal food preferences (taste or economics).

Judo Inspired Move #2: How we eat

In addition to what we eat, how we eat may also contribute to weight gain.

The body's physiologic system that regulates appetite takes time to kick in—it takes time for the body to sense that food has reached the stomach and to shut off the feeling of hunger. After eating a full meal, the satiety signals that tell us we've had enough may not kick in for a full half-hour—that's long after the blistering eleven minutes the average customer spends eating a fast-food meal at McDonald's. Thus, by eating too fast—and we do—we tend to over-stuff ourselves before our brains have the chance to slow us down.

Perhaps, then, we should learn from the French… and eat slower… much slower.

The French also serve smaller portions. And that's also significant.

While we might like to believe that people will stop eating as soon as they feel full, it doesn't work that way. Human appetite, it turns out, is surprisingly elastic, a fact that makes excellent evolutionary sense. Since our survival over the eons of human existence was more acutely threatened by starvation than by obesity, it behooved our hunter-gatherer ancestors to feast whenever the opportunity presented itself, allowing them to build up reserves of fat against future famine.

Because our appetite is elastic (a physiologic trait) and because we have an apparent "compulsion" to finish whatever food is served us (a cultural trait), we do tend to eat more when served larger portions. Back in the 1950s, the psychologist Paul S. Siegel coined the phrase "the completion compulsion" to describe his observations that people are more likely to finish what's on their plate than to stop eating because they've consumed a given amount of food. (In Chapter 12, I discussed study findings by the nutritional researchers at Penn State University that demonstrated that the presence of larger portions *in themselves* "nudged" people toward eating more.)

Hence, a plea to parents everywhere: serve smaller food portions… and take your time enjoying it. And read on.

Among the many possible strategies for curbing the innate drive to overeat in a food-rich environment, my favorite is a mealtime adage that has long been practiced by "leaner cultures" most notably Japan (the birthplace of Judo): Not to eat until hungry, and when eating to stop before feeling stuffed.

> Nowadays we think it is normal and right to eat until you are full, but many cultures specifically advise stopping well before that point is reached. The Japanese have a saying—*hara hachi bu*—counseling people to stop eating when they are 80 percent full. The Ayurvedic tradition in India advises eating until you are 75 percent full; [and] the Chinese specify 70 percent. (Note the relatively narrow range specified in all this advice: somewhere between 70 and 80 percent of capacity. Take your pick.)… That is a completely different way of thinking about satiety. So: Ask yourself not, Am I full? But: Is my hunger gone? That moment will arrive several bites sooner.[559]

The calorie gap between the point where a Japanese says he is no longer hungry and where an American says he's full is not insignificant—enough to cut the 100 kcal/day that Hill et al. are advocating.[560]

Finally, parents can do a lot to control the external cues in their home environments that can induce overeating. As I explained in my discussion of *reward*, neuroimaging studies suggest that environmental cues of palatable foods do carry motivational power and can significantly induce overeating.[561,562] This applies to both the macro-food environment (e.g., food advertising) as well as the micro-environment in our homes.

The pioneering work of Dr. Brian Wansink (who is the former Executive Director of the USDA's Center for Nutrition Policy and Promotion) and his group at Cornell University's Food and Brand Lab has helped delineate the effects of micro-environmental cues on feeding behavior. In contrast to the overwhelming emphasis (and criticism) in the literature of the obesogenic nature of our macro-environment and the role of the food industry, Wansink has argued that it is the micro-environment of our homes—what he refers to as the obesogenic nature of our "kitchenscapes" and "tablescapes"—that people have real control over and where the leverage lies as a result. A fundamental insight of his work is that visual cues in our environment—such as the way a food is presented or served—can bias our eating habits and taste preferences in ways we are unaware of. The obvious implication: a large part of eating better and eating less involves controlling our tablescape (the placement and the type of dishes, silverware, drinking glasses, and serving bowls) so our tablescape don't control us.[563] Or to use Wansink's words: it involves "learning to become illusionists." A sampling of some simple changes people can make in their homes and to their daily "mindless" (over)eating patterns are:

- Moving from a 12-inch to a 10-inch dinner plate leads people to serve and eat 22% less.
- Using tall skinny glasses rather than short wide ones causes people (even Philly bartenders) to pour 28% less (because of visual illusions).
- Because the bigger the container the more we pour, repackaging jumbo food boxes (such as cereal boxes) into smaller Ziploc bags or Tupperware containers induces people to eat less.

Judo Inspired Move #3: Burning what we Eat

Because losing weight through physical activity is usually harder and often takes longer than losing weight through dieting, exercise is rarely incorporated in people's plans for losing and/or maintaining weight. That's a mistake.

When exercise is incorporated as part of a weight-loss strategy, it tends to protect against the loss in fat-free mass (FFM). By conserving and even increasing fat-free body mass (the principal metabolically active component of total body mass), exercise partially blunts the diet-induced depression in metabolic energy expenditure that typically accompanies diet-based weight loss. It is why exercise has been shown to be key to long-term success in weight loss.

> Muscle is [our] metabolic ace in the hole… Lean body mass is the main determinant of the rate at which you burn calories at rest, so-called resting metabolic rate… So you want to keep the proportion of muscle in your body high to facilitate weight loss maintenance.

> Increasing physical activity slows the loss of lean body mass from weight loss and partly reverses the decline in (MEE). If you lose weight by reducing intake, as much as 41 percent of the weight you lose will be lean body mass. But if you restrict calories *and* exercise, only 23 percent of your weight loss will be lean body mass.[564]

Besides its metabolic benefits, there's another reason why physical activity may be indispensable (in today's appetizing environment) to weight management: It provides a substitute *reward*!

> A substantial body of science tells us that exercise engages the same neural regions as other mood-enhancing rewards and produces similar chemical responses. Just as a smoker thinks he needs a cigarette, someone who exercises regularly comes to depend on the positive effects it produces.

Exercise can also reinforce an altered self-image. You begin to identify yourself as a healthy, athletic person, someone capable of making positive choices, and that in turn gives you an incentive to maintain control. New habits begin to substitute for old ones, making it easier to stay faithful to your eating plan.[565]

Perhaps the most convincing evidence on the value of integrating physical activity and dieting—instead of choosing one over the other—to achieve and maintain weight loss comes from the National Weight Control Registry. The NWCR is the largest prospective investigation of long-term successful weight loss maintenance—consisting of approximately 10,000 individuals who have, on average, maintained weight loss for more than five years, and counting.

> Almost 100 percent of them use a combination of diet and exercise to lose weight, and about 95 percent use a combination of diet and exercise to maintain their loss. . . . How much exercise? Far more than the recommended minimum. On average they expend 2,800 kcal (12 MJ) a week through physical activity, the equivalent of walking four miles a day every day, although most use a mixture of different activities, including walking, aerobic dancing, tennis, cycling, running and lifting weights.[566]

Interestingly, when it comes to exercise and weight loss, "less may be more"! Because, for many people, the most costly aspect of exercise is the time spent doing it, there is an understandable inclination to aim at exercising at the highest possible level of intensity in order to induce the largest possible energy deficit per exercise session—i.e., trading exercise intensity for exercise time. That can be counter-productive. In (Abdel-Hamid, 2003),[567] I report the results of a study I conducted to compare weight loss of low- versus high-intensity exercising. The results were surprising: exercising more intensely induced less weight-loss. Similar results were recently reported from a study conducted by researchers at the University of Copenhagen. In that study, male experimental subjects were randomly assigned to one of three groups. The first were the non-exercisers, who served as controls. A second group undertook daily moderate workouts (consisting of jogging, cycling or otherwise sweating for about 30 minutes, or until each man had burned 300 calories). And the third group tackled a more strenuous routine of almost hour long workouts, during which each man burned 600 calories. The Danish researchers found that exercise does seem to contribute to waist-tightening, provided that the amount of exercise is neither too little nor, more strikingly, too much. At the end of 13 weeks, the members of the control group weighed the same as they had at the start, and their body fat percentages were unchanged, which is hardly surprising. The men who had exercised the most, lost an average of five pounds each. On the other hand, the volunteers who'd worked out for only 30 minutes a day did considerably better, shedding about seven pounds each.[568]

The Upshot

Managing our health—and our bodies—is not unlike managing any complex system, a task that requires skill. Motivation alone is not enough. And using Judo-like tactics to work with (not against) our body's built-in drives when "fighting" to lose weight may help.

CHAPTER 18

The Second Flowering

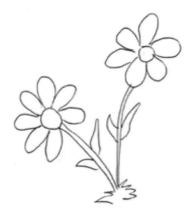

The human body, we now understand, is a conglomerate of interrelated and interdependent stock-flow-feedback processes, which together constitute a dynamic and highly complex system. Although not directly visible to us, these stock-flow-feedback processes are key governing mechanisms by which many of the body's systems are controlled and regulated. Human energy and weight regulation is no exception.

A key message of this book that is worth repeating here is that we cannot—should not—rely on intuition alone in managing such a complex system. With its many interrelated subsystems and processes (some counteracting, some reinforcing) the human body is simply too complex to effectively manage by human intuition alone. And too important. The long time delays and the many interactions between many of the body's parts and processes mean that interventions can have a multitude of consequences, some obvious and many not so obvious, some immediate and others distant in time and space (as when intervention in one part of the body affects another). To effectively manage a system as complex as our body, a reliable (and efficient) system of dynamic "bookkeeping" is required. The digital computer—a complementary innovation to systems thinking—provides that functionality.

Historians have called the late 19th century the time of the "great flowering of medicine." It was when, thanks to advances in microscopy and a deeper understanding of germs and human physiology, scientists were able to identify the cause of one infectious disease after another.[569] Today, we may be on the verge of a second flowering, one in which the growing entwinement of the healing and information sciences offers enormous possibilities for empowering people with the tools they need to more effectively manage their well-being with potentially far-reaching transformative consequences. It is a much welcomed progression in which health care becomes more personalized, more preventive, and ultimately more predictive.[570,571]

What may be driving this second flowering? And why *now*?

No one particular development, rather an array of innovations across the medical and information sciences have converged to make this happen. And that's not at all unusual. From history, we've learned that technology-based transformative leaps—whether in engineering, business, or medicine—rarely arise from the budding of a single great idea or invention. Rather, such advances typically arise from the synergetic convergence of diverse sets of "component technologies." Often, these components lay dormant for years—even decades—waiting for the right circumstances to be pulled into full development and widespread use. Taken separately, the components may offer only marginal improvement, but when they are integrated to form an "ensemble" of technologies, they induce revolutionary change. This innovation dynamic has recurred many times in diverse industries and for a wide variety of technologies. One of the classic examples is the aircraft industry of the 1930s, when five key technologies (radial air-cooled engines, retractable landing gear, monocoque bodies, wing flaps, and variable-pitch propellers) first converged and led to the development of the revolutionary DC-3 aircraft—often said to be the first airplane able to support itself both economically and aerodynamically.[572]

Similarly, the second flowering in medicine is being driven not by *one thing* but by the synergetic convergence of four *component technologies*. Together, they represent the growing entwinement of the healing and information sciences. They are: (1) Advances in molecular biology, which are expanding our understanding of the fundamental processes that underlie how the body works; (2) advances in systems and computational sciences, which are allowing us to mathematically model and predict these processes; (3) ubiquitous computing systems and intelligent sensors that can sense, analyze and communicate the physiologic data needed to personalize these models; and (4) the Internet, which provides the infrastructure to efficiently and economically deliver these capabilities to large numbers of people.

Tantalizingly Close

To-date, however, the enormous possibilities from the growing entwinement of the healing and information sciences remain just that... possibilities. Tantalizingly close-at-hand possibilities. And it is largely because so far we've done little more than use our fancy new technology to automate old ways of doing business or to deliver the (same) information faster and cheaper.

The Internet provides a good case in point. While millions of people now search the Net regularly for health and medical information— according to a Harris poll, more than 50 percent of U.S. adults do[573]—for most people, *e-health* is limited to using the Internet as a vast medical encyclopedia for health information (e.g., to search for information about things like diseases, diets, drugs and doctors).[574] And while many of the recently sprung health-oriented sites brandish sleek computerized tools for personal health management, most of these are electronic reincarnations of "legacy" tools from the pre-Internet era. For example, a de rigueur fixture on most sites is the ubiquitous caloric balance calculator. On the web, these energy calculators look faux "information-age," but in reality are just automated implementations of your mother's *energy balance equation*—the simplistic calculus that translates a 3,500 kcal energy deficit to a pound weight loss. Which, as I already noted, is not only a poor linear approximation of human energy regulation, but is also a "one-size-fits-all" model that ignores the fact that responses to weight-loss interventions vary a great deal among individuals (because of differences in body composition.)

The implicit assumption underlying such applications—and one that seems to be widely shared—is that mere automation of whatever manual processes people do "automatically" helps—somehow. But, of course, it doesn't, and it hasn't. The propensity to use our new capabilities in medical informatics to mechanize old ways of doing business (rather than enable new ones) is starkly reminiscent of the early uses of computer technology in business operations. In the 1960s and 70s, when many organizations started adopting information technology to streamline their operations, most took the path of least resistance—replacing their inefficient manual data-processing operations with automated ones. Archaic administrative processes were often left largely intact; they were simply performed faster and/or more efficiently with the fancy new technology. But making inherently inefficient processes faster didn't address their fundamental deficiencies. As a result, many of these early investments in information technology did not yield the anticipated dramatic improvements.[575]

In business, the breakthrough came when companies stopped thinking about using information technology to automate existing practices and started leveraging the power of the computer to re-engineer their business processes.

It is time to do the same in health.

The shift from "Industrial" to "Information-Age Health Care" will involve much more than just putting our current health education pamphlets up on the Web and/or using information technology to simply automate old ways of doing business. Instead of embedding outdated processes (like the ubiquitous BMI and caloric calculators) in silicon and software, we should *obliterate* them and start over.[576] It's time to use the technology not to automate existing processes but to enable new ones.

In the remaining chapters, I argue for and aim to demonstrate the feasibility and utility of a new generation of dynamic tools that support interaction and customization for personal health and wellness management. With the great advances in systems sciences, medicine, and computer technology over the last few decades, we're now in a position to put such tools into full development and widespread use. And thanks to the availability of affordable, high-quality computing capabilities and increasingly user-friendly software interfaces, ordinary people, for the first time in history, are today in a position to have access to and effectively deploy models of systems as complex as their own bodies. And the timing may be just right. The explosive growth of computer-based electronic communication is converging with another powerful trend: the increase in public initiative in taking greater responsibility for their well-being.

CHAPTER 19

Mi Model:
Devising Weight-Loss Strategies that Fit

Because of differences in body composition and/or how an energy deficit is induced (diet or exercise), responses to weight-loss interventions can vary a great deal among individuals. It is why reliance on simplistic one-size-fits-all tools—justifiable perhaps when we were computationally poor—is a bankrupt strategy that must be abandoned in favor of more intimate tools that actually fit. As consumers, we've come to expect customization in more and more of the things we buy, and now it needs to happen in health. Indeed, it is in our health and well-being where customization may return its greatest dividend.

Thanks to the great advances in medicine and computational sciences over the last few decades, we now have the models that allow us to predict with great fidelity how the human body regulates its energy and mass. And thanks to the availability of affordable, high-quality computing capabilities we can easily (and economically) tailor these tools to each person's "specs" and lifestyle preferences (what they prefer to do or not do). Perhaps best of all, increasingly user-friendly software interfaces are allowing us to "tame" these models so that lay people can use them comfortably and effectively. It is truly a new development. One that engenders enormous possibilities to empower ordinary people with the learning and decision-making tools they need to manage personal health and well-being.

Mi Model is such a tool. It is an "intimate" energy balance calculator… *and* much more. As a personal energy balance calculator, *Mi Model* can be customized to support individual planning and decision-making (e.g., determine the daily energy deficit that you require to lose "x" pounds in say three months). Unlike the energy balance equation (also known as the ubiquitous 3500 kcal per pound rule),

Mi Model does not treat energy as though it were a single currency. In *Mi Model*, how the energy deficit is induced (by dieting or exercising) partly determines what it should be. And that's not all what *Mi Model* can do. In contrast to the Energy Balance Equation which is... well an equation, *Mi Model* is a *simulation* model (of human physiology). Once "fitted," *Mi Model* can also serve as a personal learning environment (a virtual laboratory if you will) to explore and learn about the workings of one's body (for example, explore how different diet and exercise regimens affect not only body weight but also body composition).

A good metaphor for this type of model is the "flight simulator" game that many people are familiar with. These "games" are entertainment versions of the flight simulators that pilots train on when learning to fly a new aircraft. The flight simulator is a software-hardware environment that provides an artificially recreated cockpit environment within which the pilot can re-create the aircraft's controls, the environment in which to fly, and the aircraft's flight response. (At the heart of the simulator's software are replicating equations that mimic how aircraft fly, how they react to applications of flight controls and to external factors such as air speed, density, turbulence, etc.)

Flight simulators have now been acknowledged, and rightfully so, as a revolution in learning and training about flying. Rather than learning to fly an aircraft by listening to a lecture, the flight simulator aims to bring an experiential aspect to learning. On a flight simulator, pilots and prospective pilots can spend hours and hours doing something remarkably close to actual flying, experiencing all sorts of scenarios and what-ifs in terms of weather, flying conditions, and, of course, mechanical difficulties. And do so without risking either expensive planes or peoples' lives. Indeed, a great advantage of these virtual flights is that crashing hurts no one, and pilots walk away every time, better prepared for a real emergency.[577]

Beyond flying, flight-simulator type models are quickly catching on in many businesses as the preferred training environment to learn about all sorts of complex systems (engineering, managerial, economic). Likewise, in the military, the use of simulators is inducing a sea change in training. (Today, U.S. troops are practicing on simulators not only how to use their ever more complex equipment, but also the Pentagon's military strategists increasingly rely on military flight simulators to test strategic options before launching a campaign in earnest.) To educational theorists, an enticing characteristic of flight-simulator-based instruction is the active participation it requires of the learner—who is learning by making decisions, exploring and discovering.578

Mi Model extends this concept to personal health management… which, as I've argued, is precisely the setting where complexities are the most problematic and where the stakes are the highest. Analogous to a flight simulator that mimics the aerodynamics of an aircraft, *Mi Model* is essentially a simulation model of human physiology that mimics our bodies' weight/energy functions. And just as a flight simulator serves as a (safe) virtual laboratory where pilots can learn to fly (and crash) a new aircraft, *Mi Model* can serve as a personal laboratory—a virtual practice field if you will—for assessing treatment options and experience the consequences of planned interventions. [579] Metaphorically, to help you learn how to "fly" your body from where you are to where you want to be… and arrive safely at your destination. Indeed, the interface I developed for *Mi Model* is intended to give the touch and feel of flight simulator software—with their dials, buttons, and graphics.

Mi Model is the outcome of original and published research I conducted at Stanford and the Naval Postgraduate School. The overarching goal of our research program is to apply the twin innovations of systems thinking and information technology to build a new generation of decision-making and learning tools that empower ordinary people to better manage their personal health and wellbeing.

As an academic and a researcher, my goal is to demo a utilitarian yet fully functional tool—a "Model T" if you will—that is accessible and easy to use. The hope is that the concept proves enticing enough for consumers to demand these tools and for businesses to build sleeker versions with the requisite bells and whistles.

In the remainder of this chapter, I will introduce *Mi Model* and demonstrate its utility both as a customizable decision making tool as well as a laboratory for personal learning about weight management. The discussion will be somewhat brief and largely non-technical. The interested reader can find more details on the model's technical formulation in a number of articles published in the academic literature. (For example, see [Abdel-Hamid, 2002], [Abdel-Hamid, 2003] and [Abdel-Hamid, 2012].[580])

A fully functional turn-key version of the software is offered by ISEE Systems—the leading player in the Systems Thinking field—at: http://www. iseesystems.com/softwares/*Mi Model*.aspx.

Not your Mother's Energy Balance Equation

I already argued that the energy balance equation cannot faithfully project how body weight changes in response to some intervention because it ignores the body's involuntary adaptations to caloric deprivation and altered body weight (such as changes in the resting metabolic rate and the energy cost of physical activity) that can significantly dampen the rate of weight loss. And that the human energy/weight regulation system is a conglomerate of interrelated control processes and subsystems—regulating metabolism, body composition, energy intake, energy expenditure, etc. All these processes are interconnected, pushing on each other and being pushed on in return.

Unlike the simplistic single-equation energy balance equation, *Mi Model* provides an integrated holistic perspective of these interacting processes that together comprise the human weight and energy regulation system. This integrated holistic perspective allows us to capture the various interdependencies and interactions among the various subsystems and thus better assess how changes we make in one area (e.g., energy input) can be compensated for by other subsystems (e.g., energy expenditure). The benefit: much improved accuracy.

Figure 19.1 provides an overview of the model's four major subsystems: *Body Composition, Energy Intake* (EI), *Energy Expenditure* (EE), and *Energy Metabolism and Regulation*. These subsystems are not independent, stand-alone systems, but, as the interlocking gears in the figure suggest, they interact with one another.

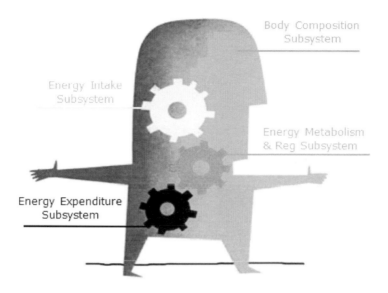

Figure 19.1: Overview of *Mi Model*'s four major Subsystems

Furthermore, the model is not limited to just providing snapshots e.g., the end result (total pounds lost) of a diet. Because it is a dynamic simulation model, it allows us to view the body's entire ("flight") path as it changes and adapts towards the end result. The benefit: deeper insight.

By properly accounting for the interactions and interdependencies between the body's many interrelated subsystems (energy intake, energy expenditure, metabolism, body composition), *Mi Model* is necessarily a highly sophisticated and complex model. Which raises an often stated concern, that the average person's knowledge and skill is grossly insufficient for properly using such a tool. *Poppycock!*

As I argued in Chapter 5, people do know enough to use such models. Thanks to the availability of affordable, high-quality computing capabilities and increasingly user-friendly software interfaces, ordinary people, for the first time in history, are today in a position to have access to and effectively deploy models of systems as complex as their own bodies.

Personalized Weight-Management

In contrast to the "one-size-fits-all" energy balance equation, *Mi Model* is a customizable tool that is tailored to each user's personal "specs." It is easily fitted by inputting three kinds of personal parameters:

1) Physical and Age related Parameters
    Such as: age, sex, current weight and body composition
2) Dietary Parameters
    Such as: daily caloric input, diet composition
3) Activity Parameters
    Such as: exercise frequency, duration and intensity

Many of the required inputs, such as age and weight, are straightforward and readily available. Others may require some digging or reflection. Nevertheless, you will find that the extra it entails tailor the model is time well spent. It becomes a valuable learning opportunity to sharpen your awareness of your own body's characteristics.

Let's consider two examples.

1. Your Body-Fat Percent

An important parameter needed to customize the model is the user's body-fat percent. It refers to the amount of fat mass as a percentage (or fraction) of total body mass i.e., to the sum of fat mass (FM) plus fat-free mass (FFM). (Clinically, human body composition can be viewed as being comprised of two compartments: fat-free mass (FFM) and fat mass (FM). Fat-free mass constitutes the skeleton, muscles, connective tissue, organ tissues, skin, bone, and water.) FM percentage varies widely among individuals, but a major determinant is a person's gender. A normal-weight man, has 12-20 percent body fat; a woman, because of her greater quantity of essential fat (in mammary glands and the pelvic region) 20-30 percent. Assessing one's FM percent as accurately as possible is critical because of the significant effects it has on weight/energy regulation.

A person's nominal maintenance energy expenditure (MEE)—which for a typical sedentary adult makes up as much as 60 to 70 percent of total energy expenditure—is determined not by their absolute body mass, but rather by their so-called metabolic mass, which is defined by the person's body composition in terms of fat mass (FM) versus fat free mass (FFM). That's because the various tissues of the body have very different qualitative and quantitative fuel requirements. Fat tissue, which is composed primarily of inert triglyceride is less metabolically active than FFM (such as muscle) and, thus, has a lower rate of fuel consumption per unit mass. (A pound of muscle burns approximately six calories a day in a resting body, compared with the two calories that a pound of fat burns.)

There is a second important reason for assessing one's FM percent as accurately as possible when attempting to lose weight. A person's body fat content at the start of a diet is an important determinant of the *composition* of the tissue that he or she will end up losing. Essentially, during weight loss, a person with more initial body fat loses more weight as fat than would a lean person, and the fatter a person is, the higher will be his or her FM loss as a percentage of total weight loss. Because initial body composition affects the composition of tissue lost during energy deprivation, it would also affect the trajectory and magnitude of the ultimate weight lost. Because fat and lean tissue are not energetically equivalent, the number of pounds or kilograms a person sheds as a result of a particular caloric deficit will vary as the mix of lost tissue (FM and FFM) changes.[581] (The energy content per kg change of body fat is 39.5 MJ and 7.6 MJ for a kg of lean mass. Thus, losing more fat from a particular caloric deficit means losing less pounds.[582])

So how to accurately assess one's body-fat percent?

Most people rely on visual inspection. But visual inspection is neither accurate nor objective. And while there are several examples of so-called body fat templates available on the Internet to use, they have not been evaluated or compared to laboratory methods and, thus, should be used with a grain of salt.[583]

Until very recently, the available options to perform an *accurate* assessment of FM % were neither particularly accessible nor affordable. They were limited to few expensive laboratory methods such as densitometry, magnetic resonance imaging (MRI), and radiography. Thankfully, better options are now becoming available.

Fat-analysis scales–which do not look much different from regular scales— can now be found in most hardware and department stores. They look like traditional bathroom scales, and, in one respect, act like them too: they weigh the body when they are stepped on. But placing your feet on a fat-analysis scale also puts them in contact with electrodes that send a small (and un-detectable) electrical current through the body. The scale compares the current entering the body with the current leaving it and calculates body fat composition using bioelectric impedance analysis, or B.I.A., which is based on the difference in the ways that an electrical current is affected by muscle and fat. Because muscle and fat have different electrical properties, the current passing through the body will be affected more or less depending on the proportions of muscle and fat. By combining this information with data like height, weight and age and comparing it with data from the general population, a body-fat percentage can be determined.

2. Daily Energy Expenditure (EE)

As a second example, consider assessing your "daily energy expenditure." Obviously you cannot expect to be able to devise a credible energy plan for losing weight if you don't know what your current (base case) daily energy expenditure level is. Yet most of us would not know it… precisely.

Well, we should. A (side) benefit of deploying a decision-support tool such as *Mi Model* is that it also serves as a learning tool that helps you—nudges you—to become better aware of how your body regulates energy.

In assessing your baseline energy expenditure level, you'll find that *Mi Model* provides considerable handholding. Figuring out one's total daily energy expenditure (EE), requires appraising its three principal components, namely, the energy expended on exercising, food processing, and (the biggest of the three) routine non-exercise physical activity. For most people, the amount of energy expended on exercise is in the range of 10-20 % of total daily energy expenditure. This discretionary component of total EE is obviously dependent on lifestyle and can vary a great deal from person to person. *Mi Model's* interface provides guidance for appraising energy expenditure levels for common exercise options such as walking, cycling, tennis, and running and includes templates for entering the information.

The second component, the thermic effect of food (TEF), typically accounts for approximately ten percent of total daily energy expenditure. TEF constitutes the various metabolic costs associated with processing food intake, which include the costs of digestion, absorption, transport, and storage of nutrients within the body. (It is referred to as the thermic effect of food because the acceleration of activity that occurs when we eat—as the GI-tract muscles speed up their rhythmic contractions, and the cells that manufacture and secrete digestive juices begin their tasks—produces heat). Daily TEF obviously depends on the amount and the composition of a person's diet—which would have been entered in the "Dietary Parameters" section. Because of that, the user does not need to calculate and enter a value for TEF, *Mi Model* has the facility to figure it out from the amount and composition of the diet entered by the user.

For most people, the largest component of total daily energy expenditure (60-70 % of it) is energy expenditure on routine activity. It is a sum of two parts. The larger component is the so called Maintenance Energy Expenditure or MEE—which is the amount of energy required to maintain the basic and essential physiological functions of the body. The second (smaller) component is the energy spent doing one's daily routines. This later part is referred to as the physical activity factor (PAF), and is typically assessed as a fraction (around 40%) of MEE. If both parts are known, total 24-hour energy expenditure on routine activity is obtained by multiplying MEE by the physical activity factor (PAF). But we are getting ahead of ourselves.

First we need to determine PAF—the multiplier to MEE needed to determine a person's routine (non-exercise) physical activity. Turns out, it is relatively straightforward—a matter of consulting tables that match work/lifestyle scenarios and energy expenditure levels and picking the appropriate value. As an example, a PAF value of 1.4 would be typical for individuals engaged in typical office and/or household daily tasks. As a frame of reference, here are other examples:

Examples PAF's:

Extremely inactive person .... less than 1.4

Office worker 1.4

Construction worker .... 1.5 - 1.7

Vigorously active agricultural worker .... 2 - 2.5

With PAF in hand, we are left with one final parameter to assess (the one most folks find mystifying): MEE. MEE, you may recall, is the amount of energy required to maintain the basic internal housekeeping functions of the body—to keep our heart beating, our lungs breathing, and our nerves transmitting. It is determined by two factors, body composition and energy balance. Body composition establishes a *nominal* MEE level that is then adjusted upwards or downwards as a function of a person's energy balance (i.e., as a function of what the person does with his or her body). With ***Mi Model***, the user has two options for how to determine MEE.

Most people can defer to the model's built-in MEE calculation (based on an empirically validated mathematical model). Using user inputs on body weight and composition (and energy balance), the model's built-in MEE calculator provides assessments of MEE that have been shown to be quite accurate (for most people). Once MEE is thus calculated, total daily energy expenditure on routine activity is assessed by multiplying MEE by the physical activity factor (PAF) supplied by the user.

Here is an example for a hypothetical dieter: a 50 year old, female office worker. We'll call her Ms. "X."

Ms. "X" personal characteristics are:

Sex: .... Female

Age: .... 50 years

Initial Weight: .... 75 kg

Height: .... 1.5 meters

BMI: 33

Fat %: 30%

Physical Activity Factor: 1.4

From that, ***Mi Model*** calculates:

- Nominal MEE: 6.7 MJ (one mega joule [MJ] is equivalent to 239 kcal).

- Daily Routine Energy Expenditure is the product of MEE and PAF.

  Thus, using her PAF of 1.4 yields:

  Daily Routine Energy Expenditure = 6.7 X 1.4 = 9.4 MJ

- From her supplied dietary input (not shown here), the model calculates:

  TEF = 1.1 MJ

- Adding the two components of energy expenditure provides:

  Ms. "X" Daily Energy Expenditure (excluding exercise) = 10.5 MJ

The analytically derived MEE calculation is the model's default option and is always automatically computed. It is built-in (and is the default option) because it provides accurate MEE assessments for most people. However, some people may opt to override it if, for example, they prefer to assess MEE by direct measurement rather than relying on (population-based) mathematical equations. Others may *need* to (e.g., because of unique metabolic circumstances say as a result of some special medical condition). To accommodate such users, the model interface allows the user to *override* its built-in MEE calculation.

To do that, the user's first order of business would be to assess his/her MEE. Today, that's not too difficult to do. Assessing MEE by direct measurement has become possible relatively recently thanks to the availability of highly portable, inexpensive indirect calorimetry devices. One example product is MedGem. It is a handheld device that assesses maintenance metabolic rate (MEE) by measuring oxygen consumption (VO_2). Devices like MedGem have been heralded as a revolutionary change in how to assess personal energy expenditure because the measurement is easy to administer and provides accurate results in only a few minutes.

When this empirical approach is pursued, the PAF adjustment factor needs to be adjusted to reconcile any differences between the actual measurement obtained (e.g., using MedGem) and *Mi Model*'s built-in MEE calculation. To demonstrate, let's extend our example for Ms. "X" to see to do that. Suppose her measurement using an indirect calorimeter such as MedGem indicates that her

MEE is 10% lower than the model's automatic calculation of 6.7 MJ (as depicted above). Rather than mess with the model's imbedded MEE equation or (worse) override/delete it (which would deprive her the opportunity to use it later if she desires), she would simply reconcile the difference by adjusting the Physical Activity Factor. In this case by decreasing it by 10 % (which would adjust it down from 1.4 to 0.9 * 1.4 = 1.26). With this simple adjustment, the model's calculation of daily routine EE (the product of its built-in MEE and the user supplied PAF) would now match the user's measured value.

Model Interface

Unlike the energy balance equation—which only provides pounds lost on a diet—Mi Model is no one-trick pony. Once personal parameters (physical, dietary and activity parameters) are input, the model can be run to design personalized weight-loss strategies and conduct what-if experiments (e.g. to compare diet versus exercise options). And because Mi Model is more than just an equation, it produces more than just a number. Indeed, its greatest utility may arguably be in utilizing it as a "learning laboratory" to gain deeper insight into how / why a diet or exercise intervention works or doesn't. For you.

It can do that because it is a holistic model that integrates the myriad physiologic/metabolic processes and subsystems that constitute the human energy/weight regulation system—such as energy intake, energy expenditure, body composition, metabolism. Which allows us to capture the various interdependencies and interactions among the various subsystems and, in turn, assess how changes we make in one area (e.g., Energy Input) can be compensated for by other subsystems (e.g., Energy Expenditure).

In terms of what the user sees, the model's interface is designed to look like a flight deck with its dials, buttons, and graphics. An example screen is shown below.

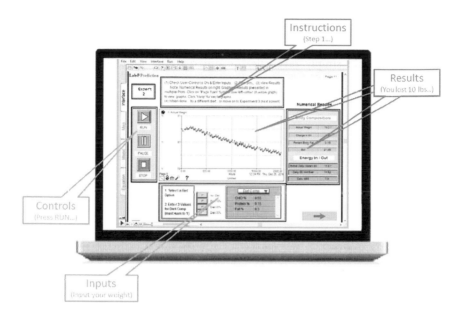

Figure 19.2: Model Interface

The figure shows one sample screen. The user can scroll through other screens to inspect a wide range of relevant variables. Example outputs that can be tracked include.

- Change in weight
- Body composition
- Energy expenditure ... MEE, exercise, thermic effect of food (TEF)
- Composition of tissue loss (FM versus FFM)
- Macronutrient energy balance: CHO/Fat caloric input versus burn rate

Notice that the model is not limited to just providing snapshots e.g., the end result (total pounds lost) of a diet. It also portrays how variables change over time e.g., over the course of a diet. Because it is a dynamic simulation model, it allows us to view the body's entire ("flight") path as it changes and adapts towards the end result.

Putting *Mi Model* to the Test

Before attempting to demonstrate *Mi Model's* utility as a tool for personal weight management, I first address the more fundamental issue of efficacy—assessing how accurate it is.

Effective prediction of treatment outcomes is crucial in managing many aspects of personal health and especially so in managing chronic-type conditions such as obesity. Without accurate predictions about the relationship between treatment interventions and outcomes, one cannot know what resources to commit to a treatment effort (e.g., the degree/longevity of a diet) nor, in retrospect, how well these resources were used. Effective prediction is also key to setting treatment goals. If one's goals are unrealistic, then failure is inevitable regardless of how hard one tries. In weight management—often a protracted endeavor—this matters a great deal because patients' expectations and the degree to which they are met (or not met) can affect their self-efficacy and long-term commitment.

The ubiquitous energy balance equation (EBE)—a.k.a. the 3500 kcal per pound rule—implies (and it is widely believed) that adherence to some diet regimen would cause body weight to drop in a straight-line (linear) fashion in direct proportion to the size of the caloric deficit. And that body weight would continue to drop as long as one adheres to the particular diet. Two assumptions underlie this simplistic model: (1) that the energy cost of lost tissue is fixed (at 3,500 kcal/lb); and (2) that the body's energy requirements remain steady, even as body size decreases.

By now you know that both of these assumptions are wrong. Let's briefly recap. Whenever significant amounts of body weight are lost (or gained), both fat-free mass (FFM) and fat mass (FM) participate in the weight loss/gain process, albeit in variable proportions. At the start of a diet, the relative contributions of these two body components to weight loss will depend, in part, on the person's initial body composition. As body composition changes with weight loss, the FM-FFM ratio also changes. For example, a dieter may start off losing 70 percent FM and 30 percent FFM for each pound of weight lost, but then progressively loses less fat as a percentage of the total as the diet progresses and his overall body fat content decreases. Because fat and lean tissue are *not* energetically equivalent, how many pounds of body weight a person sheds as a result of a particular caloric deficit will vary as the mix of lost tissue changes over the course of the diet.[584]

Second, losing weight as a result of caloric restriction affects *involuntary* energy expenditure—all three forms of it. The most obvious effect is the drop in the thermic effect of feeding (TEF), since eating less on a diet naturally lowers the metabolic cost of processing the smaller meals (captured as link 1 in Figure 19.3). This drop, however, is typically not very significant in absolute terms because TEF accounts for only ten percent of total daily energy expenditure.

A second, and slightly more delayed, response is the drop in energy expenditure on physical activity. This occurs when the dieting persists long enough for the dieter to lose an appreciable amount of weight. When this happens, the energy expended for muscular work tends to decline as a result (link 2 in Figure 19.3). The reason: as body weight drops the energy cost of weight-bearing physical activity decreases.

For most people, however, the largest adjustment to energy expenditure occurs as a result of the decline in maintenance energy expenditure (MEE). MEE drops for two reasons (captured by links 3 and 4 in Figure 19.3). The first is the loss of body mass (especially lean body tissue which is the more metabolically active component of body mass). The second factor affecting a decline in MEE is the diet's induced negative energy balance. As already explained, the body interprets caloric deficits as a deprivation "crisis" that needs to be contained. To compensate, the body decreases metabolic activity at the cellular level in order to conserve energy and restrain the rate of weight loss. Because maintenance energy expenditure for a typical sedentary adult accounts for a whopping 60-70 percent of total energy expenditure, the decline in MEE is often significant enough to alter the body's energy balance and, in turn, the rate of weight loss.

In reality, then, decreases in body weight are accompanied by continuous changes in the body's composition and in its total energy requirements. As a result, the rate of weight loss does not remain constant, but, instead, tends to decline with time—even if the prescribed diet is maintained. And so, as a diet progresses, the changes in the body's composition and in its maintenance energy requirements constantly modify the subsequent pattern of weight loss until a new equilibrium body weight is reached—often at a level substantially higher than expected. (This might help explain why even the most diligent followers of diet programs often fail to reach weight loss goals that were set by use of the static weight-loss rule.)

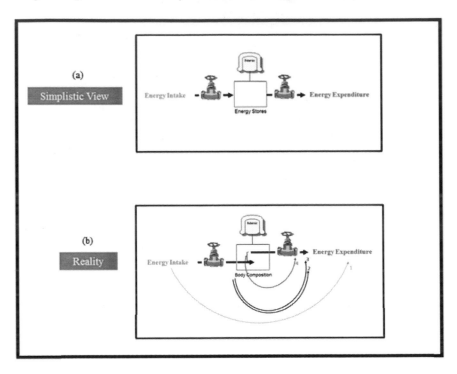

Figure 19.3: The reality of losing weight

Weight-Loss Prediction: Reality versus Fiction

To objectively assess *Mi Model*'s performance relative to the energy balance equation, the weight-loss predictions of both models were compared to actual losses by human dieters reported in a recently published empirical study. The objective of the widely cited study—conducted between March 2002 and August 2004 at the Pennington Biomedical Research Center, Baton Rouge, Louisiana—was to examine the effects of 6 months of calorie restriction in a group of forty eight overweight, non-obese (body mass index, 25 to 30) men and women.[585,586]

The forty eight participants were randomized into one of four groups: (1) 25% calorie restriction (which amounted to a 476 kcal per day reduction of energy intake); (2) calorie restriction with exercise (12.5% calorie restriction plus 12.5%

increase in energy expenditure by structured exercise); (3) a very low calorie diet until 15% reduction in body weight, followed by a weight maintenance diet; and (4) a control group (put on a weight maintenance diet). In Figure 19.4, the performances of *Mi Model* and the energy balance equation are compared to the actual results of Group 1—the group whose experimental treatment (25 % caloric restriction) was deemed the most likely to observe in real-life settings.

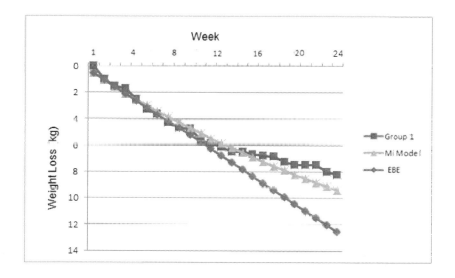

Figure 19.4: Performances of *Mi Model* and the energy balance equation compared to actual results

The energy balance equation (EBE) predicts that the 476 kcal per day reduction of energy intake would induce a linear decrease of bodyweight over time that culminates into a 12.6 kg total loss at the end of the 24 weeks. But, as you can see, that's far too optimistic. Indeed, EBE's 12.6 kg prediction is 53% greater than the 8.25 kg average weight-loss actually observed. Failure to account for the decline in maintenance energy expenditure that accompanies weight loss is what's largely responsible for this error.

By properly accounting for the decline in maintenance energy expenditure that accompanies weight loss, *Mi Model* tracks the (curvilinear) trajectory of weight loss much more closely. And for the 24 week long intervention, *Mi Model* predicts a total loss of 9.4 kg. That's appreciably closer to the actual 8.25 kg value, but is still 14 % higher. Why not even closer? One reason for the 14 % gap may be the fact that (lacking access to the participants) *Mi Model* could not be appropriately customized to each experimental subject as it should and would in practice (e.g., with each individual's body composition). If we were to do that, accuracy would be expected to improve even more.

The difference in the *shapes* of the weight-loss trajectories is an important distinction between the two models. While the rate of weight loss projected by the energy balance equation (EBE) is constant, causing weight to drop in a straight-line fashion, the *actual* trajectory of weight-loss is not. It is curvilinear. To accentuate this difference in *shapes* even more, I extended the weight-loss predictions of both models for an additional 24 weeks (Figure 19.5). As you can see, over a longer time period the gap between "fantasy" (as in the EBE projection) and "reality" (as simulated by *Mi Model*) grows and grows. Obviously, the larger the divergence, the bigger the potential disappointment by an "EBE dieter."

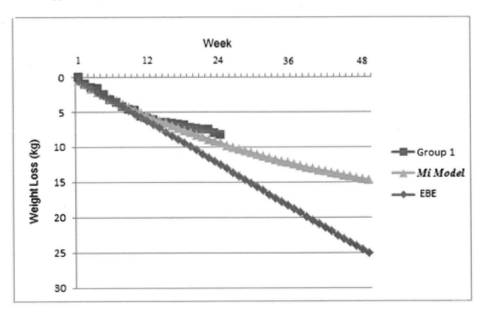

Figure 19.5: Extending weight-loss predictions to 48 weeks

Beyond the Single Number

Mi Model's utility extends beyond just predicting how many pounds or kilograms are lost on a diet. Because *Mi Model* is a holistic model that captures the myriad physiologic and metabolic processes that underlie human weight/energy regulation—unlike the *single*-equation EBE—it can portray a richer multi-dimensional picture of change. For example, *Mi Model* provides insights into:

- Not only change in total weight, but change in body composition (FM and FFM)
- Change in total energy expenditure per day and by daily activity (work, rest, exercise, eating)
- Caloric balances. For example the balance between fuel input types (carbohydrates and fats in the diet) and the fuel types expended on work and play (glucose versus free fatty acids [FFA])

To any dieter this provides added insight to more effectively assess health status and/or treatment outcomes. For a system as complex as the human body, a single metric is rarely sufficient to provide a proper assessment of health status. Weight-loss is a good case in point. The determination of the success or failure of some weight loss intervention should not be pegged on a single metric—such as pounds lost or BMI—but needs to encompass other dimensions, such as measures of body composition (how much of one's weight is fat) and fat distribution (where in one's body the fat is located).

For the experimental subjects of Group 1, as an example, *Mi Model* could predict the projected changes in body fat percent from the 25 % caloric restriction. Figure 19.6 depicts the close match between *Mi Model*'s predictions and the subjects' results. By comparison, the EBE curve is flat (no change). Why? Because the one-pony-show EBE is completely silent on how body composition changes during prolonged underfeeding!

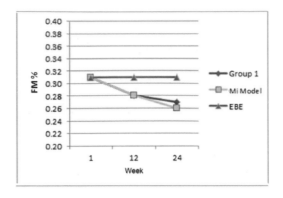

Body Fat %			
	Actual	Mi Model	EBE
	25% Cal Restriction		
Week	Group 1	Mi Model	EBE[*]
1	0.31	0.31	0.31
12	0.28	0.28	0.31
24	0.27	0.26	0.31

[*]E Bal Equ Silent

Figure 19.6: Projected changes in body fat percent

Predicting with Individual Differences in Mind

As already noted, "one-size-fits-all" energy balance calculators overlook the fact that overweight people are not a single homogenous group. An important reason why responses to weight-loss interventions can and do vary a great deal among individuals is because of differences in body composition. It turns out, a person's initial body fat content when starting a diet is an important determinant of the *composition* of tissue they end up shedding. Gilbert B. Forbes demonstrated this in a series of seminal experiments he conducted in the 1980s to investigate how human body composition affects and is affected by weight loss/gain. Based on a series of studies involving individuals of varying body fat content Forbes derived empirical relationships that predict the relative changes in body composition when body weight is gained or lost.[587] Essentially what he found was that during weight loss, obese people lose more weight as fat than do lean people, and the fatter a person is (the higher his/her FM %), the higher will be his or her FM loss as a percentage of total weight loss. Conversely, during weight gain, obese people add more weight as fat than do lean people, who add more lean tissue. (There are, of course, situations in which this does not occur. For example, exercising makes it possible to lose some weight without sacrificing FFM.[588])

By affecting the composition of tissue lost during energy deprivation, a person's initial body composition in turn affects the trajectory and magnitude of the ultimate weight that is lost. One reason tissue composition (FM or FFM) affects the amount of kilograms (or pounds) lost is that fat and lean tissue are *not* energetically equivalent. The energy content per kg change of body fat is 39.5 MJ—a lot higher than the 7.6 MJ for a kg of lean mass. Thus, losing more fat on a particular caloric deficit means losing less weight.[589] In addition, because muscle cells burn calories around three times faster than fat cells, an individual who loses proportionally more lean mass will show greater declines in energy expenditure than someone (on the *same* diet) who loses more fat. This, in turn, will affect the person's energy balance and subsequent trajectory of weight loss.

Differences in body composition are *not* the only source of variability in human energy/weight regulation. Differences among individuals have *dynamic* dimensions, as well. The ease of losing weight and keeping it off has been shown, for example, to depend not only on how overweight a person is to begin with (a static attribute), but also on the history or time course of weight gain (a dynamic one).[590,591] Though often overlooked, dynamic aspects—such as the time history of weight gain—are particularly interesting because they imply that, *for the same individual*, response to treatment can *change* over time.

Bottom line: people who are overweight are not a single homogenous group and different people—however similar they may look superficially (e.g., weigh the same) need different goals and different recipes for weight loss.[592] Reliance on simplistic one-size-fits-all tools—justifiable perhaps when we were computationally poor—is thus a bankrupt strategy that must be abandoned in favor of more intimate tools that actually fit. *Mi Model* is such a tool.

Because *Mi Model* captures individual differences—both static and dynamic—it allows us to account for the effects of individual differences in planning weight-loss interventions. To demonstrate, I'll conduct a hypothetical experiment that puts *Mi Model* through its paces and allows me to highlight the model's dual utilities: (1) To serve as a personalized decision-making tool (e.g., to predict dieting outcome); and (2) as a flight-simulator-type laboratory for learning about how and why different body compositions affect weight loss.

The Experiment

Specifically, the objective of this exercise is to gain insight into the role that individual differences—both static and dynamic—play in human weight and energy regulation *and* quantify the impact on weight-loss. To accomplish this, we play out the following scenario: that of three friends with similar weights who decide to buddy-diet. At the start of the diet, they all weigh 250 lbs. (114 kg). Their body-weight histories and body compositions, however, are quite different. The fundamental question then: What will the outcome be when the three buddies go on the *same* diet? That is, how will three subjects with similar weights but different histories of weight gain and body composition respond to an *identical* dieting intervention?

The key protagonist, we'll call him Mr. A, has been chronically overweight at the 250 lb level (114 kg) and has a body composition of 31 percent body fat. At six feet (1.83 meters) tall, this pegs his body mass index (BMI) at 30. Mr. A's relatively steady body weight is maintained on an average daily dietary input of 15.35 MJ (3,670 kcal)—his so-called *maintenance* daily energy input.

Mr. "A" convinces two friends who are equally overweight to join him on a buddy-diet. His proposal: Three months on a balanced diet of 14 MJ (3,345 kcal)—which he figures constitutes a reasonable 10 percent drop below his maintenance daily diet.

The first friend to sign on, we'll refer to him as subject "B," was originally slimmer at 100 kg (220 pounds) and 25 percent body fat but had just recently (say over the three month holidays period) put on some extra weight gaining as much as 15 percent. Now he too is 114 kg and 31 percent fat. While *statically* "A" and "B" are very similar (same weight and body composition), dynamically they are not. For subject "B," the extra 14 kg is a *recent* weight increase, while for the chronically overweight "A," the 114 kg overweight condition constitutes his normal (steady state) weight. This distinct difference in their weight time-lines has important metabolic implications.

Recall that when weight is lost on a diet the body interprets the caloric deficit as a deprivation "crisis" that needs to be contained. To compensate, the body decreases metabolic activity at the cellular level (inducing a decline in MEE) in order to conserve energy and restrain the rate of weight loss. An opposite adaptation occurs during caloric surplus and weight gain: MEE per unit of metabolic mass *increases*. These up-and-down energy-conserving and/or energy-dissipating mechanisms in MEE are the body's way to protect against the full extent of over-eating or under-eating and serve to minimize the effects of short-term fluctuations in energy balance. Specifically, in Mr. B's case, the recent gain in body weight as a result of overfeeding during the holiday season would induce an increase in his body's maintenance energy requirements.[593,594,595] A detailed calculation of the elevation in B's metabolic energy requirements as a result of his recent 14 kg gain in weight (not important here, but discussed in detail in *Thinking in Circles about Obesity*) indicates that his MEE increases from its steady state level of 9 MJ/day to 10.7 MJ/day. What *is* important here is that at that elevated level, B's MEE becomes ten-percent higher than that of his buddy Mr. "A" (at 9.7 MJ/day).[596]

This differential in energy expenditure levels between A and B is significant because it appreciably alters the effective value of the caloric imbalance the two men experience when they embark on the *same* diet. An elevation in the body's total energy expenditure (as in "B's" case) effectively expands the size of the diet's energy *deficit* and, in turn, accelerates the loss of body weight (Figure 19.7).

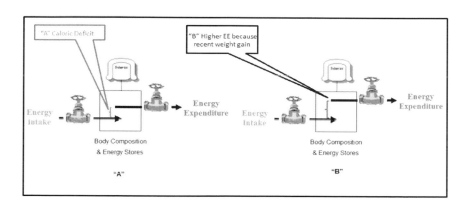

Figure 19.7: On same diet, "B'"s caloric deficit is larger

A second important individual attribute that we need to investigate is the difference in initial body composition. Body composition is particularly interesting because of the wide variability observed among people. To assess the impact of body composition, we bring in the third friend, a Mr. "C." Like "A," our third subject has been chronically overweight at 114 kg. But, unlike both "A" and "B," who have similar body compositions, C's percent FM is substantially higher, at 40 percent.

The $ 64,000 question as the three friends get set to embark on the identical die: How will three subjects with similar weights but different *histories* of weight gain and body *composition* respond to the *identical* dieting intervention?

114 kg ≠ 114 kg ≠ 114 kg!

And the answer is: the weight-loss differences among the three friends are rather dramatic!

After three months of dieting, "A" loses 3.04 kg (8.9 lbs.), dropping to a weight of 110.87 kg (244.4 pounds). In comparison, "B" experiences a larger loss of 5.68 kg (8.9 lbs.), dropping to 108.23 kg (238.6 lbs.). Not only is there a difference in the amount of weight lost—on the *same* diet—but the difference is quite substantial, with one losing half as much as the other. The reason for the difference: "B's" elevated MEE level (as a result of his recent overfeeding behavior) pushes his MEE rate to a level that's ten-percent higher than "A's" (10.73 MJ/day versus A's 9.71 MJ/day). The difference is significant because it appreciably alters the effective values of the caloric imbalance experienced by the two men. An elevation in the body's total energy expenditure (as in "B's" case) effectively expands the size of the diet's energy deficit and, in turn, accelerates the loss of body weight (Figure 19.7)

C's results are even more dramatic: "C" does not lose even a pound! The reason is body composition. "C" does not lose much weight because the 14 MJ diet (while below maintenance for Mr. "A") is very close to C's maintenance energy level—i.e., the level of caloric intake that would maintain *his* weight at its current 114 kg level (Figure 19.8). Recall that a person's nominal maintenance energy expenditure (MEE*)* is a function of metabolic mass rather than absolute body mass. Because lean body tissue is the principal metabolically active component of total body mass, the contribution of the FFM to the MEE is much greater per kilogram than that of body fat. C's relatively low maintenance energy level, compared to A's and B's, is a direct result of his body's composition—specifically, his lower percent of FFM.

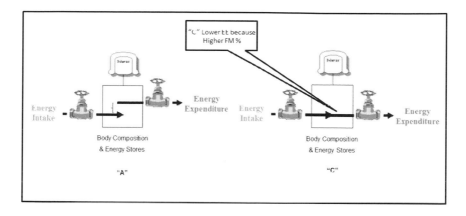

Figure 19.8: On same diet, "C"'s caloric deficit is smaller (negligible)

The dramatically different performances of the three friends on the *same* diet are plotted below in Figure 19.9.

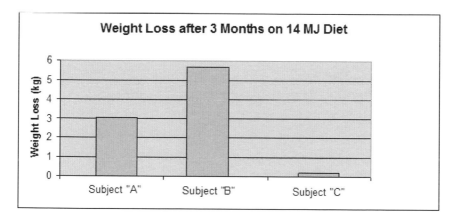

Figure 19.9

One Size Doesn't Fit All

Overall, the results of our experiment underscore the fact that overweight people are not a single homogenous group, and that different people—however similar they may look superficially (e.g., weigh the same)—need different goals and different recipes for weight loss. Static individual differences such as body composition must be considered, as should an individual's weight and dieting histories.

The results highlight the need for adopting more *personalized* models in weight management. The traditional search for the one "one-size-fits-all" model (such as the energy balance equation) that is applied en masse is a bankrupt strategy that we need to abandon.

The trend towards customization is, of course, taking root in a wide range of industries. Rather than continuing to mass produce for the increasingly elusive "average customer," many businesses are already using state-of-the-art information technology to build and deliver products and services designed to fit the precise specifications of each individual customer. As consumers, we expect that in everything else we do, and now it needs to happen in health.

Dieting versus Exercising

In managing personal health, as with most other endeavors, people typically have a spectrum of options to choose from to achieve their goals. And this is a good thing, for it allows us to choose interventions that best suit our preferences and lifestyles. However, with options comes the obligation (and challenge?) to objectively appraise alternatives and determine what works best *for us*.

A serious limitation of the energy balance equation is that it does not provide the decision-maker (you) with enough discriminatory power to compare weight-loss treatment options. The energy balance equation suggests (and it is widely held) that a decline in body weight is determined solely by the size of the energy deficit, regardless of how that deficit is induced. Energy, in other words, is treated as though it were a single currency. In reality, how an energy deficit is created *does* matter. A daily energy deficit of 500 kcal can be induced, for example, by eliminating soft drinks (two cans of Coke) and dessert (say a cheese cake) from the daily diet or by jogging four miles at a four-mile-per-hour pace. While both of these strategies would create the same caloric deficit, the trajectories of weight change that result from them could be quite different.

Specifically, the two strategies will have differing impacts on the *composition* of weight loss—fat mass versus fat-free mass—and which, in turn, will affect the body's involuntary adaptations to its maintenance energy requirements and, ultimately, energy balance. When exercise is used to create a desired energy deficit, it tends to protect against the loss in fat-free mass (FFM). (This favorable impact on body composition occurs partly because of increases in muscle size through increased protein synthesis during exercise.) By conserving and even increasing fat-free body mass (the principal metabolically active component of total body mass), exercise partially blunts the diet-induced depression in metabolic energy expenditure that typically accompanies diet-based weight loss.

But what impact do such differences have on weight loss? Are the differences only in the quality (i.e., composition) of weight loss or in quantity, as well? That's after all is the "bottom-line" question for most weight-loss seekers.

In the remainder of this section I explore these highly pertinent questions. Specifically, I'll use **Mi Model** as a vehicle to compare (and quantify) the impacts of food restriction and exercise on the amount and composition of weight loss under a number of different scenarios. My experimental subject throughout is a hypothetical overweight sedentary male with an initial weight of 100 kg and 25 percent body fat and whose maintenance daily diet computes at 14.25 MJ.

When 500 kcal ≠ 500 kcal

The first issue to settle is the basic apples-versus-oranges question: comparing the amount of weight loss on "comparable" diet and exercise regimens. Specifically, I compare changes to our subject's body weight and composition after undertaking two separate but calorically-equivalent treatments. In the first treatment, he goes on a diet by dropping his daily caloric intake by two MJ (equivalent to 478 kcal) for a twelve week period. The result of that diet is then compared to his weight loss if he participates instead in an exercise program that induces an identical daily caloric deficit of two MJ. To accommodate the fact that overweight sedentary individuals are usually physically unfit—a limitation that undoubtedly hampers their capacity to exercise—the daily two MJ (478 kcal) exercise regimen is stretched over a two-hour period. This allows for a modest intensity level of one MJ/hour (which, for example, could be achieved by leisurely walking).

A comparison of **Mi Model**'s projected changes in body weight over the 12-week period for both the dieting and exercising interventions is shown in Figure 19.10. The first thing to notice is that at the end of the three-month period, the difference in weight loss from dieting versus exercising is quite small. After twelve weeks of dieting, body weight drops by 4.9 kg (10.8 lbs) to 95.1 kg, while a calorically-equivalent daily exercise regimen causes weight to drop a comparable 4.7 kg (10.3 lbs.).

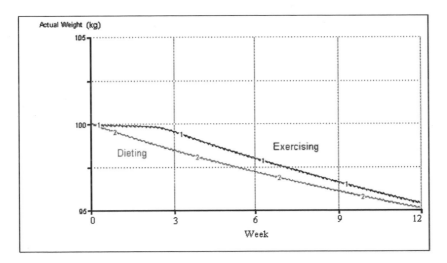

Figure 19.10: Dieting versus exercising

The weight-loss trajectories of the two interventions are quite different, however. With dieting, the subject starts losing weight almost immediately, while in the exercise scenario, body weight drops very little in the early phases. This flat start in the exercise treatment can be attributed to the increase in muscle size that our sedentary overweight subject enjoys as he embarks on the 2 MJ/day exercise regimen. The initial buildup of the subject's muscle mass (an addition to his FFM compartment) counterbalances what his body loses in FM, causing a minimal *net* change in total body weight. This exercise effect, however, is transitory. That's because the gains in muscle mass a person makes when embarking on a new exercise regimen depend on the *relative* intensity of the exercise overload—relative, that is, to the subject's fitness level. Thus, as exercise continues at the *same* intensity level, the subject's fitness invariably improves (a dynamic that's captured by **Mi**

Model), which causes this adaptive physiologic response (the gain in muscle mass) to eventually level off.

During the first few weeks of the exercise regimen, the body relies on its fat fuel reserves to compensate for both the daily caloric deficit and the initial buildup of muscle mass. While this obviously induces larger losses in FM (in comparison to dieting), it also (perhaps less obviously) precipitates less of a net loss in *total* body mass. Since FM has a much larger energy density than FFM, smaller losses in FM tissue are used to fuel larger gains in FFM. Eventually, though, as the buildup of muscle mass levels off, total weight starts to decline under the cumulative burden of the sustained two MJ daily energy deficit.

The distinctively different trajectories of weight loss from dieting versus exercising have important implications on how people interpret (or misinterpret) treatment outcomes. Consider this: If the duration of the weight-loss treatment were shorter, say four weeks long instead of twelve, our subject may conclude, as many probably do, that exercise is an ineffective weight loss strategy. But that would be both premature and wrong.

In the case of exercise, not only does size (of the caloric deficit) matter, but so does duration. Indeed, failure to properly account for this "delay effect" may help explain why published research results on the efficacy of exercise as a treatment option have been rather *mixed*. On the one hand, numerous studies have found that increased levels of physical activity are as effective as dieting (with some studies showing exercise to be more effective than dieting for long-term weight control). On the other hand, there is an equally abundant set of studies reporting just the opposite—that exercise has less (or significantly less) effect on weight loss than food restriction does.[597,598] Such mixed findings, not surprisingly, have caused confusion in the public and have led some investigators to discount the importance of exercise in the treatment of obesity.[599]

A few years ago, an American College of Sports Medicine scientific panel was assembled to review the issue. The panel concluded that the inconsistent results can be attributed, in part, to the complexity and expense of performing longer-term studies, thus limiting many experiments to relatively short durations (Grundy et al; 1999). Because significant weight changes from exercise occur *after a delay*, as the above results suggest, short-duration studies do not allow for the full estimation of the potential effects of exercise on weight loss.[600]

Difference in the time-course of weight loss is not the only difference between the exercise and diet options. The two treatment strategies also have different impacts on the composition of lost tissue (a physiologic phenomenon also captured by *Mi Model*). Figure 19.11 shows a comparison between the changes in body weight and composition (fat-free mass, fat mass and percent body fat) in dieting versus exercising. The key finding here is that, while the difference in *total* weight loss is not significant, the difference in the composition of the weight that was lost is. As the figure shows, in the exercise treatment (the dashed bars), FM drops by 4.2 kg—accounting for almost 90 percent of the total loss in weight— while FFM drops by only 0.5 kg. This contrasts with the diet treatment, in which 70 percent of the weight loss was FM and 30 percent was FFM (FM drops by 3.4 kg, while the FFM loss was 1.5 kg).[601]

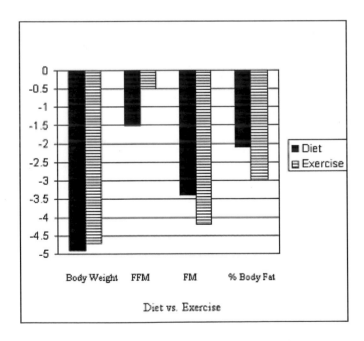

Figure 19.11: Comparing changes to body weight and composition

Overall, then, we can draw two conclusions from these results. First, given enough time, exercise—even at a moderate level—induces a comparable loss in body weight to food restriction. This should provide a more palatable option to people who would prefer exercise as a strategy to help maintain weight loss while allowing the consumption of enough calories to supply the body with adequate nutrients and energy.

Second, and perhaps more important, the experiment quantifies the significant degree to which exercise protects against the loss of fat-free mass, as well as the favorable impact it has on changes in the percent of body fat. This is potentially quite significant since maximizing fat loss yields the greatest reduction in coronary heart disease risk[602] In addition, the conservation of muscle mass during exercise-induced weight loss maintains a person's ability to perform daily tasks requiring strength and/or muscular staying power.

Trading Exercise Intensity for Exercising Time … Can More be Less?

Because, for many people, the most costly aspect of exercise is the time spent doing it, there is an understandable inclination to aim at exercising at the highest possible level of intensity in order to induce the largest possible energy deficit per exercise session and shorten exercise duration. The objective of part 2 of the experiment is to assess the viability of such a strategy—i.e., trading exercise intensity for exercise time. (Recall from Chapter 19 that *Mi Model* allows the user to specify his/her exercise duration and intensity level.)

We'll assume that the subject's time constraints allow him to exercise on only three days of the week—say Mondays, Wednesdays, and Fridays. The subject's decision task, then, is to replace the current regimen—exercising daily for two hours at the light rate of one MJ/hour—with a new exercise schedule that allows him to achieve the same weekly energy deficit of 14 MJ (3,345 kcal) in just three weekly sessions. A reasonable strategy to accomplish that would be to double the exercise intensity level from one MJ/hour to two MJ/hr and to extend the duration from two hours to two hours and twenty minutes on each of the three exercise days. (Cycling would be an exercise option that would fit that bill.)

The loss in body weight and change in percent of body fat attained after exercising for twelve weeks at this new high-intensity level are compared in Figure 19.12 to the results obtained earlier. The outcome is somewhat surprising. While exercising at the lower-intensity level caused total body weight to drop by 4.7

kg—as a combination of a modest 0.5 kg drop in FFM and a more substantial 4.2 kg drop in FM—we now see that no weight is lost when exercise intensity doubles to two MJ/hour (in fact, total body weight increases slightly from 100 to 100.37 kg).

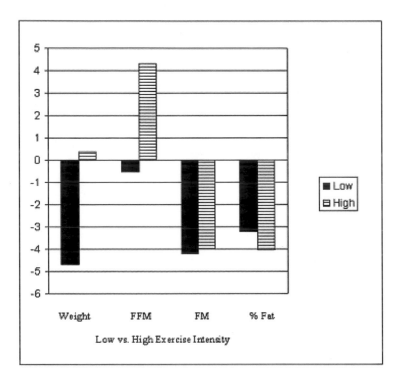

Figure 19.12: Low versus high exercise intensity

Two factors contribute to this counter-intuitive result. First, the increased level of exercise intensity induces a rather significant 4.3 kg (9.5 lb.) increase in FFM (mainly muscle mass)—a value that exceeds the simultaneous 4 kg (8.8 lb.) loss in FM. The differential induces a net increase in total body weight (albeit only a minimal 0.37 kg), but also produces a very favorable four-percent drop in our subject's body-fat percentage—lowering it from 25 percent to 21 percent.

The second factor behind the unexpected change in body weight at the higher intensity level is somewhat more subtle. When put on the high-intensity exercise regimen, our sedentary obese subject ends up expending *less* cumulative exercise energy per exercise session (and for the entire treatment period).

The cause for this unintended outcome lies in the body's selective dependence on different energy sources to fuel differing levels of exercise activity *and* a person's capacity to meet the body's specific energy needs.

During physical activity, the muscles' requirements for fuel are met by mobilization of reserves within muscle cells and from extra muscular fuel depots. How much of which fuels they use depends on an interplay among the fuels available from the diet, the intensity and duration of the activity, and the degree to which the body is conditioned to perform that activity.[603]

During low- to moderate-intensity physical activity, the lungs and circulatory system have no trouble keeping up with the muscles' need for oxygen. The individual breathes easily, and the heart beats steadily—the activity is aerobic. With the availability of oxygen, the muscles can derive their energy from both glucose and fatty acids since both can be oxidized to provide energy.[604]

Intense activity presents a different metabolic situation. Whenever a person exercises at a rate that exceeds the capacity of the heart and lungs to supply oxygen to the muscles, aerobic metabolism cannot meet energy needs. Instead, the muscles must draw more heavily on glucose (primarily in the form of muscle glycogen), which is the only fuel that can be used anaerobically—i.e., that can be metabolized to produce energy without the simultaneous use of oxygen.[605] A selective dependence on glucose metabolism during intense physical activity has an additional advantage: its rapidity of energy transfer compared to fats (about twice as fast).[606] The limitation (and it is an important one): Our glycogen reserves are rather limited—a few hundred grams amounting to about 2,500 kcal.

How much exercise can be sustained by any particular person's glycogen reserves would depend on the intensity and duration of effort, as well as on the fitness and nutritional status of the exerciser. An overweight sedentary person, such as our 100 kg subject, embarking on a new exercise regimen will not only start with more limited glycogen stores, but will also tend to use his reserves at a faster rate than will a trained athlete. (In athletes, muscle cells that repeatedly deplete their glycogen through exercise adapt by storing greater amounts of glycogen to support that work. Conditioned muscles also rely less on glycogen and more on fat for energy, so glycogen utilization occurs more slowly in trained than in untrained individuals at a given work intensity.[607]) Generally, glycogen depletion occurs within one to two hours from the onset of intense activity. As glycogen is depleted, the muscles become fatigued. This, in turn, greatly diminishes the capacity to continue exercising at a high intensity level. This dynamic is what causes our subject's energy expenditure level to drop at the higher intensity level in the experiment—the high-intensity exercise regimen collides head on with his biological limitations, and biology wins the battle.[608]

The weekly energy expenditure totals for the two intensity levels are plotted below in Figure 19.13. At the low-intensity level, the subject's actual energy expenditure matches the weekly target level of 14 MJ. In the high-intensity scenario, by contrast, he expends only 11 MJ—or 78 percent of the weekly target. This suggests that, for an overweight sedentary subject, a high-intensity-level exercise regimen can prove counterproductive as a weight-reducing strategy.

(As reported in Chapter 17, an empirical study conducted by researchers at the University of Copenhagen produced similar results. In that study, the Danish researchers found that exercise does seem to contribute to waist-tightening, provided that the amount of exercise is neither too little nor, more strikingly, too much.)

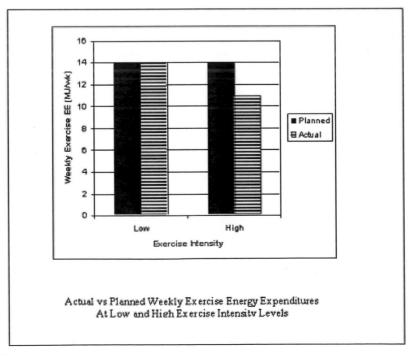

Actual vs Planned Weekly Exercise Energy Expenditures
At Low and High Exercise Intensity Levels

Figure 19.13: Weekly energy expenditure totals

For our sedentary subject, failure in the high-intensity exercise scenario occurs not because of a lack of effort, but because of pursuing what is for him a futile endeavor. This echoes a lesson we learned earlier: the importance of setting *realistic goals*. Trying harder—no matter how much harder—to attain unrealistic goals, whether for exercising or dieting, is often a recipe for failure and disappointment.

The Upshot: Don't Trade. . . . Integrate

I argued earlier that exercise is a "Judo-type move" that needs to be incorporated in people's plans for losing and/or maintaining weight. And I presented what I consider to be the most convincing data on the value of integrating physical activity and dieting—instead of choosing one over the other—to achieve and maintain weight loss. Namely, results from the National Weight Control Registry where almost 100 percent of these long-term successful "losers" use a combination of diet and exercise to lose weight, and about 95 percent use a combination of diet and exercise to maintain their loss.[609]

Granted, thermodynamic principles make it difficult for humans to lose weight quickly by exercise alone—an hour-long jog may burn 300 calories, the same 300 calories that are in a single candy bar.[610,611] This surprises and can discourage many people, but it shouldn't.

Although in comparison with weight loss from dieting, weight loss from exercise takes longer and is more work, "regular exercise appears to be one of the major factors determining the *long-term* success of weight loss programs."[612] (Due, we suspect, to its effect in conserving and even increasing fat-free body mass.) Apart from its effects on body weight and composition, regular exercise has many other potential benefits for overweight people. Indeed, a remarkable and consistent finding is that heavy people who are fit have lower risk for major killers like heart disease than thin people who are unfit.[613]

CHAPTER 20

Mi Volumetrics

When it comes to meal planning, most dieters, it seems, fall victim to a "calories-wise pounds-foolish" trap. They fret over setting weight-loss goals and calculating caloric targets, but give little thought to designing smart (satisfying) meals. For example, a common practice is to cut caloric intake by simply consuming less of the foods they are currently eating… and become resigned to feeling hungry and deprived.

It's not a recipe for success.

Successful dieting necessitates doing three things well: (1) Setting a *realistic* weight-loss goal; (2) determining the proper (*individually-tailored*) caloric deficit to achieve it; and (3) devising a palatable and *satisfying* diet that can be sustained (Figure 20.1).

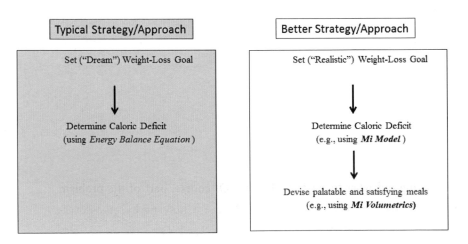

Figure 20.1 Two weight-loss strategies

I already explained how exaggerated goals (in step 1) and poor predictions (step 2) can doom weight-loss efforts. Poor food selection—our focus in this chapter—can do as well. Diets that induce deprivation almost always fail in the long run because they ignore the basic fact that people like to eat. A deprived dieter just winds up hungry and unhappy and before too long reverts back to his/her old ways.

It doesn't have to be that way. The "pounds-wise" insight of volumetrics is that, by being smart about food selection, a dieter can cut calories while staving hunger. By decreasing the energy density of foods, people can eat enough to feel satiated (sometimes even eat more than they have been) while still slimming down.

In this chapter I take this one step further. Besides juggling calories and energy densities, dieters need to compose meal plans that conform to personal preferences and needs (e.g., for things like taste, accessibility, affordability) to increase the chances of long-term success (and a healthy outcome).

Unfortunately, that's easier said than done.

It seems paradoxical, but optimal food selection in our modern environment of food abundance is no lark. The large variety of food choices available to us, while undoubtedly a blessing, can also make choosing a diet unbearably confusing. (In *The Paradox of Choice*, Barry Schwartz convincingly argues that *choice overload*, a phenomenon that applies to many common decisions not only to food selection, complicates decision-making because it tends to increase uncertainty and frustration.) Indeed, research studies of supermarket shoppers consistently show they often feel overwhelmed by the information they have to process.

"Americans Find Doing Their Own Taxes Simpler than Improving Diet and Health" blared a recent headline in *ScienceDaily*, the reputable online journal. (According to a recent study) fifty two percent of Americans think doing their taxes is easier than figuring out what to eat to be healthy. Of course, part of the problem is that we have so many food choices. Choosing becomes overwhelming. ("Americans Find Doing Their Own Taxes Simpler Than Improving Diet and Health," http://www.sciencedaily.com/releases/2012/05/120523145655.htm).

Luckily, grappling with large numbers of variables (choices) is precisely what computers are good at. Computer modeling is thus well suited to fill the gap where human cognition is taxed, allowing us to combine the strengths of the dieter with the strengths of the computer. The dieter specifies alternatives, preferences and requirements and the computer then sifts through the possibilities to help us pick the optimal choice.

In this chapter I introduce you to *Mi Volumetrics*, a computer based tool we developed to do just that—to help lay dieters optimize their meal planning.

Mi Volumetrics

Mi Volumetrics is a tool that combines two resources: a decision-support tool for optimizing meal selection and an extensive database of food options to select from. The latter is derived from the database of over 600 items compiled by Barbara Rolls and Robert Barnett in their book, *The Volumetrics Weight-Control Plan*. For each food item, Rolls and Barnett provide information on serving sizes, calories per serving, and energy density. In *Mi Volumetrics* the Rolls/Barnett data is augmented with additional metrics on total weight per serving (in grams) and macronutrient composition (fat, carbohydrate, protein and fiber) gleaned from the USDA national Nutrient Database. (The USDA National Nutrient Database for Standard Reference [SR] is the major source of food composition data in the United States. It provides the foundation for most food composition databases in the public and private sectors.)

To make the *Mi Volumetrics* tool ultra-accessible, it is built in Microsoft Excel—a software package that most people have access to and experience using. The *Mi Volumetrics* Excel model is freely available on the book's website.

Mi Volumetrics for Ms. "X"

In the remainder of this chapter, I aim to demonstrate both the utility of the *Mi Volumetrics* tool for optimizing meal selection and its layman-friendly inter-face. By optimizing I mean composing a weight-loss diet that not only meets some caloric target but is also satisfying (in both quantity and quality).

To experience the tool's entire functionality, I'll use a concrete case study: designing a diet plan for our hypothetical Ms. "X" (whom we first met in Chapter 19).

Recall, Ms. X's personal characteristics are:

Sex: .... Female
Age: .... 50 years
Initial Weight: .... 75 kg
Height: ....1.5 meters
BMI: 33
Fat %: 30%
PAF: .... 1.4 (physical activity factor)

Her base-line daily caloric intake—the current level that maintains her at 75 kg weight—is 2,500 kcal/day. We'll assume that, like many folks, Ms. "X" eats three meals a day and that her caloric allocations among the three meals are as follows:

Base-Line Meals	Calories
Breakfast	450
Lunch	900
Dinner	1150
Total =	2500

Figure 20.2 Ms. "X" caloric allocations among daily meals

With a body mass index (BMI) of 33, our hypothetical Ms. "X" realizes she is overweight and decides to go on a diet to slim down. With this book in hand, she decides to follow the three-steps of the "Better Strategy/Approach" of Figure 20.1, and proceeds as follows:

- Step 1: Set a weight-loss target to lose 7.5% of her weight in 3 months
- Step 2: Run *Mi Model* to determine the daily caloric deficit needed to achieve *her* weight-loss target.

  Upon executing *Mi Model*, she obtains the following results:

  > *Mi Model's* Recommended Intervention: A daily energy intake of 8.4 MJ = 2,000 kcal (which amounts to a 20% cut to her current food intake level)

  > *Mi Model's* Predicted Outcomes
  > Weight loss: 5.5 kg after 3 months.
  > Percent body fat drops to: 27 %
  > BMI: Drops to 30.8

- Step 3: Design palatable and satisfying meals.

To design her three palatable and satisfying meals, Ms. "X" wisely turns to *Mi Volumetrics* next. To demo *Mi Volumetrics'* application, we'll help Ms. X design one of her three meals, namely, lunch. (The process for breakfast and dinner is essentially the same.)

The first decision she needs to make is the allocation of her total daily caloric intake of 2,000 kcal among the three meals. Obviously, this is an entirely personal preference that reflects lifestyle, family circumstances, and sometimes even culture. We'll assume that she decides to follow the typical meal allocations proposed in Barbara Rolls' volumetrics books, namely, 20% to breakfast, 30% to lunch and 50% to dinner. For Ms. X's lunch, this translates to a 600 kcal meal.

Generally speaking, composing a 600 kcal lunch is no big deal. But that's not what we are after. What we seek to accomplish is much more ambitious and is much more personalized: to design the "optimal" lunch for Ms. "X." A lunch that:

- Is also satiating to *her*.
- Includes only food items that *she likes* (or can afford).

- (If needed) meets any other *personal requirements* (e.g., a ceiling on the amount of calories from fat).

Composing such a meal is not only significantly more challenging, but is also very personal. For example, what satisfies Ms. "X" might not satisfy you or me. Which is why identifying *her preferences* is where we need to start. There are several, but first and foremost we need to identify what meal size (weight) satisfies her (the top bullet above). Once we establish this important threshold (and what will be important here is the *minimum* satiation threshold), we can then proceed to compose the optimal mix of food stuffs that meet her caloric target and any other preferences or requirements.

Listen to your Gut

We've already learned that food bulk has the overriding influence on satiety—on what makes us feel full. A meal's weight, not energy content, in other words, is the key to what makes our bodies say we've eaten enough. Thus, the question for Ms. "X" (and any prospective dieter): what *is* the lunch weight that satisfies? The answer is neither obvious nor universal—it will differ from person to person. Nevertheless, it is a question we need to answer... correctly. Indeed, I'd argue, it is a piece of self-knowledge that behooves any prospective dieter to ascertain.

To help Ms. "X" answer this pertinent question, we turn to Dr. Brian Wansink and his group at Cornell University's Food and Brand Lab whose work on the issue has proved most illuminating.[614] Their research suggests that a person's satiation level is not characterized by just a single number (say 800 grams). Rather, Wansink and his team found that most people are perfectly content (and indifferent) consuming meals that fall within a gratifying margin—and which for most people is approximately 20 percent above to 20 percent below their so-called nominal satiation level. They called this range the *satiated margin*. When we eat meals that fall within that weight range—our *satiated margin*—we feel fine (content) and are indifferent of the small differences.

Figuring out one's *satiated margin* (e.g., for a lunch meal) isn't difficult. It simply requires experimenting with meal sizes that satisfy us and measuring/

recording their weights. To increase the reliability of and confidence in our assessment—and because we seek to determine a *range*—one would need to collect multiple data points, say a week's worth. After each lunch, one of two methods may be used to assess the meal's total weight: (1) physically weighing the meal (e.g., using a food scale); or (2) using **Mi Volumetrics**. With the latter approach, one would simply need to enter the food items into the **Mi Volumetrics** spreadsheet and use its built-in weight-calculator to compute the meal's total weight.

To demo, I'll assess the weight of Ms. X's pre-diet (maintenance) lunch—which at 900 kcal is 50% above her new caloric target. That pre-diet lunch is, however, what she's been eating to feel satiated.

Mi Volumetrics has separate sheets to enter food selections for each of the three meals: breakfast, lunch and dinner. To facilitate the search for/and selection of food items, the database of 600 food items is organized into food categories such as "Breads and Grains," "Cereals," "Fruits," "Beverages," etc. Each category, in turn, contains many food items. For example, the "Breads and Grains" category contains 57 entries of food items such as: bagels, French bread, rye, sourdough, etc.

As shown below (Figure 20.3), each food category has an adjacent empty cell (to its left) into which the user can enter a selection from within the category (for example, selecting French bread from the topmost "Breads and Grains" category). Notice that in the *Categories* column, some categories appear more than once. This is to allow the user to include multiple selections (such as for "Vegetables") into a meal.

LUNCH (Menu Options Below)	Categories
	Breads and Grains
	Legumes
	Milk, Yogurt, and Cheese
	Milk, Yogurt, and Cheese
	Soups
	Vegetables
	Vegetables
	Meats, Poultry, and Fish
	Meats, Poultry, and Fish
	Chips, Pretzels, and Other Snacks
	Mixed Foods
	Mixed Foods
	Fast Food
	Fast Food
	Condiments, Dressings, and Sauce
	Condiments, Dressings, and Sauce
	Beverages
	Fruit
	Fruit
	Desserts
	Desserts
	Candy

Figure 20.3: Food entry template

To compose Ms. X's base-line (pre-diet) lunch, she would enter the food items comprising her lunch into the above empty form. She obviously needs to enter food selections for only those food categories that apply to her. For food categories that do not apply, she would leave the entry cell blank. For example, if she does not eat soup for lunch, that row will be left empty.

For those categories that apply, selecting a specific food item for her lunch is straightforward. This is done by simply clicking on the *empty cell* adjacent to a category of interest. When a category's empty cell is clicked, a sub-menu showing the category's list of food options will open up from which an item may be selected. The Figure below shows the sub-menu of food options that opens up when the user clicks on the entry cell for "Breads and Grains."

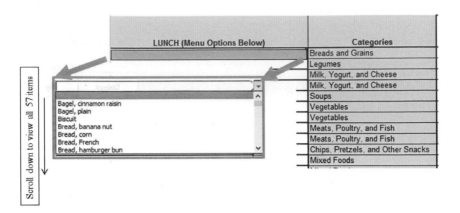

Figure 20.4: The "Breads and Grains" menu
(shown here as the Green box) opens up

The seven items shown in Figure 20.4 are just the top seven entries from a list of 57 food items within the "Breads and Grains" category. To see the rest, one simply scrolls down the list. Once the user finds the "Bread and Grains" food item they would like to select (say French bread), they would click on it to enter it as their selection.

When the selection is made, a default serving size will automatically be displayed (e.g., the default serving size for soup is "a cup of soup"). If this default serving size is the right serving size, nothing further needs to be done for that entry. If not, the user can adjust it (for example, doubling or tripling the serving size).

Below then are Ms. X's entries for her satiating (but calorically rich) pre-diet lunch (Figure 20.5).

		a. Enter value		d. Enter Value
LUNCH (Menu Options Below)	**Categories**		**Default Serving Size**	**My Serving Size**
	Breads and Grains			
	Legumes			
	Milk, Yogurt, and Cheese			
Yogurt, fruit-flavors, 99 percent fat-free	Milk, Yogurt, and Cheese		6 oz	Same
	Soups			
Lettuce, romaine	Vegetables		1 cup	Same
Potatoes, French-fried	Vegetables		1 ounce	Same
	Meats, Poultry, and Fish			
	Meats, Poultry, and Fish			
	Chips, Pretzels, and Other Snacks			
	Mixed Foods			
	Mixed Foods			
	Fast Food			
KFC, Extra Tasty Crispy Chicken breast	Fast Food		1 piece (5.9 oz.)	Same
	Condiments, Dressings, and Sauce			
Pickles, dill	Condiments, Dressings, and Sauce		1 item, 3 3/4" long	Same
	Beverages			
Orange	Fruit		1 item (medium)	Same
	Fruit			
	Desserts			
	Desserts			
	Candy			

Figure 20.5: Ms. "X" pre-diet lunch selections

Once the lunch entries are completed, *Mi Volumetrics* automatically calculates and displays the meal's total weight and caloric content:

Lunch Weight (gm)	**:**	**600**
Lunch Calories	**:**	**860**

Figure 20.6

With this, Ms. "X" has determined the weight of one (perhaps typical) pre-diet lunch—a size of lunch she's been eating to feel satiated.

To demarcate her *satiated margin*, Ms. "X" needs to repeat this exercise (at least) six more days using different lunch compositions. Let's assume she obliges and after seven lunch experiments she determines that the range of lunch sizes that satiate her are from 600-1,000 grams. (Or, using Brian Wansink's format, her satiating range is 800 grams ± 25%.) The minimum threshold of the range—600 grams—is the critical number here since it designates the minimum threshold below which she would remain hungry after consuming the meal.

Charting her New Course

At this point, Ms. "X" has delineated the key targets for her diet plan:

- Weight Loss: 7.5% of current weight in 3 months
- Daily caloric intake: 2,000 kcal (a 20% drop from her current level)
    - Lunch caloric intake: 600 kcal (30% of the daily total)
    - Lunch *satiated margin*: 600 – 1,000 grams

Before proceeding to the third and final step—designing her palatable and satisfying lunch—it may be instructive for her (indeed for any prospective dieter) to *integrate* the above set of variables into one compact graphic. *Mi EDPP* is the tool to do just that. It is a handy tool that can help Ms. "X" not only visualize where she stands but also "nudges" her towards the optimal path forward.

First, where does she stand? Ms. X's current satiating lunches lie on the (iso-caloric) 900 kcal curve on the segment between the 600 and 1,000 gram circles (Figure 20.7). The minimum threshold of her satiating margin, the 600 grams circle, is highlighted for good reason—it demarcates her critical "hungry circle." (The narrow arrow within her hungry circle designates where her *smallest* satiating pre-diet lunch would lie—at the intersection of the iso-caloric 900 kcal curve and the 600-grams-circle. The two curves intersect at the 1.5 kcal/gram energy density ray—designating the meal's *average* energy density.) Second, *Mi EDPP* also helps prescribe her optimal path forward. As depicted, she needs to "change lanes"—move from the 900 to the 600 iso-caloric hook. And once there, she needs to move along the segment of the 600 iso-caloric curve that's on the outside of the 600 gram circle (her minimum threshold for satiety). That is, she needs to compose meals that fall along the green arrow.

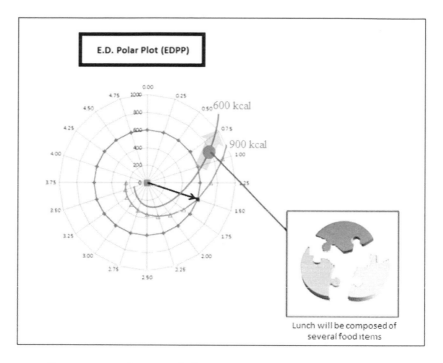

E.D. Polar Plot (EDPP)

Figure 20.7: Where Ms. "X" stands ... and where she needs to go

Designing meals that fall within the narrow band of the green arrow dramatically reduces the number of options she needs to consider and should appreciably simplify her meal planning task. Appreciably, but not totally. Why? Even within the narrow band of options demarcated by the green arrow—lunches that are above 600 grams in total weight and with an average energy density between 0.75 and 1.0 kcal/gram—she is still left with a host of variables to juggle. For example:

1) As with a jigsaw puzzle, a meal is typically composed of more than one food item—sometimes many more. This means there will be many options to mix and match when composing meals that meet particular targets such as energy density. For example, picking an energy density target within the designated range of 0.75-1.0 kcal/gram, say 0.8 kcal/gram, does *not* mean picking only food items with exactly that value. Rather, she can

pick some food items with higher energy density some with lower as long as the *average* of the entire meal is 0.8 kcal/gram. This provides flexibility, of course, but also complicates the selection task.

2) In addition to weight, caloric content, and energy density, our stated (ambitious) goal is to compose optimal meals that also reflect her *personal* preferences (e.g., for things like taste, accessibility, and affordability). This adds additional personalizing dimensions that need to be factored in. And is why **Mi Volumetrics** employs elaborate templates to enter the user's food preferences and the option to specify "Must Have" items.

3) (If needed or necessary), there could be additional requirements to satisfy (such as to limit the amount of fat or carbohydrate calories in the diet).

And she needs to accomplish all of that while sifting through a vast database of no less than 600 different food items!

Ms. X has a classic problem on her hand... a problem of *optimization*.

Meal Optimization... or what's Best?

Most succinctly, optimization is the task of seeking to select the *best* possible course of action (often from among several available to us) that maximizes some desired objective (e.g., the meal's total weight) while abiding by certain constraints (e.g., not exceed a caloric ceiling).

It is a very common type of problem that decision makers face every day. Business managers, lawmakers, engineers, investors and others who have been grappling with such complex optimization problems have long appreciated that intuition alone is unreliable in tackling them and have learned to turn to computer models for help. Today, optimization is among the most widely used applications of computer modelling.

Optimization is everywhere: Going to Disney World this summer, Optimization will be your ubiquitous companion, scheduling the crews and planes, pricing the airline tickets and hotel rooms, even helping to set capacities on the theme park rides. If you use Orbitz to book your flights, an optimization engine sifts through millions of options to find the cheapest fares. If you get directions to your hotel room from MapQuest, another optimization engine figures out the most direct route. If you ship souvenirs home, an optimization engine tells UPS which truck to put the packages on, exactly where on the truck the packages should go to make them fastest to load and unload, and what route the driver should follow to make his deliveries most efficiently.[615]

While computer-supported optimization continues to make impressive inroads in business, public policy, and the military their use in personal health management remains limited however. This needs to change—and slowly *is* changing. Few would disagree that health is precisely the setting where sub op timality is the most problematic and where the stakes are the highest. As we start assuming more responsibility for managing our health, the ability to understand and (effectively use) optimization models will (I believe) fast become a prerequisite for effectively managing our well-being. This is not to suggest that we all need to become model builders. What I am suggesting is that we all need to become capable model consumers.

So….

Does the everyday task of optimizing meal planning—an everyday activity that most people are intimately experienced with—justify computer optimization? In the next section we'll see why the answer is yes.

(When Optimizing) Don't Listen to your Gut

To demonstrate the need for and utility of optimization tools for even simple selection tasks, I'll use an introductory example I often use to kick-off the Decision Analysis course I teach at the Naval Postgraduate School. To avert a mass student exodus on the first day of class, I use a simpler variant of Ms. X's meal composition task. Rather than ask the students to select from hundreds of food items, I present them with a much smaller (a hundred times smaller) seven-item menu. Specifically, I ask them to tackle the following exercise: select from a given set of seven food items a meal that *maximizes* total meal weight without exceeding 1,500 calories.

The seven food items and their characteristics are (Figure 20.8):

	Food item	Calories	Weight
1	Pizza, thin crust, pepperoni	500	160
2	McDonald's French Fries	250	80
3	McDonald's apple Pie, baked	350	100
4	KFC Chicken Breast	600	200
5	Ice Cream cone, Choc Covered	700	220
6	Fish, King Salmon	450	120
7	White Cake with Frosting	300	80

Figure 20.8 Seven food options

What would be that optimal meal? (A note to the reader: before proceeding, I suggest you take a few minutes to derive your own optimal meal composition. It could be instructive—and maybe even fun!)

Over the years my students' performances have been remarkably consistent and, I suspect, representative of what most folks would do. What I have found (and is consistent with what other researchers have as well) is that in dealing with such seemingly simple "what's best" problems, decision-makers invariably rely on "rules of thumb" or "heuristics" rather than cumbersome math. Heuristics are convenient (occasionally sufficient) mental short-cuts we routinely rely on in many judgmental tasks we face to simplify our world. Indeed, it almost seems to be part of human nature. ("The technical definition of *heuristic* is a simple procedure that helps find adequate, though often imperfect, answers to difficult questions. The word comes from the same root as eureka."[616]) These mental shortcuts are an efficient quick-and-dirty strategy that helps us reduce mental effort and speed up the process of finding satisfactory solutions... most of the time. Unfortunately, these "short-cuts" can lead to systematic errors in certain cases. As they do here.

Going back to our class exercise: For many of my students, a common (and perfectly reasonable) approach is to sort the foods in the list (some sort by calories others by weight or energy density) and then go through the list top-to-bottom picking food items until the total caloric target is reached.

Below (Figure 20.9) I show the solution that would be selected when the seven food items are sorted by energy-density (the most common approach):

	Food item	Calories	Weight	E.D.	cum cal		Cum wt
4	KFC Chicken Breast	600	200	3.00	600		200
1	Pizza, thin crust, pepperoni	500	160	3.13	1,100		360
2	McDonald's French Fries	250	80	3.13	1,350	←	440
5	Ice Cream cone, Choc Covered	700	220	3.18	2,050		
3	McDonald's apple Pie, baked	350	100	3.50	2,400		
6	Fish, King Salmon	450	120	3.75	2,850		
7	White Cake with Frosting	300	80	3.75	3,150		

Figure 20.9: Solution when sorting by energy density

Not bad… but it is *not* the best (optimal) meal. Nor are the solutions derived when the food items are sorted by weight or calories. To understand why, let's take a closer look at the above solution. In this case, the student/dieter sorts the seven food items by energy density (from the lowest item #4 to highest item #7) and then, starting at the top, proceeds to select foods on the list (while cumulatively adding the total number of calories) until they hit the caloric ceiling. This leads to the selection of food items # 4, 1, and 2.

- It produces a meal with a total weight = 440 grams and with 1,350 total calories

- The meal's weight cannot be increased further without exceeding the 1,500 caloric target since all remaining food items (# 5, 3, 6, and 7) pack more than 150 calories.

Again, not bad… but (as noted) there is a *better* solution which uses the caloric budget more effectively!

But it requires a proper optimization tool (such as **Mi Volumetrics**) to derive it. The optimal solution (Figure 20.10) selects food item 3 instead of item 2. By selecting food items 4, 1, 3 we compose the *optimal* (most satisfying) meal for the dieter: with a total weight of 460 grams and a total caloric content of 1,450 kcal. Here is the solution:

	Food item	Calories	Weight		cum cal		Cum wt
1	Pizza, thin crust, pepperoni	500	160		500		160
3	McDonald's apple Pie, baked	350	100		850		260
4	KFC Chicken Breast	600	200		1,450	⬅	460
2	McDonald's French Fries	250	80		1,700		
7	White Cake with Frosting	300	80		2,000		
6	Fish, King Salmon	450	120		2,450		
5	Ice Cream cone, Choc Covered	700	220		3,150		

Figure 20.10: Optimal Solution

In the table below (Figure 20.11), I compare my students' three "intuitive" solutions to the optimal one.

Rule of Thumb	Meal Total Weight (grams)
Sort by Calories	380
Sort by Weight	420
Sort by Energy Density	440
Optimal Solution	460

Figure 20.11: Comparing Solutions

In this class exercise, the three suboptimal solutions are not that far off, but that's only because the problem is overly simplified with only seven food items (not 600). As the problem gets bigger, the divergence between what's optimal and what's not grows… and the stakes will be higher.

The bottom-line "lesson:" *when it comes to optimization-type problems, better not to listen to your gut.* The intuitive approach often fails us.

Luckily, as already noted, that's precisely where computer tools can help. Utilizing these models, dieters, like managers, business analysts, policy makers, and engineers now have a decision-support tool to search through a messy maze of food options and learn quickly and cost-effectively answers that would seldom be obtainable through raw intuition.

With this in mind, let's now return to our non-academic scenario of 600-plus food items and demo the application of *Mi Volumetrics* to design the optimal lunch for Ms. "X." Specifically, helping her select food items that maximize her lunch's bulk without exceeding the caloric target she set for losing weight.

Optimizing Meal Selection using *Mi Volumetrics*

At this point, Ms. "X" has already accomplished two necessary preparatory steps:

1) Set a weight-loss target to lose 7.5% of her weight in 3 months.

2) Determined her daily energy intake target at 2,000 calories (using *Mi Model*). And based on that, determined her desired caloric allocations among the three meals to be: 400 calories for breakfast, 600 for lunch and 1,000 for dinner.

To compose her optimal "palatable and satisfying" lunch (the remaining third step), she has also determined that her *minimum* satiating threshold for lunch is 600 grams (and her satiating margin: 600 – 1,000 grams).

With this in hand, she is now ready to deploy *Mi Volumetrics* to design her optimal meal. This third step has three sub-steps (A, B and C):

A. Using the *Mi Volumetrics'* food selection templates, she needs to enter desirable food candidates. In this first sub-step, it is important to note, she is not yet designing *the* meal, rather she is casting a wide net to include all desirable food *candidates* that may be used to compose her lunch. The more food candidates she enters here, the wider the net she casts and the more helpful the program will be. (Users are, thus, advised to take the time to fill the entire selection-template and not leave any cells blank.)

To accomplish this, Ms. X would go through the list of food categories one at a time and,

   o From each category, pick the food item she would like to be considered (e.g. Plain Bagel in "Breads and Grains" or Diet Cola in "Beverages").

o If she's O.K. with the default serving size for a selection, she would do nothing, and move to the next category. If her desired serving size is different, she can override the default value (e.g., selecting a serving size that is double or triple the default value).

o She may (but doesn't have to) designate up to 3 food entries as "MUST HAVES." The program will oblige by forcing these to be included in the optimal solution.

B. In the second sub-step, she specifies the constraints that her optimal meal needs to satisfy. Constrains are certain performance criteria that the optimal meal must meet. There are two:

(a) The meal's total *weight* needs to equal or exceed her minimal satiating threshold. In this case, her meal needs to equal or exceed 600 grams.

(b) The meal's total *caloric content* needs to equal or be less than her caloric target. In this case be equal to or less than 600 kcal.

When done entering her food selections and constrains, Ms. X could then proceed to run the Optimization function.

C. In the third and final sub-step, she runs the *Mi Volumetrics'* optimization function to compose her optimal lunch. This is accomplished by clicking the "Run Optimization" button.

In a few milliseconds, *Mi Volumetrics*, will oblige and display an optimal solution. Below (Figure 20.12)is an example optimal meal composed by the model (showing the meal's six selected food items and their servings).

RESULTS

Proposed Lunch Entries	Servings
Cream of mushroom soup, condensed, canned, prepared with 2 percent milk	1
Lettuce, romaine	1
Chili, vegetarian with three beans	1
Pickles, dill	1
Wine, red	1
Orange	1

569	Calories
836	Wt (gm)

Lunch Weight (gm): 836

Lunch Calories: 569

Figure 20.12: Optimal meal

As shown, the optimal lunch's total weight is 836 grams (smack in the middle of her satiating margin) and its total caloric content is 569 (below her target ceiling of 600 kcal). Furthermore, it is a meal composed of food items *she* likes. Ms. "X" has just composed her optimal lunch. *Mission accomplished!*

Because the **Mi Volumterics'** database (and model) has been augmented to incorporate additional nutritional data elements, Ms. "X" can utilize the tool to accomplish even more. For example, **Mi Volumetrics** can provide Ms. "X" with a breakdown of the macronutrient content of her optimal meal as shown in Figure 20.13. Proper nutrient composition is paramount to maximize energy level, well-being, and overall health. Which is why tracking the nutritional composition of our food intake is always important—but is *especially so when dieting.* On a diet we are eating less, thus we are at a higher risk of not getting an adequate amount of nutrients. Below is the macronutrient composition of Ms. X's optimal meal.

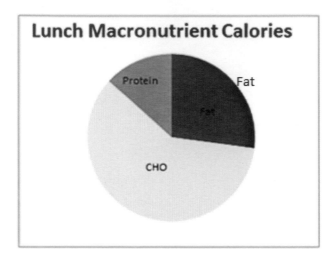

Figure 20.13: Macronutrient composition of Ms. X's optimal meal

Upon displaying the macronutrient composition, Ms. "X" can then re-deploy *Mi Volumetrics* to customize her optimal meal even further e.g., to design meals that achieve *additional* objectives. Indeed, that's precisely where optimization-type models are really at their best—allowing us to explore (and devise) new and better strategies when pursuing our goals. For example, the *Mi Volumterics* tool can be utilized to design meals that do not exceed targets for fat- or carbohydrate-derived calories or that include a minimum amount of fiber (e.g., to satisfy health-related dictates).

Mi Volumetrics versus the "Old ways"

Finally, it may be instructive to compare the *Mi Volumetrics* approach to the traditional way of meal planning. To do that, I'll compare Ms. X—our sophisticated user of *Mi Model* and *Mi Volumetrics*—to a Ms. "Old-ways," a friend of Ms. "X" who also starts at the same weight (75 kg) and base-line diet (2,500 kcal) and who has also decided to go on a diet to lose weight. I'll also assume that her satiated threshold is similar to Ms. X (600 grams for lunch). Her base-line (pre-diet) satiating lunch (again, just like Ms. "X") is a 900 kcal lunch and at 600 grams yields an average energy density of 1.5 kcal/gram.

That's where the similarities between the two friends end. Moving forward, Ms. "Old ways" approaches her weight-loss effort in manner that's very different from that of Ms. "X":

- Rather than picking a realistic goal, she goes for her "dream" goal: To lose 10 kg (equivalent to 22 pounds) in 3 months

- Rather than using **Mi Model**, she relies on the energy balance equation (the 3,500 kcal per pound rule) Her calculus, thus, proceeds as follows:
  - 22 pounds are worth: $22*3,500 = 77,000$ kcal
  - 77,000 kcal deficit over 3 months (90 days) translates to $77,000 / 90 = 855$ kcal/day
  - This means she needs to reduce her daily caloric intake from 2,500 kcal to $2500 - 855 = 1,645$ kcal
  - Using the same meal allocations as Ms. "X," her lunch's caloric content $= 0.3 * 1,645 = 493$ kcal

- Rather than using **Mi Volumetrics** to compose an optimal lunch, we'll assume she uses the common (though naïve) strategy of simply eating smaller portions of the foods she is currently eating. This means that while her lunch's bulk will decrease, the meal's energy density (of 1.5 kcal/gram) stays the same. From this we can calculate that her 493 kcal lunch will weigh approximately 330 grams

The table below compares the two dieters' situations.

	Ms. "X"	Ms. "Old-ways"
Current Weight	75 kg (BMI: 33)	75 kg (BMI: 33)
Current SS Daily Food Intake	2,500 kcal	2,500 kcal
Current Lunch	900 kcal, 600 grams	900 kcal, 600 grams
Weight-Loss target	5.5 kg in 3 months	10 kg in 3 months
Diet Caloric Intake	2,000 kcal (Lunch: 600 kcal)	1,645 kcal (Lunch: 493 kcal)
Lunch (optimal)	600 kcal, 836 grams	493 kcal, 330 grams

Figure 20.14

The striking differences between the two dieting friends' meal plans are nicely manifested when plotted on **Mi EDPP**. As Figure 20.15 clearly indicates, Ms. X is meeting her caloric target and does so on a meal plan that does not leave her feeling hungry and deprived—her optimal meal falls outside the 600 gram "hungry circle." Ms. "Old ways" lunch, on the other hand, falls within the hungry circle (because it is below the 600 gram threshold) leaving her feeling hungry and deprived. Which doesn't bode well for her long-term prospects. In all likelihood, she'll just wind up hungry and unhappy and most probably will go back to her old ways.

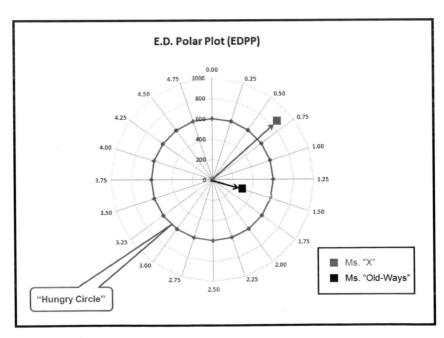

Figure 20.15: Comparison of the two friends

CHAPTER 21

Mi Analytics

What's measured improves.

Peter F. Drucker

Mi Model and **Mi Volumetrics** are tools we developed to help dieters devise better (more customized) plans and strategies for achieving their weight-loss goals. That's good and well, but it is important to remember that without effective execution, even the best of plans won't amount to much. It will just be fantasy. Peter F. Drucker, the management guru, put it best: "Plans are only good intentions unless they immediately degenerate into hard work."

For many dieters, the Achilles heel to successful execution is *measurement*. According to John Jakicic, a professor at the University of Pittsburgh and a researcher in the field of long-term weight control, there is a simple reason for why most people have trouble succeeding in losing weight: "While everyone understands they have to burn more calories than they take in, most people don't know how many calories they burn a day... they have no clue."[617] Well... it *is* important to have a clue.

In managing personal health, the importance of accurate monitoring and timely feedback cannot be overstated. Continuous feedback about how one is doing is essential in sustaining the process of change—especially in chronic conditions such as obesity. Self-monitoring provides the feedback needed for evaluating one's progress, assessing and (if needed) revising strategies, and increasing one's sense of self-regulatory efficacy. Which may explain why self-monitoring has been found, in numerous studies, to be substantially associated with greater weight loss and maintenance and why it has been described as the "cornerstone" of behavioral treatments of obesity.[618, 619,620]

Accurate and timely self-monitoring, however, can be hard work. On the energy expenditure side, getting a clue—or at least a reasonable estimate—of energy expenditure often required the use of complex scientific equipment or a visit to a laboratory. Guess how often people took that approach? On the input side of the equation, monitoring energy intake can be similarly burdensome. Until recently, the most often used method of tracking food intake was the paper record. As anyone who's ever tried to keep a regular journal knows, use of a paper record and its associated work of looking up nutrient content of foods and calculating totals can become tedious and time-consuming.

Thankfully, things are changing. Digital self-tracking devices designed to accurately gauge physical activity and track calories burned are significantly lessening the burden of self-monitoring by taking the effort out of recording and compiling.

It is truly a *new* development.

The *Third* Digital Transformation

After the mainframe and the personal computing eras, we now stand at the brink of a *third* digital transformation. This so-called third wave in computing is all about *ubiquitous computing*—in which (intelligent) information-processing technologies diffuse into our everyday objects and activities. An array of innovations across the technology landscape are converging to make smart, connected *ubiquitous computing* devices technically and economically feasible. These include breakthroughs in the performance, miniaturization, and energy efficiency of sensors and batteries; highly compact, low-cost computer processing power and data storage (which make it feasible to add intelligence to wearable products); and low-cost wireless connectivity.

Already, an ambitious breed of behavior tracking devices and apps are becoming an integral accessory to our daily lives. These affordable, wearable computing capabilities promise to transform their owners into personal data collectors, able to analyze and improve the minutiae of their daily lives—what they eat and how much they move and play. They include sensors and tracking devices that will enable us to easily monitor an enormous number of diverse (physiologic) states— including weight, blood pressure, movement (steps taken), body fat levels, caloric intake, etc. The prodigious amount of personal data these smart connected products will generate, many believe, will alter the nature of personal health management and transform health self-regulation.

In the remainder of this chapter I discuss in more detail some of these promising technologies and their functionality.

Self-Knowledge through Self-Tracking

The new breed of behavior-tracking devices are benefiting greatly from the development and deployment of small, non-invasive sensors that can autonomously and continually monitor biologic characteristics that are of vital concern to anyone trying to slim down. The overarching goal of such mobile-wearable systems is to provide us with personal tools to enhance the way our bodies communicate their needs to us so that we can respond promptly to our shifting interior landscapes and ultimately transform personal health regulation into an information science, where data and computing are marshaled to revolutionize health monitoring and decision-making.

"Watch" this

I started writing this chapter on March 9th, 2015, the day Apple officially launched their Apple Watch. It is the latest entry into the nascent segment of wearable fitness tracking devices and apps that aim to enhance the capacity (and convenience) to gather and analyze personal health data. According to an Apple video, Apple Watch has the features of an "all-day fitness tracker." An accelerometer measures movement, while an "activity app" captures various metrics, including calories burned, daily exercise time and number of times the wearer stands up during the day, all "with the goal of helping you sit less, move more and get some exercise."

While the Apple Watch is not the first fitness tracker on the market, Apple's size and influence as a trendsetter is expected to focus attention on the potential of this blossoming genre of wearable (computing) devices. Some market observers (Juniper Research) are already predicting that broader-use wearable devices, like the Apple Watch, will eventually eclipse the simpler fitness-oriented devices currently on the market. We'll see.

For now, though, the "hottest" market niche is unquestionably those *simpler* personal activity-tracking bracelets whose (apparent) attraction is that they provide all the computing functionality wherever the user might be. The benefit: making us constantly aware of how active we are (or aren't). The research firm ABI estimates that 42 million fitness and heath wearable devices were shipped in 2014, up from 32 million in 2013. It's a steep upward trend that is showing no signs of slowing down. (Juniper Research predicts unit sales will approximately double to more than 70 million by 2018). [621]

Among the current generation leaders of *personal activity-tracking bracelets* are: the Jawbone Up band, Nike's FuelBand and Fitbit (the current market share leader).

All three devices incorporate sensors—called accelerometers—that collect information about movement in three directions (up and down, side to side, and forward and back), which is then fed into algorithms that analyze that movement to determine whether someone is walking, jumping or sleeping restfully. The devices rely on mathematical equations that were developed using popular activities, such as brisk walking or jogging. (Light-intensity activities or more subtle movements, such as gently pedaling a stationary bicycle are not detected as well. But we can expect this to improve quickly.[622])

In terms of design, all three are in the form of textured rubber bracelets. Nike's Fuelband and Fitbit incorporate a built-in screen but jawbone's UP does not. The screen makes a powerful difference. It means that you can see how you're doing without needing a smart phone. On Nike's FuelBand, as an example, with each press of the adjacent button, the word "Steps" or "Calories" or "Time" scrolls by on a matrix of very bright LED lights.[623]

Most activity trackers can also connect—through a wireless (Bluetooth) connection or using USB cable—to apps running on a smartphone or computer to upload activity information (such as a day's worth of activity or a consumed meal) into applications that can crunch the numbers to provide more detailed analyses. The analytical apps can be as basic as a Facebook-style timeline of daily activities or more advanced software that spins activity data to generate elaborate charts and graphics (e.g., to show trends in daily behavior and/or provide feedback on how one stands in relation to personal targets). And with a continuously expanding capacity to store historical statistics, some of these applications are now allowing users to compare a day's results with performances from past weeks and even months.

When combined with a smartphone, additional types and forms of personal data (besides physical activity) may be collected and analyzed. For example, smartphone apps allow users to track food intake by scanning bar codes on food items in a supermarket or by choosing from a categorized list of common foodstuffs in a database. These food-tracker apps can then provide a food log and analyze how caloric intake stacks up against calories burned, as well as the percentage of fats, carbohydrates and proteins eaten. By significantly reducing the burden of recording and compiling—effectively "liberating" users from having to look up foods in a nutrient booklet and calculating the nutrient content of foods consumed—these food-tracking tools should help dieters become more aware of their eating behaviors, improve adherence to self-monitoring and to dietary goals, and improve long-term dietary changes.

The Upshot

The point of self-tracking isn't just to accumulate data. Easily accessible feedback about physical activity and food intake, it is hoped, will provide users with the agency needed to begin or maintain healthy behavior change. Self-trackers, in other words, want to convert that data into better behavior, better habits—in short, better health.[624,625] And, indeed, they seem to being doing just that. For example, "…studies have shown that if there's some visible, omnipresent monitor of your negative behavior—spending too little energy, eating too much food—you're far more likely to correct it."[626]

Towards that end, the latest iteration of self-tracking devices are adding several new motivational "arrows" to their quiver. Many, for example, now incorporate social networking motivational components. By adding new comparatives, they let users compare their data with friends (or to the average of their age group) online, establishing a friendly rivalry or at least guilt.

Even more proactively, many of the latest devices now brandish vibrating alarms that can wake users from naps, or nudge its wearer at intervals throughout the day to remind them to stay active. (Apple Watch calls its functionality a "taptic engine," which taps users on the wrist with a tactile sensation to induce a nudge.) Simply donning one of these devices works as a fancier version of a string tied around one's finger: a reminder to get up and move.

All this should serve to improve self-regulation and increase dieter compliance (e.g., to the *Mi Model* and *Mi Volumetrics* plans). But there is also a second, perhaps less apparent, beneficial effect. By receiving personalized feedback data that are accurate, complete, relevant, and readily accessible in a format that can be used for performance analysis, one invariably learns a great deal about oneself. Eventually, wearable devices will help people understand more of their bodies' behaviors and help them find better ways to tweak them. And ultimately, by advancing self-knowledge through self-tracking with technology people can find a better route to self-improvement and develop their capacities so that their human potential finds its optimal expression.

CHAPTER 22

Smarter Than We Think

[In 1998,] the year after his defeat by Deep Blue, Garry Kasparov set out to see what would happen if he paired a machine and a human chess player in a collaboration. Like a centaur, the hybrid would have the strength of each of its components: the processing power of a large logic circuit and the intuition of a human brain's wetware. The result: human-machine teams, even when they didn't include the best grandmasters or most powerful computers, consistently beat teams composed solely of human grandmasters or superfast machines.[627]

This is one of the many interesting examples in Clive Thompson's new book *Smarter Than You Think; How Technology Is Changing Our Minds For The Better* of how human-computer symbiosis is enlarging our intellect. In the book, Thompson convincingly makes the case that "intelligence amplification"—the symbiotic smarts that occur when human cognition is augmented by a close interaction with computers—will allow us to perform at higher levels, accomplishing acts of reasoning that are impossible for us alone.

Nowhere is this more essential, and potentially more rewarding, than in managing our health and wellbeing. Personal health, after all, is precisely the setting where complexities are the most problematic and where the stakes are the highest.

A good case in point: managing human weight and energy regulation. As argued in this book, managing our weights—and our bodies—is not unlike managing any complex system, a task that requires skill and the right tools. Motivation alone is not enough. With its many interrelated subsystems and feedback processes (some counteracting, some reinforcing), the human energy and weight regulation system is simply too complex to effectively manage by human intuition alone. The system's complexities are neither capricious nor mysterious, and (as we learned) have a lot to do with the body's homeostatic processes—its adaptive (and defensive) mechanisms that continuously aim to maintain the body's internal stability in the face of internal or external threats to that stability. Our bodies cannot leave energy metabolism to chance; lack of energy means failure to thrive, and often, failure to survive.[628]

The redundancy and complex compensatory interactions that characterize human energy regulation are what make it difficult to interrupt and manage. Luckily, that's where "intelligence amplification"—the symbiotic smarts that occur when human cognition is augmented by a close interaction with computers—can help. Unlike a mental model, computer models can reliably and efficiently trace through time the implications of a messy maze of interactions. And they can do so efficiently and reliably and without stumbling over cognitive bias or gaps in intuition. Computer models can, thus, help us fill the gap where human cognition is most suspect.

It's why many in public health increasingly believe that the growing—and synergistic—entwinement of the healing and information sciences is our ticket not just to cure disease but to develop our capacities to prevent it. When fully unleashed, an expanding repertoire of personal information technologies will empower ordinary people with the learning and *tailored* decision-making tools they need to more effectively manage personal well-being—with potentially far-reaching transformative consequences.

This is no futuristic vision or wishful thinking. All the technological building-blocks to provide a new generation of tailored tools for personal health management are available… here and now. For example, thanks to the great advances in medical and computational sciences, we already have the models to predict with greater fidelity how the human body regulates its energy and mass (**Mi Model** is an example). And thanks to the availability of ubiquitous computing elements—already imbedded in our phones, homes, and even cloths—we can capture, analyze and communicate the physiologic data needed to personalize these models.

Finally, the Internet provides the infrastructure to efficiently and economically deliver these tools to large numbers of people.

But for that to happen, individuals—consumers—will need to step up and lead the way. Without the active participation of consumers in this revolution, the process will be inexorably slowed.[629] The stakes riding on our success/failure obviously are enormous, not only for individual well-being but for the nation's economic health as well.

REFERENCES

1   Cutler, D.M., Glaeser, E.L. and Shapiro, J.M. (2003). Why Have Americans Become More Obese? *Journal of Economic Perspectives,* 17(3), 93-118.

2   Grady, D. (2003, November 11). What Should we Eat? *New York Times,* p. D6.

3   Pool, R. (2001). *Fat: Fighting the Obesity Epidemic.* Oxford: Oxford University Press.

4   Shell, E.R. (2002). *The Hungry Gene: The inside story of the obesity industry.* New York: Grove Press.

5   In some sub-populations the problem is worse than in others. For example, data from the National Health and Nutrition Examination Surveys clearly show that the rates of obesity in the United States follows a socio-economic gradient, such that the burden of the disease falls disproportionately on people with limited resources, racial-ethnic minorities, and the poor. (The data show that the lowest educated groups having a prevalence of obesity that runs about 5 percent higher than more educated sub-populations). Reference: Speakman, J.R. (2003). Obesity: Part one- The greatest health threat facing mankind. Biologist, 50(1), 11-14.

6   Reuters News Service, May 29, 2003.

7   Children are obese if their body mass index is equal to or greater than the 95th percentile of the age and gender-specific body mass charts compiled by the Centers for Disease Control & Prevention. A child who is in the 85th percentile is overweight and at risk for obesity.

8   Brownell, K.D. & Horgen, K.B. (2004). *Food Fight.* Chicago: Contemporary Books.

9   Pollan, M. (2003, October 26). The (Agri)Cultural Contradictions Of Obesity. *New York Times Magazine,* p. 41.

10   Schlosser, E. (2002). *Fast Food Nation: The Dark Side of the All-American Meal.* New York: Perennial.

11   Analysis of recent data from the National Health and Nutrition Examination Surveys—conducted by CDC's National Center for Health Statistics—suggests

obesity rates have been leveling off since 1999-2003. At this point, however, no one knows whether the pause will become permanent or whether it is simply a temporary reprieve, perhaps a statistical aberration, before the rates start upward again. Researchers need to see a few more years of data before declaring whether this is a true plateau in prevalence or just a temporary lull. In the meantime, most agree, it remains critical to help those who are already overweight and work to reduce the number of overweight Americans. Far too many children and adults are still overweight and at risk of illness and death unless we commit to reversing not just stabilizing the epidemic.

12   Mullainathan, S. (2013, November 10). The Co-Villains Behind Obesity's Rise. New York Times.

13   *Wall Street Journal.* (2003, November 14), p. W1.

14   "Dogs and cats are classified as overweight when their body weight is 15 percent above what is deemed 'optimal' for their breed, and they are considered obese when their weight exceeds 30 percent above optimal" (Brody, J.E. [2006, July 18]. Wonder Where That Fat Cat Learned to Eat? *New York Times*).

15   Hill, J.O. and Peters, J.C. (1998). Environmental Contributions to the Obesity Epidemic. *Science,* 280, 1371-1374.

16   Brownell, K.D. & Horgen, K.B. (2004). *Food Fight.* Chicago: Contemporary Books.

17   *Ibid.*

18   McKinsey Global Institute (2014). Overcoming obesity: An initial economic analysis.

19   World Health Organization (2002). *The World Health Report 2002: Reducing Risks, Promoting Healthy Life.* Geneva: World Health Organization.

20   Easterbrook, G. (2004, March 14). The Nation: Wages of Wealth; All This Progress Is Killing Us, Bite by Bite. *New York Times, p. 5.*

21   Brody, J.E. (2013, July 2). A Label Calls Attention To Obesity. New York Times.

22   McKinsey Global Institute (2014). Overcoming obesity: An initial economic analysis.

23   Manson, J.E. and Bassuk, S.S. (2003). Obesity in the United States: A fresh look at its high toll. *JAMA,* 289(2), 229-230.

24   *Ibid.*

25   Cohen, P. (2004, May 15). Forget Lonely. Life Is Healthy at the Top. *New York Times.*

26   Hill, J.O. and Peters, J.C. (1998). Environmental Contributions to the Obesity Epidemic. *Science*, 280, 1371-1374.

27   Wall Street Journal (2000, January 11). Being Overweight in Midlife Boosts Heart Risks. *Wall Street Journal.*

28   Brownell, K.D. & Horgen, K.B. (2004). *Food Fight.* Chicago: Contemporary Books.

29   Carlos Poston, W.S. and Foreyt, J.P. (2000). Successful management of the obese patient. *American Family Physician*, 61(12), 3615-3622.

30   McKay, B. (2004, August 24). Obesity is linked to cancer risk. *Wall Street Journal.*

31   Brownell, K.D. & Horgen, K.B. (2004). *Food Fight.* Chicago: Contemporary Books.

32   O'Neil, J. (2005, January 25). Testing: Obesity May Skew Prostate Test. *New York Times.*

33   Brody, J.E. (2003, May 6). Another study finds a link between excess weight and cancer. *New York Times,* p. D7.

34   Brownell, K.D. & Horgen, K.B. (2004). *Food Fight.* Chicago: Contemporary Books.

35   Rundle, R.L. (2004, March 9). Obesity issues for elderly may rise. *Wall Street Journal*, p. D3.

36   Wall Street Journal (2004, April 22). Weight Loss May Ease Arthritis. *Wall Street Journal*, p. D2.

37   Fackelmann, K. (2005, August 25). Does diabetes lurk behind Alzheimer's? *USA Today,* p. 1D.

38   Kumanyika, S.K. (2001). Minisymposium on Obesity: Overview and some strategic considerations. *Annu. Rev. Public Health*, 22, 293-308.

39   Kirschenbaum, D.S. and Fitzgibbon, M.L. (1995). Controversy about the treatment of obesity: Criticisms or challenges? *Behavior Therapy*, 26, 43-68.

40   Battle, E.K. and Brownell, K.D. (1996). Confronting a rising tide of eating disorders and obesity: Treatment vs. prevention and policy. *Addictive Behaviors*, 21(6), 755-765.

41   Rand, D.S.W. & Macgregor, A.M.C. (1991). Successful weight loss following obesity surgery and the perceived liability of morbid obesity. *International Journal of Obesity*, 15, 577-579.

42   Brownell, K.D. & Fairburn, C.G. (Eds.). (1995). *Eating Disorders and Obesity: A Comprehensive Handbook.* New York: The Guilford Press.

43   Bray, G.A, Bouchard, C., and James, W.P.T. (Eds.). (1998). *Handbook of Obesity*. New York: Marcel Dekker, Inc.

44   Wadden, T.A. & Stunkard, A.J. (Eds.). (2002). *Handbook of Obesity Treatment*. New York: The Guilford Press.

45   *Ibid.*

46   Cassell, J.A. (1995). Social anthropology and nutrition: A different look at obesity in America. *J. of the Am. Dietetic Ass.*, 95(4), 424-427.

47   Dietz, W.H. (1998). Health consequences of obesity in youth: childhood predictors of adult disease. *Pediatrics*, 101, 518-525.

48   Wadden, T.A. & Stunkard, A.J. (Eds.). (2002). *Handbook of Obesity Treatment*. New York: The Guilford Press.

49   Shils, M.E., Olson, J.A., Shike, M., and Ross, A.C. (Eds.). (1999). *Modern Nutrition in Health and Disease*. Baltimore, Maryland: Williams & Wilkins.

50   Hellmich, N. (2002, October 9). By the millions, kids keep gaining weight. *USA Today*, p. 9D.

51   Shils, M.E., Olson, J.A., Shike, M., and Ross, A.C. (Eds.). (1999). *Modern Nutrition in Health and Disease*. Baltimore, Maryland: Williams & Wilkins.

52   Wadden, T.A. & Stunkard, A.J. (Eds.). (2002). *Handbook of Obesity Treatment*. New York: The Guilford Press.

53   Allison, D.B. and Saunders, S.E. (2000). Obesity in North America: An Overview. *Medical Clinics of North America*, 84(2), 305-333.

54   Epperson, S. (2003, September 8). The Obesity Charge. *Time*, 162 (10), p. 100.

55   Wing, R.R. & Greeno, C.G. (1994). Behavioral and psychosocial aspects of obesity and its treatment. *Baillière Clinical Endocrinology and Metabolism*, 8(3), 689-703.

56   Seidell, J.C. (1998). Societal and personal costs of obesity. *Exp Clin Endocrinol Diabetes*, 106(suppl 2), 7-9.

57   Speakman, J.R. (2003). Obesity: Part one- The greatest health threat facing mankind. *Biologist*, 50(1), 11-14.

58   Bjorntorp, P. (2001). Thrifty genes and human obesity. Are we chasing ghosts? *Lancet*, 358, 1006-1008.

59   Porter, R. ed. (1996). *The Cambridge Illustrated History of Medicine*. Cambridge, UK: Cambridge University Press.

60   Lawrence, P.R. & Nohria, N. (2002). *Driven: How Human Nature Shapes our Choices*. San Francisco, CA: Jossey-Bass.

61   Pool, R. (2001). *Fat: Fighting the Obesity Epidemic.* Oxford: Oxford University Press.

62   Lawrence, P.R. & Nohria, N. (2002). *Driven: How Human Nature Shapes our Choices.* San Francisco, CA: Jossey-Bass.

63   *Ibid.*

64   *Ibid.*

65   Eaton, S.B. (1992). Humans, Lipids and Evolution. *Lipids,* 27(10), 814-820.

66   Pi-Sunyer, X. (2003). A clinical view of the obesity problem. *Science,* 299, 859-860.

67   Peters, J.C., Wyatt, H.R., Donahoo, W.T., and Hill, J.O. (2002). From instinct to intellect: the challenge of maintaining healthy weight in the modern world. *Obesity Reviews,* 3, 69-74.

68   Brownell, K.D. & Horgen, K.B. (2004). *Food Fight.* Chicago: Contemporary Books.

69   Lawrence, P.R. & Nohria, N. (2002). *Driven: How Human Nature Shapes our Choices.* San Francisco, CA: Jossey-Bass.

70   *Ibid.*

71   Bray, G.A, Bouchard, C., and James, W.P.T.(Eds.). (1998). *Handbook of Obesity.* New York: Marcel Dekker, Inc.

72   Wansink, B. and Huckabee, M. (2005). De-Marketing Obesity. *California Management Review,* 47(4), 6-18.

73   Brown, P.J. (1998). Culture, Evolution, and Obesity. In G.A. Bray, C. Bouchard, and W.P.T. James (Eds.). *Handbook of Obesity.* New York: Marcel Dekker, Inc.

74   Pool, R. (2001). *Fat: Fighting the Obesity Epidemic.* Oxford: Oxford University Press.

75   Bray, G.A, Bouchard, C., and James, W.P.T.(Eds.). (1998). *Handbook of Obesity.* New York: Marcel Dekker, Inc.

76   Eaton, S.B., Eaton, S.B., Konner, M.J., and Shostak, M. (1996). An Evolutionary Perspective Enhances Understanding of Human Nutritional Requirements. *J. Nutr.* 126, 1732-40.

77   Pool, R. (2001). *Fat: Fighting the Obesity Epidemic.* Oxford: Oxford University Press.

78   *Ibid.*

79   Flier, J.S. (2004). Obesity wars: Molecular progress confronts an expanding epidemic. *Cell,* 116, 337-350.

80   The robber crab (birgus latro), shows amazing transitions between asymme-
      try and symmetry as adaptive responses to different stages of its life cycle. It
      begins its post-larval existence with a symmetrical abdomen. It then occupies
      a dextral gastropod shell (i.e. one with a left-banded spiral) and adapts to this
      change in habitat by developing an asymmetric abdomen. Once it has out-
      grown its adopted protective shell shelter and becomes free-living once more,
      it reverts back to its original symmetric design.

81   Lawrence, P.R. & Nohria, N. (2002). *Driven: How Human Nature Shapes our
      Choices*. San Francisco, CA: Jossey-Bass.

82   Lawrence, P.R. & Nohria, N. (2002). *Driven: How Human Nature Shapes our
      Choices*. San Francisco, CA: Jossey-Bass.

83   Pool, R. (2001). Fat: Fighting the Obesity Epidemic. Oxford: Oxford University
      Press.

84   Eaton, S.B., Eaton, S.B., Konner, M.J., and Shostak, M. (1996). An Evolutionary
      Perspective Enhances Understanding of Human Nutritional Requirements. J.
      Nutr. 126, 1732-40.

85   Brownell, K.D. & Horgen, K.B. (2004). Food Fight. Chicago: Contemporary
      Books.

86   McKinsey Global Institute (2014). Overcoming obesity: An initial economic
      analysis.

87   Brownell, K.D. & Horgen, K.B. (2004). *Food Fight*. Chicago: Contemporary
      Books.

88   O'Keefe, J.H. et al. (2010). Achieving Hunter-gatherer Fitness in the 21st
      Century: Back to the Future. *Am J Med*. 123(12):1082-6.

89   *Ibid.*

90   Nestle, M. (2002). *Food Politics: How the food industry influences nutrition and
      health*. Berkeley, CA: University of California Press.

91   Brownell, K.D. & Horgen, K.B. (2004). *Food Fight*. Chicago: Contemporary
      Books.

92   Philipson, T.J. and Posner, R.A. (2003). The long-run growth in obesity as a
      function of technological change. *Perspectives in Biology and Medicine*, 46(3),
      S87-S107.

93   Brownell, K.D. & Horgen, K.B. (2004). *Food Fight*. Chicago: Contemporary
      Books.

94   Postrel, V. (2001, March 22). Americans' waistlines have become the victims of
      economic progress. *New York Times*, p. C2.

95   Franklin, B.A. (2001). The downside of our technological revolution? An obesity-conducive environment. *The Am J of Cardiology*, 87, 1093-1095.

96   Eaton, S.B., Eaton, S.B., Konner, M.J., and Shostak, M. (1996). An Evolutionary Perspective Enhances Understanding of Human Nutritional Requirements. J. Nutr. 126, 1732-40.

97   Pool, R. (2001). *Fat: Fighting the Obesity Epidemic.* Oxford: Oxford University Press.

98   *Ibid.*

99   Blundell, J.E. & King, N.A. (1996). Overconsumption as a cause of weight gain: behavioral-physiological interactions in the control of food intake (appetite). In Ciba Foundation Symposium ed. The Origins and Consequences of Obesity (pp. 138-154). Hoboken, NJ: John Wiley & Sons.

100   Mattes, R.D., Pierce, C.B., and Friedman, M.I. (1988). Daily caloric intake of normal-weight adults: response to changes in dietary energy density of a luncheon meal. *Am. J. Clin. Nutr.* 48, 214-9.

101   Grady, D. (2002, November 26). Why we Eat (and Eat and Eat). *New York Times,* p. D1.

102   French, S. and Castiglione, K. (2002). Recent advances in the physiology of eating. *Proceedings of the Nutrition Society,* 61, 489-496.

103   Pi-Sunyer, F.X. (1999). Obesity. In M.E. Shils, J.A. Olson, M. Shike, and A.C. Ross (Eds.). Modern Nutrition in Health and Disease. Baltimore, MD: Williams & Wilkins.

104   Pool, R. (2001). Fat: Fighting the Obesity Epidemic. Oxford: Oxford University Press.

105   Marx, J. (2003). Cellular warriors at the battle of the bulge. Science, 299, 846-849.

106   Bell, C.G., Walley, A.J., and Froguel, P. (2005). The genetics of human obesity. Nature Reviews Genetics, 6, 221-234.

107   Marx, J. (2003). Cellular warriors at the battle of the bulge. Science, 299, 846-849.

108   Blundell, J.E. & King, N.A. (1996). Overconsumption as a cause of weight gain: behavioral-physiological interactions in the control of food intake (appetite). In Ciba Foundation Symposium ed. *The Origins and Consequences of Obesity (pp. 138-154).* Hoboken, NJ: John Wiley & Sons.

109   Whitney, E.N. and Rolfes, S.R. (1999). *Understanding Nutrition.* Belmont, CA: West/Wadsworth.

110   Peters, J.C., Wyatt, H.R., Donahoo, W.T., and Hill, J.O. (2002). From instinct to intellect: the challenge of maintaining healthy weight in the modern world. *Obesity Reviews*, 3, 69-74.

111   Polivy, J. and Herman, P. (1985). Dieting and Binging: A causal analysis. *American Psychologist*, 40(2), 193-201.

112   Shetty, P.S. (1990). Physiological mechanisms in the adaptive response of metabolic rates to energy restriction. *Nutrition Research Reviews* 3, 49-74.

113   Parker-Pope, T. (2012, January 1). The Fat Trap. New York Times.

114   Pi-Sunyer, X. (2003). A clinical view of the obesity problem. *Science,* 299, 859-860.

115   *Ibid.*

116   McArdle, W.D., Katch, F.I., and Katch, V.L. (1996). *Exercise Physiology: Energy, Nutrition, and Human Performance.* Baltimore, MD: Williams & Wilkins.

117   Dalton, S. ed. (1997). *Overweight and Weight Management: The Health Professional's Guide to Understanding and Practice.* Gaithersburg, Maryland: An Aspen Publication.

118   Pi-Sunyer, F.X. (1999). Obesity. In M.E. Shils, J.A. Olson, M. Shike, and A.C. Ross (Eds.). *Modern Nutrition in Health and Disease.* Baltimore, MD: Williams & Wilkins.

119   Whitney, E.N. and Rolfes, S.R. (1999). *Understanding Nutrition.* Belmont, CA: West/Wadsworth.

120   Vasselli, J.R. and Maggio, C.A. (1988). Mechanisms of appetite and body-weight regulation. In R.T. Frankle and M. Yang (Eds.). Obesity and Weight Control: The Health Professional's Guide to Understanding and Treatment. Rockville, Maryland: Aspen Publishers, Inc.

121   Eaton, S.B., Eaton, S.B., Konner, M.J., and Shostak, M. (1996). An Evolutionary Perspective Enhances Understanding of Human Nutritional Requirements. *J. Nutr.* 126, 1732-40.

122   Pool, R. (2001). *Fat: Fighting the Obesity Epidemic.* Oxford: Oxford University Press.

123   Pool, R. (2001). *Fat: Fighting the Obesity Epidemic.* Oxford: Oxford University Press.

124   New York Times (2013, May 11). Heat Trapping Gas Passes Milestone Raising Fears. New York Times.

125   Blundell, J.E. & King, N.A. (1996). Overconsumption as a cause of weight gain: behavioral-physiological interactions in the control of food intake (appetite).

In Ciba Foundation Symposium ed. *The Origins and Consequences of Obesity (pp. 138-154)*. Hoboken, NJ: John Wiley & Sons.

126   Zernike, K. (2003, November 9). Food Fight; Is Obesity the Responsibility of the Body Politic? *New York Times.*

127   Hunt, E. (1989). Cognitive Science: Definition, Status, and Questions. *Ann. Rev. Psychol,* 40, 603-29.

128   Ann Chapman J. & Ferfolja, T. (2001). Fatal Flaws: The acquisition of imperfect mental models and their use in hazardous situations. *Journal of Intellectual Capital,* (2), 398-409.

129   Sterman, J. D. (2002) All Models are Wrong: Reflections on Becoming a Systems Scientist. *System Dynamics Review,* 18, 501-531.

130   Ann Chapman J. & Ferfolja, T. (2001). Fatal Flaws: The acquisition of imperfect mental models and their use in hazardous situations. *Journal of Intellectual Capital,* (2), 398-409.

131   Eaton, S.B., Eaton, S.B., Konner, M.J., and Shostak, M. (1996). An Evolutionary Perspective Enhances Understanding of Human Nutritional Requirements. *J. Nutr.* 126, 1732-40.

132   Lobstein, T. (2006). Comment: Preventing child obesity-an art and a science. *Obesity Reviews,* 7(suppl 1), 1-5.

133   Spake, A. (2003). The science of slimming: Getting rid of all those unwanted pounds is as simple as calories in, calories out. *U.S. News & World Report,* 134(21), 34-38.

134   *Ibid.*

135   Taylor, S.E. & Brown, J.D. (1988). Illusion and Well-Being: A Social Psychological Perspective on Mental Health. *Psychological Bulletin,* 103, 193-210.

136   Peterson, C. & Stunkard, A.J. (1989). Personal Control and Health Promotion. *Soc. Sci. Med.,* 28, 819-828.

137   Clarke, V.A., Lovegrove, H., Williams, A., and Macpherson, M. (2000). Unrealistic Optimism and the Health Belief Model. *Journal of Behavioral Medicine,* 23, 367-376.

138   McKenna, F. P. (1993), "It won't happen to me: Unrealistic optimism or illusion of control?", British Journal of Psychology (British Psychological Society) 84 (1): 39–50

139   Whalen, C.K., Henker, B., O'Neil, R., Hollingshead, J., Holman, A., and Moore, B. (1994). Optimism in Children's Judgments of Health and Environmental Risks. *Health Psychology,* 13, 319-325.

140   Taylor, S.E. & Brown, J.D. (1988). Illusion and Well-Being: A Social Psychological Perspective on Mental Health. *Psychological Bulletin,* 103, 193-210.

141   Kuchler, F. and Variyam, J.N. (2003). Mistakes were made: misperception as a barrier to reducing weight. International J of Obesity, 27, 856-861.

142   Robinson, E. and Kirkham, TC (2013). Is he a healthy weight? Exposure to obesity changes perception of the weight status of others. International Journal of Obesity, 1–5.

143   Etelson, D., Brand, D.A., Patrick, P.A., and Shirali, A. (2003). Childhood obesity: Do parents recognize this health risk? Obesity Research, 11(11), 1362-1368.

144   Rietmeijer-Mentink, M. et al. (2012). Difference between parental perception and actual weight status of children: a systematic review. Maternal and Child Nutrition, 9, pp. 3–22.

145   De La O, Angela et al. (2009). Do Parents Accurately Perceive Their Child's Weight Status? Journal of Pediatric Health Care, 23(4), 216-221.

146   Pickstone, J.V. (2000). *Ways of Knowing: A new history of science, technology and medicine.* Chicago: The University of Chicago Press,

147   Oliver, J.E. and Lee, T. (2005). Public Opinion and the Politics of Obesity in America. *Journal of Health Politics, Policy and La,*30(5), 923-954.

148   Pool, R. (2001). *Fat: Fighting the Obesity Epidemic.* Oxford: Oxford University Press.

149   Nestle, M. et al. (1998). Behavioral and social influences on food choice. *Nutrition Reviews,* 56(5), S50-S74.

150   Skelton, J.A. & Croyle, R.T. (Eds.). (1991). *Mental representation in health and illness.* New York: Springer-Verlag.

151   Nestle, M. and Jacobson, M.F. (2000). Halting the obesity epidemic: A public health policy approach. *Public Health Reports,* 115, 12-24.

152   Jeffery, R.W. (2001). Public health strategies for obesity treatment and prevention. *Am J Health Behav,* 25(3), 252-259.

153   A quote by Andrew Wang in E.J. Huth and T.J. Murray (2000). *Medicine in Quotations: Views of Health and Disease through the Ages.* Philadelphia: American College of Physicians.

154 Hammond, J.S, Keeney, R.L., and Raiffa, H. (1998). The Hidden Traps in Decision Making. *Harvard Business Review*, 76(5), 47-58.

155 Brody, J. (2004, March 23). Sane Weight Loss in a Carb-Obsessed World: High Fiber and Low Fat. *New York Times*.

156 Sterman, J. D. (1994). Learning In and About Complex Systems. *System Dynamics Review*, 10, 291-330.

157 Norman, D.A. (1993). *Things that make us smart: Defending human attributes in the age of the machine*. Reading, MA: Addison-Wesley.

158 *Ibid.*

159 According to the United Nations' Second Assembly on Ageing, a million people now turn 60 every month, a demographic revolution that will mean older people will soon outnumber the young for the first time in history. Reference: Daly, E. (2002, April 9). U.N. Says Elderly Will Soon Outnumber Young for First Time. *New York Times*.

160 Topol, E. (2012). The Creative Destruction of Medicine. New York: Basic Books.

161 Einhorn, H. J. and Hogarth, R. M. (1987). Decision making: Going forward in reverse. Harvard Business Review, 65(1): 66-70.

162 Sterman, J.D. (2000). Business Dynamics: Systems Thinking and Modeling for a Complex World. Boston, Massachusetts: Irwin McGraw-Hill.

163 Sterman, J.D. and Booth Sweeney, L. Cloudy Skies: Assessing Public Understanding of Global Warming. System Dynamics Review 2002; 18, 207-240.

164 Senge, P.M. (1990). *The Fifth Discipline: The Art & Practice of the Learning Organization*. New York: Doubleday/Currency.

165 Wilson, E.O. (1998). *Consilience: The Unity of Knowledge*. New York: Alfred A. Knopf.

166 Diez-Roux, A.V. (1998). On genes, individuals, society, and epidemiology. *Am J. of Epidemiology*, 148(11), 1027-1032.

167 Ackoff, R.L. (1994). Systems thinking and thinking systems. *System Dynamics Review*, 19(2-3), 175-188.

168 Jervis, R. (1997). *System Effects: Complexity in Political and Social Life*. Princeton, NJ: Princeton University Press.

169 Capra, F. (1996). *The Web of Life: A scientific understanding of living systems*. New York: Anchor Books.

170   Ackoff, R.L. (1994). Systems thinking and thinking systems. *System Dynamics Review*, 19(2-3), 175-188.

171   Capra, F. (1996). *The Web of Life: A scientific understanding of living systems.* New York: Anchor Books.

172   Institute of Medicine (2010). Bridging The Evidence Gap In Obesity Prevention: A Framework To Inform Decision Making. Institute of Medicine.

173   Brownell, K.D. & Fairburn, C.G. (Eds.). (1995). *Eating Disorders and Obesity: A Comprehensive Handbook.* New York: The Guilford Press

174   Pool, R. (2001). *Fat: Fighting the Obesity Epidemic.* Oxford: Oxford University Press.

175   Senge, P.M. (1990). *The Fifth Discipline: The Art & Practice of the Learning Organization.* New York: Doubleday/Currency.

176   Capra, F. (1996). *The Web of Life: A scientific understanding of living systems.* New York: Anchor Books.

177   Laszlo, E. (1996). *The Systems View of the World: A Holistic Vision for Our Time (Advances in Systems Theory, Complexity, and the Human Sciences).* Cresskill, NJ: Hampton Press.

178   Senge, P.M. (1990). *The Fifth Discipline: The Art & Practice of the Learning Organization.* New York: Doubleday/Currency.

179   High Performance Systems (1997). An Introduction to Systems Thinking. Hanover, NH: High Performance Systems.

180   Gonzalez C and Wong H. 2012. Understanding stocks and flows through analogy. System Dynamics Review 28(1):3-27.

181   Cronin MA, Gonzalez C, and Sterman JD. 2009. Why don't well-educated adults understand accumulation? A challenge to researchers, educators, and citizens. Organizational Behavior and Human Decision Processes 108:116-130.

182   Khare A and Inman J.J. 2009. Daily, Week-Part, and Holiday Patterns in Consumers' Caloric Intake. J. of Public Policy & Marketing 28(2):234-252.

183   Wansink B. 2004. Environmental Factors that Increase the Food Intake and Consumption Volume of Unknown Consumers. Annu. Rev. Nutrition 24:455-79.

184   Cronin MA, Gonzalez C, and Sterman JD. 2009. Why don't well-educated adults understand accumulation? A challenge to researchers, educators, and citizens. Organizational Behavior and Human Decision Processes 108:116-130.

185   Parker-Pope T. 2005. The Skinny on Holiday Weight Gain: It's Not as Bad as You Think, but it Sticks. Wall Street Journal, December 13; p. D1.

186   Yanovski, J.A. et al. A prospective study of holiday weight gain. The New England J of Med. 2000; 342(12), 861-7.

187   Sterman, J.D. and Booth Sweeney, L. Cloudy Skies: Assessing Public Understanding of Global Warming. System Dynamics Review 2002; 18, 207-240.

188   *Ibid.*

189   Richardson, G.P. and Pugh, G.L. (1981). Introduction to System Dynamics Modeling and Dynamo. Cambridge, MA:The MIT Press.

190   Meadows, D. (1999). Leverage Points: Places to Intervene in a System. The Sustainability Institute, Hartland, Vermont.

191   Brownell, K.D. & Fairburn, C.G. (Eds.). (1995). *Eating Disorders and Obesity: A Comprehensive Handbook*. New York: The Guilford Press

192   Johnson, L.R. (1998). *Essential Medical Physiology*. Philadelphia, PA: Lippincott-Raven Publishers.

193   Polivy, J. and Herman, P. (1985). Dieting and Binging: A causal analysis. *American Psychologist*, 40(2), 193-201.

194   McArdle, W.D., Katch, F.I., and Katch, V.L. (1996). Exercise Physiology: Energy, Nutrition, and Human Performance. Baltimore, MD: Williams & Wilkins.

195   Hargrove, J.L. (1998). Dynamic Modeling in the Health Sciences. New York: Springer.

196   Vasselli, J.R. & Maggio, C.A. (1997). Mechanisms of Appetite and Body Weight Regulation. In A. Dalton (ed.). Overweight and weight Management: The Health Professional's Guide to Understanding and Practice. Gaithersburg, Maryland: Aspen Publishers, Inc.

197   Pool, R. (2001). *Fat: Fighting the Obesity Epidemic*. Oxford: Oxford University Press.

198   Shell, E.R. (2002). *The Hungry Gene: The inside story of the obesity industry*. New York: Grove Press.

199   Koopmans, H.S. (1998). Experimental studies on the control of food intake. In G.A. Bray, C. Bouchard, and W.P.T. James (Eds.). *Handbook of Obesity* (pp. 273-311). New York: Marcel Dekker, Inc.

200   Flier, J.S. and Maratos-Flier, E. (2007). What fuels fat. *Scientific American*, 297(3), 72-81.

201 Flier, J.S. and Maratos-Flier, E. (2007). What fuels fat. *Scientific American*, 297(3), 72-81.

202 Jéquier, E. and Tappy, L. (1999). Regulation of body weight in humans. Physiological Reviews, 79(2), 451-480.

203 Flier, J.S. and Maratos-Flier, E. (2007). What fuels fat. Scientific American, 297(3), 72-81.

204 *Ibid.*

205 Bell, C.G., Walley, A.J., and Froguel, P. (2005). The genetics of human obesity. Nature Reviews Genetics, 6, 221-234.

206 Jéquier, E. and Tappy, L. (1999). Regulation of body weight in humans. Physiological Reviews, 79(2), 451-480.

207 Woods, S.C., Schwartz, M.W., Baskin, D.G., and Seeley, R.J. (2000). Food Intake and the Regulation of Body Weight. Annu. Rev. Psychol. 51, 255-277.

208 Schwartz, M.W., Baskin, D.G., Kaiyala, K.J., and Woods, S.C. (1999). Model for the regulation of energy balance and adiposity by the central nervous system. Am J Clin Nutr., 69, 584-96.

209 Woods, S.C., Schwartz, M.W., Baskin, D.G., and Seeley, R.J. (2000). Food Intake and the Regulation of Body Weight. Annu. Rev. Psychol. 51, 255-277.

210 Schwartz, M.W. & Seeley, R.J. (1997). The new biology of body weight regulation. J Am Diet Assoc., 97, 54-58.

211 Baumeister, R.F. & Heatherton, T.F. (1996). Self-Regulation Failure: An Overview. *Psychological Inquiry*, 7(1), 1-15.

212 Blundell, J.E. & Tremblay, A. (1995). Appetite control and energy (fuel) balance. *Nutrition Research Reviews*, 8, 225-242.

213 Baumeister, R.F., Heatherton, T.F., and Tice, D.M. (1994). *Losing Control: How and why people fail at self-regulation*. San Diego, CA: Academic Press.

214 Muraven, M., Tice, D. M., & Baumeister, R. F. (1998). Self-control as a limited resource: Regulatory depletion patterns. *Journal of Personality and Social Psychology*, 74, 774- 89.

215 Muraven, M., & Baumeister, R. F. (2000). Self-regulation and depletion of limited resources: Does self-control resemble a muscle? *Psychological Bulletin*, 126, 247-259.

216 *Ibid.*

217 Vasselli, J.R. & Maggio, C.A. (1997). Mechanisms of Appetite and Body Weight Regulation. In A. Dalton (ed.). Overweight and weight Management:

The Health Professional's Guide to Understanding and Practice. Gaithersburg, Maryland: Aspen Publishers, Inc.

218   Parker-Pope, T. (2012, January1). The Fat Trap. New York Times.

219   Novotny, J.A. & Rumpler, W.V. (1998). Modeling of energy expenditure and resting metabolic rate during weight loss in humans. In A.J. Clifford and H.G. Muller (Eds.). Mathematical Modeling in Experimental Nutrition. New York: Plenum Press.

220   Meadows, D.H. (2008). Thinking in systems: A Primer. White River Junction, Vermont: Chelsea Green Publishing.

221   Buckmaster, L. and Brownell, K.D. (1988). Behavior Modification: The state of the art. In R.T. Frankle and M. Yang (Eds.). Obesity and Weight Control: The Health Professional's Guide to Understanding and Treatment. Rockville, Maryland: Aspen Publishers, Inc.

222   Sjöström, L. (1980). Fat cells and body weight. In A.J. Stunkard (Ed.). *Obesity*. Philadelphia: W.B. Saunders Company.

223   Shils, M.E., Olson, J.A., Shike, M., and Ross, A.C. (Eds.). (1999). *Modern Nutrition in Health and Disease*. Baltimore, Maryland: Williams & Wilkins.

224   A µg is a microgram, or one-millionth (10^{-6}) of a gram.

225   McArdle, W.D., Katch, F.I., and Katch, V.L. (1996). *Exercise Physiology: Energy, Nutrition, and Human Performance*. Baltimore, MD: Williams & Wilkins.

226   Whitney, E.N. and Rolfes, S.R. (1999). *Understanding Nutrition*. Belmont, CA: West/Wadsworth.

227   Vasselli, J.R. and Maggio, C.A. (1988). Mechanisms of appetite and body-weight regulation. In R.T. Frankle and M. Yang (Eds.). Obesity and Weight Control: The Health Professional's Guide to Understanding and Treatment. Rockville, Maryland: Aspen Publishers, Inc.

228   Whitney, E.N. and Rolfes, S.R. (1999). *Understanding Nutrition*. Belmont, CA: West/Wadsworth.

229   Stipp, D. (2003, February 3). The quest for the antifat pill nature programmed us to overeat. Fen-Phen helped that, until it backfired. Safer drugs may be coming soon. *Fortune Magazine,* pp. 66-7.

230   Buckmaster, L. and Brownell, K.D. (1988). Behavior Modification: The state of the art. In R.T. Frankle and M. Yang (Eds.). Obesity and Weight Control: The Health Professional's Guide to Understanding and Treatment. Rockville, Maryland: Aspen Publishers, Inc.

231   Vasselli, J.R. and Maggio, C.A. (1988). Mechanisms of appetite and body-weight regulation. In R.T. Frankle and M. Yang (Eds.). *Obesity and Weight Control: The Health Professional's Guide to Understanding and Treatment.* Rockville, Maryland: Aspen Publishers, Inc.

232   There is now evidence that the induction of *ob* mRNA is a function of fat cell size, with larger fat cells expressing more *ob* mRNA than smaller cells. See: Jebb, S.A. et al. (1996). Changes in macronutrient balance during over- and underfeeding assessed by 12-d continuous whole-body calorimetry. *Am J Clin Nutr.*, 64, 259-66.).

Fat cell size may also be signaled through enzymatic mechanisms mounted on fat cell membranes. One such mechanism involves the enzyme lipoprotein lipase (LPL), which plays a key role in the process of lipid deposition in the adipose tissue. See: Whitney, E.N. and Rolfes, S.R. (1999). Understanding Nutrition. Belmont, CA: West/Wadsworth.

233   Jéquier, E. and Tappy, L. (1999). Regulation of body weight in humans. *Physiological Reviews,* 79(2), 451-480.

234   Sterman, J.D. (2000). *Business Dynamics: Systems Thinking and Modeling for a Complex World.* Boston, Massachusetts: Irwin McGraw-Hill.

235   Weick, K. (1979). *The Social Psychology of Organizing.* New York: Addison-Wesley.

236   Sterman, J.D. (2000). *Business Dynamics: Systems Thinking and Modeling for a Complex World.* Boston, Massachusetts: Irwin McGraw-Hill.

237   Sterman, J.D. (2000). *Business Dynamics: Systems Thinking and Modeling for a Complex World.* Boston, Massachusetts: Irwin McGraw-Hill.

238   Hensrud, Donald D. Mayo Clinic on Healthy Weight. Rochester, Minnesota: Mayo Clinic Health Information. 2000: p. 79.

239   McArdle, W.D., Katch, F.I., and Katch, V.L. (1996). Exercise Physiology: Energy, Nutrition, and Human Performance. Baltimore, MD: Williams & Wilkins.

240   Weinsier, R.L., Bracco, D., and Schutz, Y. (1993). Predicted effects of small decreases in energy expenditure on weight gain in adult women. International J. of Obesity, 17, 693-699.

241   Hall, K.D. et al. (2011). Quantifi cation of the eff ect of energy imbalance on bodyweight. Lancet; 378: 826–37.

242   Wier, L.T. et al. (2001). Determining the amount of physical activity needed for long-term weight control. *International J of Obesity,* 25, 613-621.

243 Foster, G.D., Wadden, T.A., Vogt, R.A., and Brewer, G. (1997). What Is a Reasonable Weight Loss? Patients' Expectations and Evaluations of Obesity Treatment Outcomes. *Journal of Consulting and Clinical Psychology,* 65, 79-85.

244 Anderson, G.H. (1993). Regulation of food intake. In M.E. Shils, J.A. Olson, and M. Shike (Eds.). *Modern Nutrition in Health and Disease (8th edition).* Philadelphia: Lea & Febiger.

245 Diez-Roux, A.V. (1998). On genes, individuals, society, and epidemiology. *Am J. of Epidemiology,* 148(11), 1027-1032.

246 Mela, D.J. (2006). Eating for pleasure or just wanting to eat? Reconsidering sensory hedonic responses as a driver of obesity. Appetite, 47: 10-17.

247 Pollan, M. (2006). The Omnivore's Dilemma. New York: The Penguin Press.

248 Cornier, M., Von Kaenel, S., Bessesen, D.H. and Tregellas, J.R. (2007). Effects of overfeeding on the neuronal response to visual food cues. Am J Clin Nutr, 86: 965–71.

249 Bellisari, A. (2007). Evolutionary origins of obesity. Obesity Reviews, 9: 165-180.

250 Heitman, B.L. and Garby, L. (2002). Composition (lean and fat tissue) of weight changes in adult Danes. Am J Clin Nutr, 75: 840-7.

251 Pinel, J.P., Assanand, S. and Lehman, D.R. (2000). Hunger, Eating, and Ill Health. American Psychologist, 55(10), 1105 1116.

252 Saper, C.B., Chou, T.C. and Elmquist, J.K. (2002). The Need to Feed: Homeostatic and Hedonic Control of Eating. Neuron, 36:199–211.

253 *Ibid.*

254 Pinel, J.P., Assanand, S. and Lehman, D.R. (2000). Hunger, Eating, and Ill Health. American Psychologist, 55(10), 1105 1116.

255 Kessler, D.A. (2009). The end of overeating. New York: Rodale.

256 Pinel, J.P., Assanand, S. and Lehman, D.R. (2000). Hunger, Eating, and Ill Health. American Psychologist, 55(10), 1105 1116.

257 Pelchat, M.L. (2002). Of human bondage: Food craving, obsession, compulsion, and addiction. Physiology & Behavior, 76:347– 352.

258 Erlanson-Albertsson, C. (2005). How Palatable Food Disrupts Appetite Regulation. Basic & Clinical Pharmacology & Toxicology, 97: 61–73.

259 Saper, C.B., Chou, T.C. and Elmquist, J.K. (2002). The Need to Feed: Homeostatic and Hedonic Control of Eating. Neuron, 36:199–211.

260 *Ibid.*

261 Kessler, D.A. (2009). The end of overeating. New York: Rodale.

262 Erlanson-Albertsson, C. (2005). How Palatable Food Disrupts Appetite Regulation. Basic & Clinical Pharmacology & Toxicology, 97: 61–73.

263 Pinel, J.P., Assanand, S. and Lehman, D.R. (2000). Hunger, Eating, and Ill Health. American Psychologist, 55(10), 1105 1116.

264 Parker-Pope, T. (2009, June 23). How the Food Makers Captured Our Brains. New York Times.

265 Lowe, M.R. et al. (2009). The Power of Food Scale. A new measure of the psychological influence of the food environment. Appetite 53:114–118.

266 Kessler, D.A. (2009). The end of overeating. New York: Rodale.

267 Senge, P.M. (1990). The Fifth Discipline: The Art & Practice of the Learning Organization. New York: Doubleday/Currency.

268 Weick, K. (1979). The Social Psychology of Organizing. New York: Addison-Wesley.

269 Senge, P.M. (1990). The Fifth Discipline: The Art & Practice of the Learning Organization. New York: Doubleday/Currency.

270 Senge, P.M. (1990). *The Fifth Discipline: The Art & Practice of the Learning Organization*. New York: Doubleday/Currency.

271 Sterman, J.D. (2000). *Business Dynamics: Systems Thinking and Modeling for a Complex World*. Boston, Massachusetts: Irwin McGraw-Hill.

272 Nestle, M. (2002). *Food Politics: How the food industry influences nutrition and health*. Berkeley, CA: University of California Press.

273 Nielsen, S.J. and Popkin, B.M. (2004). Changes in beverage intake between 1977 and 2001. *Am J Prev Med*, 27(3), 205-210.

274 Sanger-Katz, M. (2015, July 26). America Starts to Push away from the Plate. New York Times, p. 1.

275 Brownell, K.D. & Horgen, K.B. (2004). *Food Fight*. Chicago: Contemporary Books.

276 Cutler, D.M., Glaeser, E.L. and Shapiro, J.M. (2003). Why Have Americans Become More Obese? *Journal of Economic Perspectives,* 17(3), 93-118.

277 Dunn, D. (1997). Introduction to the study of women and work. In D. Dunn (ed.) *Workplace/Women's Place: An Anthology*. Los Angeles: Roxbury Publishing Company.

278 Nestle, M. (2002). *Food Politics: How the food industry influences nutrition and health*. Berkeley, CA: University of California Press.

279 Cutler, D.M., Glaeser, E.L. and Shapiro, J.M. (2003). Why Have Americans Become More Obese? *Journal of Economic Perspectives,* 17(3), 93-118.

280 Chou, S., Grossman, M. and Saffer, H. (2001). An economic analysis of adult obesity: Results from the behavioral risk factor surveillance system. *Third Int'l Health Economics Assoc. Conf.* York, England, Jul 23-25, 2001.

281 Burke, J. (1995). *Connections.* Boston: Little, Brown and Company.

282 Cutler, D.M., Glaeser, E.L. and Shapiro, J.M. (2003). Why Have Americans Become More Obese? *Journal of Economic Perspectives,* 17(3), 93-118.

283 *Ibid.*

284 Philipson, T. (2001). The world-wide growth in obesity: An economic research agenda. *Health Economics,* 10, 1-7.

285 Cutler, D.M., Glaeser, E.L. and Shapiro, J.M. (2003). Why Have Americans Become More Obese? *Journal of Economic Perspectives,* 17(3), 93-118.

286 Bowers, D.E. (2000). Cooking trends echo changing roles of women. *Food Review,* 23(1), 23-29.

287 French, S.A., Story, M., and Jeffery, R.W. (2001). Environmental influences on eating and physical activity. *Annu. Rev. Public Health,* 22, 309-35.

288 Cutler, D.M., Glaeser, E.L. and Shapiro, J.M. (2003). Why Have Americans Become More Obese? *Journal of Economic Perspectives,* 17(3), 93-118.

289 Bowers, D.E. (2000). Cooking trends echo changing roles of women. *Food Review,* 23(1), 23-29.

290 Brownell, K.D. & Horgen, K.B. (2004). *Food Fight.* Chicago: Contemporary Books.

291 Mitka, M. (2003). Economist takes aim at "big fat" US lifestyle. *JAMA,* 289(1), 33-34.

292 Hill, J.O. et al. (2003). Obesity and the environment: Where do we go from here? *Science,* 299, 853-855.

293 Philipson, T.J. and Posner, R.A. (2003). The long-run growth in obesity as a function of technological change. *Perspectives in Biology and Medicine,* 46(3), S87-S107.

294 Raeburn, P. et al. (2002, October 21). Why we're so fat. *Business Week,* pp. 112-114.

295 French, S.A., Story, M., and Jeffery, R.W. (2001). Environmental influences on eating and physical activity. *Annu. Rev. Public Health,* 22, 309-35.

296 Philipson, T. (2001). The world-wide growth in obesity: An economic research agenda. *Health Economics,* 10, 1-7.

297 Cutler, D.M., Glaeser, E.L. and Shapiro, J.M. (2003). Why Have Americans Become More Obese? *Journal of Economic Perspectives,* 17(3), 93-118.

298   *Laigh, A. (2003, May 15).* Increasing obesity: slim hopes for a culture that lacks self-control. *The Sydney Morning Herald.*

299   Critser, G. (2003). *Fat Land: How Americans became the fattest people in the world.* Boston: Mariner Books.

300   Cutler, D.M., Glaeser, E.L. and Shapiro, J.M. (2003). Why Have Americans Become More Obese? *Journal of Economic Perspectives,* 17(3), 93-118.

301   Oliver, J.E. (2006). *Fat Politics: The real story behind America's obesity epidemic.* Oxford, UK: Oxford University Press.

302   McCrory, M.A., Suen, V.M.M., and Roberts, S.B. (2002). Biobehavioral influences on energy intake and adult weight gain. *The Journal of Nutrition,* 132, S3830-S3836.

303   Franklin, B.A. (2001). The downside of our technological revolution? An obesity-conducive environment. *The Am J of Cardiology,* 87, 1093-1095.

304   Zizza, C. et al. (2001). Significant increase in young adults' snacking between 1977-1978 and 1994-1996 represents a cause for concern! *Preventive Medicine,* 32, 303-310.

305   Kenney, J.J. (2004). To snack or not to snack, that is the question. www.foodandhealth.com.

306   *Ibid.*

307   McCrory, M.A., Suen, V.M.M., and Roberts, S.B. (2002). Biobehavioral influences on energy intake and adult weight gain. *The Journal of Nutrition,* 132, S3830-S3836.

308   Oliver, J.E. (2006). *Fat Politics: The real story behind America's obesity epidemic.* Oxford, UK: Oxford University Press.

309   McCrory, M.A., Suen, V.M.M., and Roberts, S.B. (2002). Biobehavioral influences on energy intake and adult weight gain. *The Journal of Nutrition,* 132, S3830-S3836.

310   French, S.A., Story, M., and Jeffery, R.W. (2001). Environmental influences on eating and physical activity. *Annu. Rev. Public Health,* 22, 309-35.

311   Oliver, J.E. (2006). *Fat Politics: The real story behind America's obesity epidemic.* Oxford, UK: Oxford University Press.

312   Schlosser, E. (2002). *Fast Food Nation: The Dark Side of the All-American Meal.* New York: Perennial.

313   DiMeglio, D.P. and Mattes, R.D. (2000). Liquid versus solid carbohydrate: Effects on food intake and body weight. *International Journal of Obesity,* 24, 794-800.

314 McCrory, M.A., Suen, V.M.M., and Roberts, S.B. (2002). Biobehavioral influences on energy intake and adult weight gain. *The Journal of Nutrition*, 132, S3830-S3836.

315 Sanger-Katz, M. (2015, July 26). America Starts to Push away from the Plate. New York Times, p. 1.

316 Schlosser, E. (2002). *Fast Food Nation: The Dark Side of the All-American Meal.* New York: Perennial.

317 Critser, G. (2003). *Fat Land: How Americans became the fattest people in the world.* Boston: Mariner Books.

318 *Ibid.*

319 Taras, H. et al. (2004). Soft drinks in school. *Pediatrics*, 113(1), 152-154.

320 Critser, G. (2003). *Fat Land: How Americans became the fattest people in the world.* Boston: Mariner Books.

321 Ludwig, D.S., Peterson, K.E., and Gortmaker, S.L. (2001). Relation between consumption of sugar-sweetened drinks and childhood obesity: a prospective, observational analysis. *The Lancet*, 357, 505-508.

322 Brownell, K.D. & Horgen, K.B. (2004). *Food Fight.* Chicago: Contemporary Books.

323 Popkin, B.M. (2007). The World is Fat. *Scientific American*, 297(3), 88-95.

324 DiMeglio, D.P. and Mattes, R.D. (2000). Liquid versus solid carbohydrate: Effects on food intake and body weight. *International Journal of Obesity*, 24, 794-800.

325 A measure of the potential of water molecules to move between regions of differing concentrations across a water-permeable membrane.

326 Bowers, D.E. (2000). Cooking trends echo changing roles of women. *Food Review*, 23(1), 23-29.

327 McCrory, M.A., Suen, V.M.M., and Roberts, S.B. (2002). Biobehavioral influences on energy intake and adult weight gain. *The Journal of Nutrition*, 132, S3830-S3836.

328 Brody, J. (2002, July 16). How to eat Without Tipping the Scale. *New York Times*, p. D7.

329 Schlosser, E. (2002). *Fast Food Nation: The Dark Side of the All-American Meal.* New York: Perennial.

330 Shell, E.R. (2002). *The Hungry Gene: The inside story of the obesity industry.* New York: Grove Press.

331 Barboza, D. (2003, August 3). If you Pitch It, They Will Eat. *New York Times*.

332   Story, M., Neumark-Sztainer, D., and French, S. (2002). Individual and environmental influences on adolescent eating behaviors. *Supplement to the J of the Am Dietetic Ass*, 102(3), S40-S51.

333   Buckley, N. (2003, February 18). Unhealthy food is everywhere, 24 hours a day, and inexpensive. *Financial Times*, p. 13.

334   Bowers, D.E. (2000). Cooking trends echo changing roles of women. *Food Review*, 23(1), 23-29.

335   Rothman Morris, B. (2005, October 26). Eating, Drinking, Cooking and, Oh Yes, Driving, Too. *New York Times*.

336   Shell, E.R. (2002). *The Hungry Gene: The inside story of the obesity industry.* New York: Grove Press.

337   Critser, G. (2003). *Fat Land: How Americans became the fattest people in the world.* Boston: Mariner Books.

338   Bowman, S.A. et al. (2004). Effects of fast-food consumption on energy intake and diet quality among children in a national household survey. *Pediatrics*, 113(1), 112-118.

339   French, S.A. et al. (2001). Fast food restaurant use among adolescents: associations with nutrient intake, food choices and behavioral and psychosocial variables. *International J of Obesity*, 25, 1823-1833.

340   McCrory, M.A., Suen, V.M.M., and Roberts, S.B. (2002). Biobehavioral influences on energy intake and adult weight gain. *The Journal of Nutrition*, 132, S3830-S3836.

341   McCrory, M.A. et al. (1999). Overeating in America: Association between restaurant food consumption and body fatness in healthy adult men and women ages 19 to 80. *Obesity Research*, 7(6), 564-571.

342   Bowman, S.A. et al. (2004). Effects of fast-food consumption on energy intake and diet quality among children in a national household survey. *Pediatrics*, 113(1), 112-118.

343   Wansink, B. (2006). Mindless Eating: Why We Eat More Than We Think. New York: Bantam Books.

344   Moss, M. (2013). Salt, Sugar, Fat: How the Food Giants Hooked Us.New York: Random House.

345   French, S.A. et al. (2001). Fast food restaurant use among adolescents: associations with nutrient intake, food choices and behavioral and psychosocial variables. *International J of Obesity*, 25, 1823-1833.

346   French, S.A., Story, M., and Jeffery, R.W. (2001). Environmental influences on eating and physical activity. *Annu. Rev. Public Health*, 22, 309-35.

347   Drewnowski, A. (2003). Fat and Sugar: An economic analysis. *J. of Nutrition*, 133, 838S-840S.

348   Critser, G. (2003). *Fat Land: How Americans became the fattest people in the world*. Boston: Mariner Books.

349   French, S.A., Story, M., and Jeffery, R.W. (2001). Environmental influences on eating and physical activity. *Annu. Rev. Public Health*, 22, 309-35.

350   Poppitt, S.D. and Prentice, A.M. (1996). Energy density and its role in the control of food intake: Evidence from metabolic and community studies. *Appetite*, 26, 153-174.

351   Blundell, J.E. (1995). The Psychbiological approach to appetite and weight control. In K.D. Brownell & C.G. Fairburn, C.G. (Eds.). *Eating Disorders and Obesity: A Comprehensive Handbook* (pp. 13-20). New York: The Guilford Press.

352   Drenowski, A. and Specter, S.E. (2004). Poverty and obesity: the role of energy density and energy costs. *Am J Clin Nutr*, 79, 6-16.

353   *Ibid.*

354   Hill, J.O., Wyatt, H.R., and Melanson, E.L. (2000). Genetic and environmental contributions to obesity. *Medical Clinics of North America*, 84(2), 333-346.

355   Stubbs, R.J., Prentice, A.M., and James, W.P.T. (1997). Carbohydrates and energy balance. *Annals New York Academy of Sciences*, 819(1), 44-69.

356   Blundell, J.E. & King, N.A. (1996). Overconsumption as a cause of weight gain: behavioral-physiological interactions in the control of food intake (appetite). In Ciba Foundation Symposium ed. *The Origins and Consequences of Obesity (pp. 138-154)*. Hoboken, NJ: John Wiley & Sons.

357   *Ibid.*

358   Poppitt, S.D. and Prentice, A.M. (1996). Energy density and its role in the control of food intake: Evidence from metabolic and community studies. *Appetite*, 26, 153-174.

359   Drenowski, A. and Specter, S.E. (2004). Poverty and obesity: the role of energy density and energy costs. *Am J Clin Nutr*, 79, 6-16.

360   Brody, I. (2004, October 5). With Fruits and Vegetables, More can be less. *New York Times*, p. D8.

361   Critser, G. (2003). *Fat Land: How Americans became the fattest people in the world*. Boston: Mariner Books.

362   Hazab, G. (2004, July 6). You are how you eat. *New York Times*.

363   Winter, G. (2002, July 7). America rubs its stomach, and says bring it in. *New York Times*, p. 5.

364   Shell, E.R. (2002). *The Hungry Gene: The inside story of the obesity industry.* New York: Grove Press.

365   Whitney, E.N. and Rolfes, S.R. (1999). *Understanding Nutrition*. Belmont, CA: West/Wadsworth.

366   Brownell, K.D. & Horgen, K.B. (2004). *Food Fight*. Chicago: Contemporary Books.

367   Franklin, B.A. (2001). The downside of our technological revolution? An obesity-conducive environment. *The Am J of Cardiology*, 87, 1093-1095.

368   *Ibid.*

369   Brownell, K.D. & Horgen, K.B. (2004). *Food Fight*. Chicago: Contemporary Books.

370   Nielsen, S.J. and Popkin, B.M. (2004). Changes in beverage intake between 1977 and 2001. *Am J Prev Med*, 27(3), 205-210.

371   Critser, G. (2003). *Fat Land: How Americans became the fattest people in the world*. Boston: Mariner Books.

372   Brownell, K.D. & Horgen, K.B. (2004). *Food Fight*. Chicago: Contemporary Books.

373   Brody, J. (2006, July 11). Forget the Second Helpings. It's the First Ones That Count. *New York Times*.

374   Spencer, M. (2004, November 7). Let them eat cake. *The Guardian Weekly*.

375   Goode, E. (2003, July 22). The gorge-yourself environment. *New York Times*, p. F1

376   Winter, G. (2002, July 7). America rubs its stomach, and says bring it in. *New York Times*, p. 5.

377   Brody, J. (2006, July 11). Forget the Second Helpings. It's the First Ones That Count. *New York Times*.

378   Martin, A. (2007, March 25). Will Diners Still Swallow This? *New York Times*.

379   Brownell, K.D. & Horgen, K.B. (2004). *Food Fight*. Chicago: Contemporary Books.

380   Young, L.R. and Nestle, M. (2002). The contribution of expanding portion sizes to the US obesity epidemic. *Am J of Public Health*, 92(2), 246-249.

381   Brownell, K.D. & Horgen, K.B. (2004). *Food Fight*. Chicago: Contemporary Books.

382 Winter, G. (2002, July 7). America rubs its stomach, and says bring it in. *New York Times*, p. 5.

383 Pollan, M. (2003, October 26). The (Agri)Cultural Contradictions Of Obesity. *New York Times Magazine*, p. 41.

384 Martin, A. (2007, March 25). Will Diners Still Swallow This? *New York Times*.

385 Young, L.R. and Nestle, M. (2002). The contribution of expanding portion sizes to the US obesity epidemic. *Am J of Public Health*, 92(2), 246-249.

386 McCrory, M.A., Suen, V.M.M., and Roberts, S.B. (2002). Biobehavioral influences on energy intake and adult weight gain. *The Journal of Nutrition*, 132, S3830-S3836.

387 Critser, G. (2003). *Fat Land: How Americans became the fattest people in the world*. Boston: Mariner Books.

388 Rolls, B.J., Engell, D., and Birch, L.L. (2000). Serving portion size influences 5-year-old but not 3-year-old children's food intakes. *J of the Am Dietetic Ass.*, 100(2), 232-234.

389 French, S.A., Story, M., and Jeffery, R.W. (2001). Environmental influences on eating and physical activity. *Annu. Rev. Public Health*, 22, 309-35.

390 Critser, G. (2003). *Fat Land: How Americans became the fattest people in the world*. Boston: Mariner Books.

391 *Ibid.*

392 Rolls, B.J., Engell, D., and Birch, L.L. (2000). Serving portion size influences 5-year-old but not 3-year-old children's food intakes. *J of the Am Dietetic Ass.*, 100(2), 232-234.

393 Critser, G. (2003). *Fat Land: How Americans became the fattest people in the world*. Boston: Mariner Books.

394 Rolls, B.J., Morris, E., and Roe, L.S. (2002). Portion size of food affects energy intake in normal-weight and overweight men and women. *Am J Clin Nutr*, 76, 1207-13.

395 *Ibid.*

396 *Ibid.*

397 Pollan, M. (2006). *The Omnivore's Dilemma: A natural history of four meal*. New York: The Penguin Press.

398 Eaton, S.B., Eaton, S.B., Konner, M.J., and Shostak, M. (1996). An Evolutionary Perspective Enhances Understanding of Human Nutritional Requirements. *J. Nutr.* 126, 1732-40.

399   Eaton, S. B., Eaton, S. B., III & Cordain, L. (2002) Evolution, diet, and health. In P.S. Ungar. & M.F. Teaford (Eds.). *Human Diet: Its Origin and Evolution.* pp. 7-17. Westport, CT: Bergin & Garvey.

400   Philipson, T.J. and Posner, R.A. (2003). The long-run growth in obesity as a function of technological change. *Perspectives in Biology and Medicine,* 46(3), S87-S107.

401   Franklin, B.A. (2001). The downside of our technological revolution? An obesity-conducive environment. *The Am J of Cardiology,* 87, 1093-1095.

402   French, S.A., Story, M., and Jeffery, R.W. (2001). Environmental influences on eating and physical activity. *Annu. Rev. Public Health,* 22, 309-35.

403   Dunn, D. (1997). Introduction to the study of women and work. In D. Dunn (ed.) *Workplace/Women's Place: An Anthology.* Los Angeles: Roxbury Publishing Company.

404   Nestle, M. and Jacobson, M.F. (2000). Halting the obesity epidemic: A public health policy approach. *Public Health Reports,* 115, 12-24.

405   French, S.A., Story, M., and Jeffery, R.W. (2001). Environmental influences on eating and physical activity. *Annu. Rev. Public Health,* 22, 309-35.

406   McArdle, W.D., Katch, F.I., and Katch, V.L. (1996). *Exercise Physiology: Energy, Nutrition, and Human Performance.* Baltimore, MD: Williams & Wilkins.

407   French, S.A., Story, M., and Jeffery, R.W. (2001). Environmental influences on eating and physical activity. *Annu. Rev. Public Health,* 22, 309-35.

408   Brownell, K.D. & Horgen, K.B. (2004). *Food Fight.* Chicago: Contemporary Books.

409   Philipson, T.J. and Posner, R.A. (2003). The long-run growth in obesity as a function of technological change. *Perspectives in Biology and Medicine,* 46(3), S87-S107.

410   Brownell, K.D. & Horgen, K.B. (2004). *Food Fight.* Chicago: Contemporary Books.

411   Postrel, V. (2001, March 22). Americans' waistlines have become the victims of economic progress. *New York Times,* p. C2.

412   Franklin, B.A. (2001). The downside of our technological revolution? An obesity-conducive environment. *The Am J of Cardiology,* 87, 1093-1095.

413   Brownell, K.D. & Horgen, K.B. (2004). *Food Fight.* Chicago: Contemporary Books.

414   Shell, E.R. (2002). *The Hungry Gene: The inside story of the obesity industry.* New York: Grove Press.

415   *Ibid.*

416   Bray, G.A, Bouchard, C., and James, W.P.T.(Eds.). (1998). *Handbook of Obesity.* New York: Marcel Dekker, Inc.

417   Forrester, J.W. (1979). System Dynamics: Future Opportunities. Paper D-3108-1, The System Dynamics Group, Sloan School of Management, Massachusetts Institute of Technology.

418   Nestle, M. and Jacobson, M.F. (2000). Halting the obesity epidemic: A public health policy approach. *Public Health Reports*, 115, 12-24.

419   Shell, E.R. (2002). *The Hungry Gene: The inside story of the obesity industry.* New York: Grove Press.

420   French, S.A., Story, M., and Jeffery, R.W. (2001). Environmental influences on eating and physical activity. *Annu. Rev. Public Health*, 22, 309-35.

421   Hall, K.D. et al. (2011). Quantifi cation of the eff ect of energy imbalance on bodyweight. Lancet; 378: 826–37.

422   Koplan, J.P. and Dietz, W.H. (1999). Caloric Imbalance and public health policy. *JAMA*, 282(16), 1579-1581.

423   Hill, J.O. et al. (2003). Obesity and the environment: Where do we go from here? *Science*, 299, 853-855.

424   Shell, E.R. (2002). *The Hungry Gene: The inside story of the obesity industry.* New York: Grove Press.

425   French, S.A., Story, M., and Jeffery, R.W. (2001). Environmental influences on eating and physical activity. *Annu. Rev. Public Health*, 22, 309-35.

426   http://www.cnbc.com/id/100762511.

427   Moore, M. (2003, April 23). City, suburban designs could be bad for your health. *USA Today*, p. 1.

428   Shell, E.R. (2002). *The Hungry Gene: The inside story of the obesity industry.* New York: Grove Press.

429   Spors, K. (2003, October 21). Don't Just Sit there. *Wall Street Journal*, p. R8.

430   Franklin, B.A. (2001). The downside of our technological revolution? An obesity-conducive environment. *The Am J of Cardiology*, 87, 1093-1095.

431   *Ibid.*

432   French, S.A., Story, M., and Jeffery, R.W. (2001). Environmental influences on eating and physical activity. *Annu. Rev. Public Health*, 22, 309-35.

433   Schlosser, E. (2002). *Fast Food Nation: The Dark Side of the All-American Meal.* New York: Perennial.

434 Brody, J. (2004, August 3). TV's Toll on Young Minds and Bodies. *New York Times*.

435 French, S.A., Story, M., and Jeffery, R.W. (2001). Environmental influences on eating and physical activity. *Annu. Rev. Public Health*, 22, 309-35.

436 Elias, M. (2005, March 9). Electronic world swallows up kids' time, study finds. *USA TODAY*.

437 Schlosser, E. (2002). *Fast Food Nation: The Dark Side of the All-American Meal*. New York: Perennial.

438 Dalton, S. ed. (1997). *Overweight and Weight Management: The Health Professional's Guide to Understanding and Practice*. Gaithersburg, Maryland: An Aspen Publication.

439 Brownell, K.D. & Horgen, K.B. (2004). *Food Fight*. Chicago: Contemporary Books.

440 McArdle, W.D., Katch, F.I., and Katch, V.I.. (1996). *Exercise Physiology: Energy, Nutrition, and Human Performance*. Baltimore, MD: Williams & Wilkins.

441 Wadden, T.A. & Stunkard, A.J. (Eds.). (2002). *Handbook of Obesity Treatment*. New York: The Guilford Press.

442 McArdle, W.D., Katch, F.I., and Katch, V.L. (1996). *Exercise Physiology: Energy, Nutrition, and Human Performance*. Baltimore, MD: Williams & Wilkins.

443 Markoff, J. (2004, December 30). Internet Use Said to Cut Into TV Viewing and Socializing. *New York Times*.

444 Hu, F.B. et al. (2003). Television watching and other sedentary behaviors in relation to risk of obesity and Type 2 Diabetes Mellitus in women. *JAMA*, 289(14), 1785-1791.

445 French, S.A., Story, M., and Jeffery, R.W. (2001). Environmental influences on eating and physical activity. *Annu. Rev. Public Health*, 22, 309-35.

446 Racette, S.B., Deusinger, S.S., and Deusinger, R.H. (2003). Obesity: Overview of prevalence, etiology, and treatment. *Physical Therapy*, 83(3), 276-288.

447 Nestle, M. (2002). *Food Politics: How the food industry influences nutrition and health*. Berkeley, CA: University of California Press.

448 Brody, J. (2004, January 20). The Widening of America, or How Size 4 Became a Size 0. *New York Times*, p. D7.

449 Nestle, M. and Jacobson, M.F. (2000). Halting the obesity epidemic: A public health policy approach. *Public Health Reports*, 115, 12-24.

450 Critser, G. (2003). *Fat Land: How Americans became the fattest people in the world*. Boston: Mariner Books.

451 McArdle, W.D., Katch, F.I., and Katch, V.L. (1996). *Exercise Physiology: Energy, Nutrition, and Human Performance.* Baltimore, MD: Williams & Wilkins.

452 Pool, R. (2001). *Fat: Fighting the Obesity Epidemic.* Oxford: Oxford University Press.

453 Forrester, J.W. (1979). System Dynamics: Future Opportunities. Paper D-3108-1, The System Dynamics Group, Sloan School of Management, Massachusetts Institute of Technology.

454 Brownell, K.D. & Horgen, K.B. (2004). *Food Fight.* Chicago: Contemporary Books.

455 Shils, M.E., Olson, J.A., Shike, M., and Ross, A.C. (Eds.). (1999). *Modern Nutrition in Health and Disease.* Baltimore, Maryland: Williams & Wilkins.

456 Mulvihill, M.L. (1995). *Human Diseases: A Systemic Approach.* Stamford, Connecticut: Appleton & Lange.

457 Brown, G. (1999). *The Energy of Life: The science of what makes our minds and bodies work.* New York: The Free Press.

458 Brooks, G.A., Fahey, T.D., White, T.P., and Baldwin K.M. (2000). *Exercise Physiology: Human Bioenergetics and its Applications.* Mountain View, Ca: Mayfield Publishing Company.

459 Jairath, N. (1999). *Coronary Heart Disease & Risk Factor Management: A Nursing Perspective.* Philadelphia: W.B. Saunders Company.

460 Swinburn, B., Egger, G., and Raza, F. (1999). Dissecting obesogenic environments: The development and application of a framework for identifying and prioritizing environmental interventions for obesity. *Preventive Medicine*, 29, 563-570.

461 Larkin, M. (2003). Can cities be designed to fight obesity? *The Lancet*, 362, 1046-1047.

462 Roberts, N., Andersen, D., Deal, R., Garet, M., and Shaffer, W. (1983). *Introduction to Computer Simulation: A System Dynamics Modeling Approach.* Reading, MA: Addison-Wesley Publishing Company.

463 Forrester, J.W. (1979). System Dynamics: Future Opportunities. Paper D-3108-1, The System Dynamics Group, Sloan School of Management, Massachusetts Institute of Technology.

464 Wegner, D.M. (2002). The Illusions of Conscious Will. Cambridge, MA: Bradford Books.

465 McArdle, W.D., Katch, F.I., and Katch, V.L. (1996). *Exercise Physiology: Energy, Nutrition, and Human Performance.* Baltimore, MD: Williams & Wilkins.

466   Sterman, J.D. & Booth Sweeney, L. (2002). Cloudy Skies: Assessing Public Understanding of Global Warming. *System Dynamics Review,* 18, 207-240.

467   Richardson, G.P. and Pugh, G.L. (1981). Introduction to System Dynamics Modeling and Dynamo. Cambridge, MA:The MIT Press.

468   Sterman, J. D. (1991). A Skeptic's Guide to Computer Models. In G.O. Barney, W.B. Kreutzer, and M.J. Garrett (Eds.) *Managing a Nation.* 2 ed. Boulder, CO: Westview Press.

469   Gustafson, D.H. et al. (1999). Impact of a patient-centered, computer-based health information/support system. *Am J Prev Med,* 16(1), 1-9.

470   Jeffery, R.W. (1998). Prevention of Obesity. In G.A. Bray, C. Bouchard, and W.P.T. James (Eds.). *Handbook of Obesity.* New York: Marcel Dekker, Inc.

471   Kalota, G. (2005, April 17). The Body Heretic: It Scorns Our Efforts. *New York Times.*

472   Sterman, J.D. (2000). *Business Dynamics: Systems Thinking and Modeling for a Complex World.* Boston, Massachusetts: Irwin McGraw-Hill.

473   Kalota, G. (2005, April 17). The Body Heretic: It Scorns Our Efforts. *New York Times.*

474   Szabo, L. (2005, December 19). Will the Sins of your past catch up with you? *USA Today,* p. 5d.

475   **Ibid.**

476   Kalota, G. (2005, April 17). The Body Heretic: It Scorns Our Efforts. *New York Times.*

477   Kumanyika, S.K. (2001). Minisymposium on Obesity: Overview and some strategic considerations. *Annu. Rev. Public Health,* 22, 293-308.

478   Blundell, J.E. & King, N.A. (1996). Overconsumption as a cause of weight gain: behavioral-physiological interactions in the control of food intake (appetite). In Ciba Foundation Symposium ed. *The Origins and Consequences of Obesity (pp. 138-154).* Hoboken, NJ: John Wiley & Sons.

479   Glanz, K., Rimer, B.K., Lewis, F.M. (Eds.). (2002). *Health Behavior and Health Education: Theory, Research, and Practice.* San Francisco, CA: Jossey-Bass.

480   Pickstone, J.V. (2000). *Ways of Knowing: A new history of science, technology and medicine.* Chicago: The University of Chicago Press,

481   Oliver, J.E. and Lee, T. (2005). Public Opinion and the Politics of Obesity in America. *Journal of Health Politics, Policy and La,*30(5), 923-954.

482   Pool, R. (2001). *Fat: Fighting the Obesity Epidemic.* Oxford: Oxford University Press.

483   Nestle, M. et al. (1998). Behavioral and social influences on food choice. *Nutrition Reviews*, 56(5), S50-S74.

484   Skelton, J.A. & Croyle, R.T. (Eds.). (1991). *Mental representation in health and illness*. New York: Springer-Verlag.

485   Bjorntorp, P. (2001). Thrifty genes and human obesity. Are we chasing ghosts? *Lancet*, 358, 1006-1008.

486   American College of Sports Medicine. (1995). *ACSM's Guidelines for Exercise Testing and Prescription*. Baltimore, Maryland: Williams & Wilkins.

487   Wadden, T.A. & Stunkard, A.J. (Eds.). (2002). *Handbook of Obesity Treatment*. New York: The Guilford Press.

488   Brownell, K.D. & Fairburn, C.G. (Eds.). (1995). *Eating Disorders and Obesity: A Comprehensive Handbook*. New York: The Guilford Press.

489   *Ibid.*

490   Plous, S. (1993). *The Psychology of Judgment and Decision Making*. New York: McGraw Hill.

491   Tierney, J. (2008, January 1). A 100 Percent Chance of Alarm. *New York Times*.

492   *Ibid.*

493   Krieger, N. (1994). Epidemiology and the web of causation: Has anyone seen the spider? *Soc. Sci. Med.,* 39(7), 887-903.

494   Wadden, T.A. & Stunkard, A.J. (Eds.). (2002). *Handbook of Obesity Treatment*. New York: The Guilford Press.

495   Wadden, T.A. & Stunkard, A.J. (Eds.). (2002). *Handbook of Obesity Treatment*. New York: The Guilford Press.

496   Diez-Roux, A.V. (1998). On genes, individuals, society, and epidemiology. *Am J. of Epidemiology*, 148(11), 1027-1032.

497   Shell, E.R. (2002). The Hungry Gene: The inside story of the obesity industry. New York: Grove Press.

498   Hall, K.D. et al. (2011). Quantifi cation of the eff ect of energy imbalance on bodyweight. Lancet; 378: 826–37.

499   GazianoJ, J.M. (2010). Fifth Phase of the Epidemiologic Transition The Age of Obesity and Inactivity. JAMA; 303(3):275-276.

500   Polivy, J. and Herman, C.P. (2002). If at first you don't succeed: False hopes of self-change. American Psychologist, 57(9).

501   Foster, G.D., Wadden, T.A., Vogt, R.A., and Brewer, G. (1997). What Is a Reasonable Weight Loss? Patients' Expectations and Evaluations of Obesity Treatment Outcomes. *Journal of Consulting and Clinical Psychology*, 65, 79-85.

502   Wadden, T.A., Brownell, K.D., and Foster, G.D. (2002). Obesity: Responding to the Global epidemic. *J of Consulting and Clinical Psychology*, 70(3), 510-525.

503   Foster, G.D., Wadden, T.A., Vogt, R.A., and Brewer, G. (1997). What Is a Reasonable Weight Loss? Patients' Expectations and Evaluations of Obesity Treatment Outcomes. Journal of Consulting and Clinical Psychology. 65, 79-85.

504   Dutton, G.R. et al. (2010). Weight loss goals of patients in a health maintenance organization. Eating Behaviors; 11, 74–78.

505   Dalle Grave, R. et al. (2004). Weight Loss Expectations in Obese Patients Seeking Treatment at Medical Centers. *Obesity Research*, 12 (12), 2005-12.

506   Sterman, J.D. (2000). *Business Dynamics: Systems Thinking and Modeling for a Complex World*. Boston, Massachusetts: Irwin McGraw-Hill.

507   Muraven, M., Tice, D. M., & Baumeister, R. F. (1998). Self-control as a limited resource: Regulatory depletion patterns. *Journal of Personality and Social Psychology*, 74, 774- 89.

508   Muraven, M., & Baumeister, R. F. (2000). Self-regulation and depletion of limited resources: Does self-control resemble a muscle? *Psychological Bulletin*, 126, 247-259

509   Baumeister, R.F., Heatherton, T.F., and Tice, D.M. (1994). *Losing Control: How and why people fail at self-regulation*. San Diego, CA: Academic Press.

510   Baumeister, R.F., Heatherton, T.F., and Tice, D.M. (1994). *Losing Control: How and why people fail at self-regulation*. San Diego, CA: Academic Press.

511   Muraven, M., Tice, D. M., & Baumeister, R. F. (1998). Self-control as a limited resource: Regulatory depletion patterns. *Journal of Personality and Social Psychology*, 74, 774- 89.

512   *Ibid.*

513   Muraven, M., & Baumeister, R. F. (2000). Self-regulation and depletion of limited resources: Does self-control resemble a muscle? *Psychological Bulletin*, 126, 247-259.

514   Muraven, M., & Slessareva, E. (2003). Mechanisms of self-control failure: Motivation and limited resources. *Personality and Social Psychology Bulletin*, 29, 894-90.

515   Muraven, M., Tice, D. M., & Baumeister, R. F. (1998). Self-control as a limited resource: Regulatory depletion patterns. *Journal of Personality and Social Psychology*, 74, 774- 89.

516   Freud, S. (1930). *Civilization and its discontents.* London: Hogarth.

517 Tangney, J.P., Baumeister, R.F., and Boone, A.L. (2004). High self-control pre-dicts good adjustment, less pathology, better grades, and interpersonal success. *J of Personality*, 72(2), 271-322.

518 Roizen, M.F. & Oz, M.C. (2006). *You on a Diet: The owner's manual for waist management.* New York: Free Press.

519 Muraven, M., Tice, D. M., & Baumeister, R. F. (1998). Self-control as a limited resource: Regulatory depletion patterns. *Journal of Personality and Social Psychology*, 74, 774- 89.

520 *Ibid.*

521 Muraven, M., & Baumeister, R. F. (2000). Self-regulation and depletion of limited resources: Does self-control resemble a muscle? *Psychological Bulletin*, 126, 247-259.

522 Muraven, M., Tice, D. M., & Baumeister, R. F. (1998). Self-control as a limited resource: Regulatory depletion patterns. *Journal of Personality and Social Psychology*, 74, 774- 89.

523 *Ibid.*

524 Muraven, M. (2003). Blowing your diet: Models of self-control. *Contemporary Psychology*, 48(6), 742-44.

525 Muraven, M., Tice, D. M., & Baumeister, R. F. (1998). Self-control as a limited resource: Regulatory depletion patterns. *Journal of Personality and Social Psychology*, 74, 774- 89.

526 Tangney, J.P., Baumeister, R.F., and Boone, A.L. (2004). High self-control pre-dicts good adjustment, less pathology, better grades, and interpersonal success. *J of Personality*, 72(2), 271-322.

527 Muraven, M., & Baumeister, R. F. (2000). Self-regulation and depletion of limited resources: Does self-control resemble a muscle? *Psychological Bulletin*, 126, 247-259.

528 Innate individual differences can now be measured. Tangney et al developed an instrument (based on 36 dimensions) to measure self-control strength. See: Tangney, J.P., Baumeister, R.F., and Boone, A.L. (2004). High self-control pre-dicts good adjustment, less pathology, better grades, and interpersonal success. J of Personality, 72(2), 271-322.

529 Muraven, M., Tice, D. M., & Baumeister, R. F. (1998). Self-control as a limited resource: Regulatory depletion patterns. *Journal of Personality and Social Psychology*, 74, 774- 89.

530 *Ibid.*

531   Muraven, M. (2003). Blowing your diet: Models of self-control. *Contemporary Psychology*, 48(6), 742-44.

532   Muraven, M., Tice, D. M., & Baumeister, R. F. (1998). Self-control as a limited resource: Regulatory depletion patterns. *Journal of Personality and Social Psychology*, 74, 774- 89.

533   Baumeister, R.F., Heatherton, T.F., and Tice, D.M. (1994). *Losing Control: How and why people fail at self-regulation*. San Diego, CA: Academic Press.

534   Kiley, D. (2005, September 19). My Dinner With NutriSystem. *Business Week*.

535   Wing, R.R. and Hill, J.O. (2001). Successful weight loss maintenance. *Annual Review of Nutrition*, 21, 323-341.

536   Hill, J.H. and Wing, R. (2003). The National Weight Control Registry. *The Permanente Journal*, 7(3), 34-37.

537   Hill, J.O. and Billington, C.J. (2002). It's time to start treating obesity. *The Am J of Cardiology*, 89, 969-970.

538   Brownell, K.D. & Rodin, J. (1994). Medical, Metabolic, and Psychological Effects of Weight Cycling. *Arch Intern Med*, 154, 1325-1330.

539   Foreyt, J.P. and Poston, W.S.C. (1998). Obesity: A never-ending cycle? *Int J Fertil*, 43(2), 111 116.

540   Wing, R.R. and Hill, J.O. (2001). Successful weight loss maintenance. *Annu. Rev. Nutr.*, 21, 323-41.

541   Kolata, G. (2007, May 8). Genes Take Charge, and Diets Fall by the Wayside. *New York Times*.

542   Muraven, M., & Baumeister, R. F. (2000). Self-regulation and depletion of limited resources: Does self-control resemble a muscle? *Psychological Bulletin*, 126, 247-259.

543   Friedman, J.M. (2003). A war on obesity, not the obese. *Science*, 299, 856-863.

544   Baumeiter, R.F. and Tierney, J. (2011). Willpower, New York: The Penguin Press.

545   Neel, J.V. (1999). The "thrift genotype" in 1998. *Nutrition Reviews*, 57(5), S2-S9.

546   Winter, G. (2000, October 29). Search for an easy solution fuels an industry rooted in gullibility. *New York Times*, p. 1.

547   Bruni, F. (2014, May 27). Diet Lures and Diet Lies. New York Times.

548   *USA Today*, (2005, January 13). p. 1A.

549   Russell, S.A. (2005). *Hunger: An Unnatural History*. New York: Basic Books.

550 Brooks, F.P. (1987). No Silver Bullet: Essence and Accidents of Software Engineering. *Computer,* 20(4), 10-19.

551 Wansink, B. (2006). Mindless Eating: Why We Eat More Than We Think. New York: Bantam Books.

552 Rolls, B.J. (2009). The relationship between dietary energy density and energy intake. Physiology & Behavior; 97, 609–615.

553 Larkin, M. (2003). Can cities be designed to fight obesity? *The Lancet,* 362, 1046-1047.

554 Hill, J.O. et al. (2003). Obesity and the environment: Where do we go from here? *Science,* 299, 853-855.

555 Rolls, B.J. (2009). The relationship between dietary energy density and energy intake. Physiology & Behavior; 97, 609–615.

556 Blatt, A.D., Roe, L.S. and Rolls, B.J. (2011). Hidden Vegetables: An effective strategy to reduce energy intake and increase vegetable intake in adults. Am J Clin Nutrition, 93:756-63

557 McCrory, M.A., Suen, V.M.M., and Roberts, S.B. (2002). Biobehavioral influences on energy intake and adult weight gain. The Journal of Nutrition, 132, S3830-S3836.

558 Critser, G. (2003). Fat Land: How Americans became the fattest people in the world. Boston: Mariner Books.

559 Pollan, M. (2009). Food Rules: An Eater's Manual. London: Penguin Books.

560 Hill, J.O. et al. (2003). Obesity and the environment: Where do we go from here? Science, 299, 853-855.

561 Cornier, M., Von Kaenel, S., Bessesen, D.H. and Tregellas, J.R. (2007). Effects of overfeeding on the neuronal response to visual food cues. Am J Clin Nutr, 86: 965–71.

562 Lowe, M.R. and Butryn, M.L. (2007). Hedonic hunger: A new dimension of appetite? Physiology & Behavior. 91, 432–439.

563 Wansink, B. (2006). Mindless Eating: Why We Eat More Than We Think. New York: Bantam Books.

564 Rolls, B. and Barnett, R.A. (2000). The Volumetrics Weight-Control Plan. New York: Harper.

565 Kessler, D.A. (2009). The End of Overeating: Taking Control of the Insatiable American Appetite. New York: Rodale.

566 Brody, J.E. (2000, October 17). One-two punch for losing pounds: Exercise and careful diet. New York Times.

567   Abdel-Hamid, T.K. (2003). Exercise and Diet in Obesity Treatment: An Integrative System Dynamics Perspective. Medicine & Science in Sports & Exercise, 35(3), 400-413.

568   Rosenkilde, M. et al. (2012). Body fat loss and compensatory mechanisms in response to different doses of aerobic exercise - a randomized controlled trial in overweight sedentary males. American Journal of Physiology, 303(6):R571-9.

569   Capell, K., Arndt, M. and Carey, J.(2005, September 5). Drugs Get Smart. *Business Week.*

570   Millenson, M.L. (2006). The promise of personalized medicine: A conversation with Michael Svinte. *Health Affairs*, published online 14 February, pp. w54-w60.

571   Baker, S. and Leak, B. (2006, January 23). Math Will Rock Your World. *Business Week.*

572   Senge, P.M. (1990). *The Fifth Discipline: The Art & Practice of the Learning Organization.* New York: Doubleday/Currency.

573   Lohr, S. (2007, August 14). Dr Google and Dr Microsoft. *New York Times.*

574   Neuhauser, L. and Kreps, G.L. (2003). Rethinking communication in the E-health era. *Journal of Health Psychology,* 8(1), 7-23.

575   Hammer, M., (1990). Reengineering Work: Don't Automate, Obliterate. *Harvard Business Review,* July/August, pp. 104-112.

576   Phrase first coined by Michael Hammer.

577   Sterman, J.D. (2006). Learning from evidence in a complex world. *American Journal of Public Health,* 96(3), 505-514.

578   De Kler, R. (1998). Clinical simulations: A pedagogical and chronological perspective. In J.G. Anderson and M. Katzper (Eds.). Proceedings of the 1998 Medical Sciences Simulation Conference (pp. 181-6). San Diego, CA: Society for Computer Simulation International.

579   Sterman, J. D. (1992). Teaching Takes Off: Flight Simulators for Management Education. *OR/MS Today,* 40-44.

580   Abdel-Hamid, T.K. (2002). Modeling the Dynamics of Human Obesity. *System Dynamics Review,* Vol. 18, No. 4, 431-471. Abdel-Hamid, T.K. (2003). Exercise and Diet in Obesity Treatment: An Integrative System Dynamics Perspective. *Medicine & Science in Sports & Exercise,* 35(3), 400-413. Abdel-Hamid, T.K.. (2012). EUREKA: Insights into Human Energy and Weight Regulation from Simple—Bathtub-like—Models. *Int. J. of System Dynamics Applications,* Volume 1, No. 3.

581 Stipanuk, M.H. (Ed.). (2000). Biochemical and Physiological aspects of Human Nutrition. Philadelphia: W.B. Saunders Company.

582 Hall, K.D. et al. (2011). Quantifi cation of the eff ect of energy imbalance on bodyweight. Lancet; 378: 826–37.

583 Peele, L. Body Fat Percentage. http://www.leighpeele.com/body-fat-pictures-and-percentages.

584 Stipanuk, M.H. (Ed.). (2000). Biochemical and Physiological aspects of Human Nutrition. Philadelphia: W.B. Saunders Company.

585 Hall, K.D. et al. (2011). Quantifi cation of the eff ect of energy imbalance on bodyweight. Lancet; 378: 826–37.

586 Heilbronn, L.K. et al. (2006). Effect of 6-Month Calorie Restriction on Biomarkers of Longevity, Metabolic Adaptation, and Oxidative Stress in Overweight Individuals A Randomized Controlled Trial. JAMA, 295(13), 1539-49.

587 Stipanuk, M.H. (Ed.). (2000). *Biochemical and Physiological aspects of Human Nutrition*. Philadelphia: W.B. Saunders Company.

588 Ballor, D.L. & Poehlman, E.T. (1994). Exercise-training enhances fat-free mass preservation during diet-induced weight loss: a meta-analytical finding. *International Journal of Obesity,* 18, 35-40.

589 Hall, K.D. et al. (2011). Quantifi cation of the eff ect of energy imbalance on bodyweight. Lancet; 378: 826–37.

590 Keesey, R.E. (1993). Physiological Regulation of Body Energy: Implications for Obesity. In A.J. Stunkard and T.A. Wadden. Obesity: Theory and Therapy. New York: Raven Press, Ltd.

591 Saltzman, E. & Roberts, S.B. (1995). The Role of Energy Expenditure in Energy Regulation: Findings from a Decade of Research. Nutrition Reviews 53, 209-220.

592 Uma, G. & Siva Perraju, T. (2000). Services on the Net: an agent based approach. Database and Expert Systems Applications, Proceedings of the 11th International Workshop (pp. 770 - 774). London, UK.

593 Keesey, R.E. (1993). Physiological Regulation of Body Energy: Implications for Obesity. In A.J. Stunkard and T.A. Wadden. Obesity: Theory and Therapy. New York: Raven Press, Ltd.

594 Saltzman, E. & Roberts, S.B. (1995). The Role of Energy Expenditure in Energy Regulation: Findings from a Decade of Research. Nutrition Reviews 53, 209-220.

595   Forbes, G.B. (1987). Human body composition: Growth, Aging, Nutrition and Activity. New York: Springer-Verlag.

596   Westerterp et al's (1995) empirically derived formulation is used to calculate nominal REE as follows: Nominal REE = 0.024*FM + 0.102*FFM + 0.85 (MJ/day).

597   McArdle, W.D., Katch, F.I., and Katch, V.L. (1996). Exercise Physiology: Energy, Nutrition, and Human Performance. Baltimore, MD: Williams & Wilkins.

598   Andrews, J. F. (1991). Exercise for slimming. Proceedings of the Nutrition Society. 50: 459-471.

599   Melby, C.L., Commerford, S.R., and Hill, J.O. (1998). Exercise, Macronutrient Balance, and Weight Control. In D.R. Lamb and R. Murray (Eds.) *Perspectives in Exercise Science and Sports Medicine (Volume II): Exercise, Nutrition, and Weight Control.* Carme, IN: Cooper Publishing Group.

600   Kirk, E.P., Jacobsen, D.J., Gibson, C., Hill, J.O., and Donnelly, J.E. (2003). Time course for changes in aerobic capacity and body composition in overweight men and women in response to long-term exercise: the Midwest Exercise Trial (MET). International J. of Obesity, 27, 912-919.

601   The composition of weight loss is clearly a function of the type of exercise. Resistance training, for example, tends to preserve more of the fat-free mass component than does aerobic exercise.

602   Ballor, D.L. & Poehlman, E.T. (1994). Exercise-training enhances fat-free mass preservation during diet-induced weight loss: a meta-analytical finding. International Journal of Obesity, 18, 35-40.

603   Whitney, E.N. and Rolfes, S.R. (1999). Understanding Nutrition. Belmont, CA: West/Wadsworth.

604   *Ibid.*

605   *Ibid.*

606   McArdle, W.D., Katch, F.I., and Katch, V.L. (1996). Exercise Physiology: Energy, Nutrition, and Human Performance. Baltimore, MD: Williams & Wilkins.

607   Whitney, E.N. and Rolfes, S.R. (1999). Understanding Nutrition. Belmont, CA: West/Wadsworth.

608   Brown, G. (1999). *The Energy of Life: The science of what makes our minds and bodies work.* New York: The Free Press.

609   Brody, J.E. (2000, October 17). One-two punch for losing pounds: Exercise and careful diet. New York Times.

610   Pool, R. (2001). Fat: Fighting the Obesity Epidemic. Oxford: Oxford University Press.

611   Leermakers, E.A., Dunn, A.L., and Blair, S.N. (2000). Exercise management of obesity. Medical Clinics of North America, 84(2), 419-440.

612   van Baak, M.A. (1999). Exercise training and substrate utilization in obesity. J Obes Relat Metab Disord, 23, S11–S17.

613   Brownell, K.D. & Horgen, K.B. (2004). Food Fight. Chicago: Contemporary Books.

614   Wansink, B. (2006). Mindless Eating: Why We Eat More Than We Think. New York: Bantam Books.

615   Ragsdale, C.T. (2008). Spreadsheet Modeling and Decision Analysis, Mason, Ohio: South-Western Cengage Learning.

616   Kahneman, D. (2013). *Thinking, Fast and Slow*. New York: Farrar, Straus and Giroux.

617   Furchgott, R. (2012, January 5). Devices to Keep Track of Calories, Lost or Gained. New York Times.

618   Bandura, A. (1997). *Self-Efficacy: The Exercise of Control*. New York: W.H. Freeman and Company.

619   Acharya, S. D. et al. (2011). Using a Personal Digital Assistant for Self-Monitoring Influences Diet Quality in Comparison to a Standard Paper Record among Overweight/Obese Adults. J Am Diet Assoc. 111: 583-588.

620   Baker, R.C. (1993). Self-monitoring may be necessary for successful weight control. *Behavior Therapy*. 24, 377-394.

621   Gibbs, N. (ed). (2014). *Your Body: the Science of Keeping it Healthy*. New York, Time Books.

622   Brustein, J. (2013, March 14). Tool Kit, Walking, Jumping and Resting, for the Record. New York Times.

623   Pogue, D. (2012, November 15). Wristbands Keep Tabs on Fitness. New York Times.

624   Gibbs, N. (ed). (2014). *Your Body: the Science of Keeping it Healthy*. New York, Time Books.

625   Tate, E.B. et al. (2013). mHealth approaches to child obesity prevention: successes, unique challenges, and next directions. TBM; 3:406–415.

626   Pogue, D. (2012, November 15). Wristbands Keep Tabs on Fitness. New York Times.

627   Isaacson, W. (2013, November 3). Brain Gain: (Book Review: Smarter Than You Think by Clive Thompson). New York Times, Book Review.

628   Hargrove, J.L. (1998). *Dynamic Modeling in the Health Sciences.* New York: Springer.

629   Topol, E. (2012). *The Creative Destruction of Medicine.* New York: Basic Books

INDEX

A

B

C

D

E